Cultural Diversity
in Health and Illness

CULTURALCARE

There is something that transcends all of this
I am I ... You are you
Yet. I and you
Do connect
Somehow, sometime.

To understand the "cultural" needs
Samenesses and differences of people
Needs an open being
See—Hear—Feel
With no judgment or interpretation
Reach out
Maybe with that physical touch
Or eyes, or aura
You exhibit your openness and willingness to
Listen and learn
And, you tell and share
In so doing—you share humanness
It is acknowledged and shared
Something happens—
Mutual understanding

—Rachel E. Spector

Cultural Diversity in Health and Illness

NINTH EDITION

Rachel E. Spector, PhD, RN, CTN-A, FAAN

Needham, MA 02494

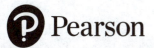 Pearson

330 Hudson Street, New York, NY 10013

Publisher: Julie Levin Alexander
Publisher's Assistant: Sarah Henrich
Executive Editor: Katrin Beacom
Editorial Assistant: Erin Sullivan
Content Producer: Erin Rafferty
Director, Publishing Operations: Paul DeLuca
Managing Content Producer: Melissa Bashe
Development Editor: Adelaide McCulloch
Vice President of Sales and Marketing: David Gesell
Vice President, Director of Marketing: Margaret Waples

Senior Product Marketing Manager: Christopher Barry
Field Marketing Manager: Brittany Hammond
Manufacturing Manager: Maura Zaldivar-Garcia
Composition: Lumina Datamatics, Inc.
Full-Service Project Management: Saraswathi Muralidhar, Lumina Datamatics, Inc.
Interior Designer: Lumina Datamatics, Inc.
Cover Image: agsandrew/Fotolia
Printer/Binder: RR Donnelley & Sons
Cover Printer: RR Donnelley & Sons

Credits and acknowledgments borrowed from other sources and reproduced, with permission, in this textbook appear on pages 286–289.

All photos courtesy Rachel Spector unless otherwise noted.

Notice: Care has been taken to confirm the accuracy of information presented in this book. The author, editors, and the publisher, however, cannot accept any responsibility for errors or omissions or for consequences from application of the information in this book and make no warranty, express or implied, with respect to its contents.

The authors and publisher have exerted every effort to ensure that drug selections and dosages set forth in this text are in accord with current recommendations and practice at time of publication. However, in view of ongoing research, changes in government regulations, and the constant flow of information relating to drug therapy and drug reactions, the reader is urged to check the package inserts of all drugs for any change in indications of dosage and for added warnings and precautions. This is particularly important when the recommended agent is a new and/or infrequently employed drug.

Library of Congress Cataloging-in-Publication Data
Names: Spector, Rachel E., author.
Title: Cultural diversity in health and illness / Rachel E. Spector, PhD, RN, CTN-A, FAAN, Needham, MA.
Description: Ninth edition. | Boston : Pearson, [2017] | Includes bibliographical references and index.
Identifiers: LCCN 2016026577 | ISBN 9780134413310 | ISBN 0134413318
Subjects: LCSH: Transcultural medical care—United States. | Health attitudes—United States. | Transcultural nursing—United States.
Classification: LCC RA418.5.T73 S64 2017 | DDC 362.1/0425—dc23 LC record available at https://lccn.loc.gov/2016026577

2   16

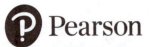

ISBN-13: 978-0-13-441331-0
ISBN-10:   0-13-441331-8

I would like to dedicate this text to

My husband, Manny;
Sam, Hilary, Julia, and Emma;
Becky, Perry, Naomi, Rose, and Miriam;
the memory of my parents, Joseph J. and Freda F. Needleman,
and my in-laws, Sam and Margaret Spector;
and the memory of my beloved mentor, Irving Kenneth Zola.

Contents

Preface

Every book, every volume you see here, has a soul. The soul of the person who wrote it and of those who read it and lived and dreamed with it.

—*Carlos Ruiz Zafon,*
The Shadow of the Wind, *2001*

In 1977—nearly 40 years ago—I prepared the first edition of *Cultural Diversity in Health and Illness*. Now, as I begin the ninth edition of this book—the eighth revision—I realize that this is an opportunity to reflect on an endeavor that has filled a good deal of my life for the past 39 years. I believe this book has a soul and it, in turn, has become an integral part of my soul. I have lived—through practice, teaching, consulting, and research—this material since 1974 and have developed many ways of presenting this content. In addition, I have tracked for countless years:

1. The U.S. Census
2. Immigration—numbers and policies
3. Poverty—figures and policies
4. Healthcare—costs and policies
5. Morbidity and mortality rates
6. Nursing and other healthcare manpower issues, and
7. The emergence and growth of the concepts of health disparities and cultural and linguistic competence.

My concepts are *HEALTH*, defined as "the balance of the person, both within one's being—physical, mental, and spiritual—and in the outside world—natural, communal, and metaphysical"; *ILLNESS*, "the imbalance of the person, both within one's being—physical, mental, and spiritual—and in the outside world—natural, communal, and metaphysical"; and *HEALING*, "the restoration of balance, both within one's being—physical, mental, and spiritual—and in the outside world—natural, communal, and metaphysical." I have learned over these years that within many traditional heritages (defined as "old," not contemporary or modern), people tend to define *HEALTH*, *ILLNESS*, and *HEALING* in this manner. Imagine a kaleidoscope—the tube can represent *HEALTH*, *ILLNESS*, and *HEALING*. The objects within the kaleidoscope reflect the traditional tools used to care for a given person. If you love kaleidoscopes, you know what I am describing and that the patterns that emerge are infinite.

In addition, I have had the unique opportunity to travel to countless places in the United States and abroad. I make it a practice to visit the traditional markets, pharmacies, and shrines and dialogue with the people who work in or patronize those settings, and I have gathered invaluable knowledge and unique items and images. My tourist dollars are invested in amulets and remedies, and my collection is large. Digital photography has changed my eyes; I may be a "digital immigrant," rather than a "digital native," but the camera has proven to be my most treasured companion. I have been able to use the images of sacred objects and sacred places to create HEALTH Traditions Imagery. The opening images for each chapter and countless images within the chapters are the results of these explorations. Given that there are times when we do not completely understand a concept or an image, several images are slightly blurred or dark to represent this wonderment.

The first edition of this book was the outcome of a *promesa*—a promise— I once made. The promise was made to a group of Asian, Black, and Hispanic students I taught in a medical sociology course in 1973. In this course, the students wound up being the teachers, and they taught me to see the world of healthcare delivery through the eyes of the healthcare consumer rather than through my own well-intentioned eyes. What I came to see, I did not always like. I did not realize how much I did not know; I believed I knew a lot. I promised the students that I would take what they taught me regarding HEALTH and teach it to students and colleagues. I have held on to the *promesa*, and my experiences over the years have been incredible. I have met people and traveled. At all times I have held on to the idea and goal of attempting to help nurses, other healthcare providers, and, as often as possible, laypeople be aware of and sensitive to the HEALTH, ILLNESS, and HEALING beliefs and needs of people from varied backgrounds.

I know that looking inside closed doors carries with it a risk. I know that people prefer to think that our society is a "melting pot" and that the traditional beliefs and practices have vanished with the expected acculturation and assimilation into mainstream North American modern life. Many people, however, have continued to carry on the traditional customs and culture from their native lands and heritage, and HEALTH, ILLNESS, and HEALING beliefs are deeply entwined within the cultural and social beliefs that people have. To understand HEALTH and ILLNESS beliefs and practices, it is necessary to see each person in his or her unique sociocultural world. The theoretical knowledge that has evolved for the development of this text is cumulative, and much of the "old" material is relevant *today* as many HEALTH, ILLNESS, and HEALING beliefs do not change. However, many beliefs and practices do go underground.

The purpose of each edition has been to increase awareness of the dimensions and complexities involved in caring for people from diverse cultural backgrounds. I wished to share my personal experiences and thoughts concerning the introduction of cultural concepts into the education of healthcare professionals. The books represented my answers to the questions:

- How does one effectively expose a student to cultural diversity?
- How does one examine healthcare issues and perceptions from a broad social viewpoint?

As I have done in the classroom over the years, I attempt to bring you, the reader, into direct contact with the interaction between providers of care within the North American healthcare system and the consumers of healthcare. The staggering issues of healthcare delivery are explored and contrasted with the choices that people may make in attempting to deal with healthcare issues.

When I began this journey in nursing, there were limited resources available to answer my questions and to support me in my passion for knowledge. The situation has dramatically changed, and today there is almost more information than one can absorb! Not only is this information being sought by nurses, but all stakeholders in the healthcare industry are struggling with this concept. The demographics of America, and the world, have changed, and perhaps this challenge of building bridges between cultural groups can be seen as a way to open opportunities to do this in many disciplines. Indeed, the content is readily available:

- Countless books and articles have been published in nursing, medicine, public health, and the popular media over the past 40 years that contain invaluable information relevant to CULTURALCOMPETENCY.
- Innumerable workshops and meetings have been and are available where the content is presented and discussed.
- "Self-study" programs on the internet have been developed that provide continuing education credits to nurses, physicians, and other providers.

However, *the process of becoming* CULTURALLYCOMPETENT is not generally provided for. Issues persist, such as:

- Demographic disparity exists in the profile of healthcare providers and in health status.
- Patient needs, such as modesty, space, and gender-specific care, are not universally met.
- Religious-specific needs are not met in terms of meal planning, procedural planning, conference planning, and so forth.
- Communication and language barriers exist.

As you build a base of knowledge and experiences, you begin making your way to CULTURALCOMPETENCY. As your base of knowledge and experience matures and grows, you become an advocate of CULTURALCARE, as it will be described in Chapter 1.

■ Overview

Unit I focuses on the background knowledge that healthcare providers must recognize as the foundation for developing CULTURALCOMPETENCY.

- Chapter 1 presents an overview of the significant content related to the ongoing development of the concepts of cultural and linguistic competency as it is described by several different organizations.

■ Chapter 2 explores the concept of cultural heritage and history and the roles they play in one's perception of health and illness. This exploration is first outlined in general terms: What is culture? How is it transmitted? What is ethnicity? What is religion? How do they affect a person's health? What major sociocultural events occurred during the life trajectory of a person that may influence his or her personal health beliefs and practices?

■ Chapter 3 presents a discussion of the diversity—demographic, immigration, and poverty—that impacts on the delivery of and access to healthcare. The backgrounds of each of the U.S. Census Bureau's categories of the population, an overview of immigration, and an overview of issues relevant to poverty are presented.

■ Chapter 4 reviews the provider's knowledge of his or her own perceptions, needs, and understanding of health and illness.

Unit II explores the domains of HEALTH, blends them with one's personal heritage, and contrasts them with the allopathic philosophy.

■ Chapter 5 introduces the concept of HEALTH and develops the concept in broad and general terms. The HEALTH Traditions Model is presented, as are natural methods of HEALTH maintenance and protection.

■ Chapter 6 explores the concept of HEALTH restoration or HEALING and the role that faith plays in the context of HEALING, or magico-religious, traditions. This is an increasingly important issue, which is evolving to a point where the healthcare provider must have some understanding of this phenomenon.

■ Chapter 7 discusses family heritage and explores personal and familial HEALTH traditions. It includes an array of familial health/HEALTH beliefs and practices shared by people from many different heritages.

■ Chapter 8 focuses on the healthcare provider culture and the allopathic healthcare delivery system.

Once the study of each of these components has been completed, Unit III (Chapters 9 to 13) moves on to explore selected population groups in greater detail, to portray a panorama of traditional HEALTH and ILLNESS beliefs and practices, and to present relevant healthcare issues.

Chapter 14 is devoted to an overall analysis of the book's contents and how best to apply this knowledge in healthcare delivery, health planning, and health education, for both the patient and the healthcare professional.

Each chapter in the text opens with images relevant to the chapter's topic. They may be viewed in the CULTURALCARE Museum on the accompanying Web page. The CULTURALCARE Museum is cumulative, and the images from earlier versions of this text are included.

These pages cannot do full justice to the richness of any one culture or any one health/HEALTH belief system. By presenting some of the beliefs and practices and suggesting background reading, however, the book can begin to inform and sensitize the reader to the needs of a given group of people. It can also serve as a model for developing cultural knowledge of populations that are not included in this text. The template used for Chapters 9–13 presents each community's background; traditional definitions of HEALTH and ILLNESS; traditional methods of HEALTH maintenance and protection, and restoration; traditional methods of HEALING and HEALERS; and current health problems. This template can be followed in doing research in the populations you may be working with. The template is also practical in other countries.

There is so much to be learned. Countless books and articles are now available that address these problems and issues. It is not easy to alter attitudes and beliefs or stereotypes and prejudices, to change a person's philosophy. Some social psychologists state that it is almost impossible to lose all of one's prejudices; yet changes can be made. I believe the healthcare provider *must* develop the ability to deliver CULTURALCARE and knowledge regarding personal fundamental values regarding health/HEALTH and illness/ILLNESS. With acceptance of one's own values come the framework and courage to accept the existence of differing beliefs and values. This process of realization and acceptance can enable the healthcare provider to be instrumental in meeting the needs of the consumer in a collaborative, safe, and professional manner.

This book is written primarily for the student in allied health professional programs, nursing, medical, social work, and other healthcare provider disciplines. I believe it will be helpful also for providers in all areas of practice, especially community health, long-term oncology, chronic care settings, and geriatric and hospice centers. I am attempting to write in a direct manner and to use language that is understandable by all. The material is sensitive, yet I believe that it is presented in a sensitive manner. At no point is my intent to create a vehicle for stereotyping. I know that one person will read this book and nod, "Yes, this is how I see it," and someone else of the same background will say, "No, this is not correct." This is the way it is meant to be. It is incomplete by intent. It is written in the spirit of open inquiry, so that an issue may be raised and so that clarification of any given point will be sought *from the patient* as healthcare is provided.

The deeper I travel into this world of cultural diversity, the more I wonder at the variety. It is wonderfully exciting. By gaining insight into the traditional attitudes that people have toward HEALTH and HEALTHCARE, I found my own nursing practice was enhanced, and I was better able to understand the needs of patients and their families. It is thrilling to be able to meet, to know, and to provide care to people from all over the world and every walk of life. It is the excitement of nursing. As we go forward in time, I hope that these words will help you, the reader, develop CULTURALCARE skills and help you provide the best care to all.

You don't need a masterpiece to get the idea.

—*Pablo Picasso*

■ Features

- ■ The *HERITAGECHAIN* links the chapters and concepts to one another (see pages 1, 67, and 147).
- ■ *Research on Culture and Health.* As evidence-based practice grows in importance, its application is expected in all aspects of healthcare. This special feature spotlights how current research informs and impacts cultural awareness and competence.
- ■ *Unit and Chapter Objectives.* Each unit and chapter opens with objectives to direct the reader when studying.
- ■ *Unit Exercises and Activities.* The beginning of each unit provides exercises and activities related to the topic. Questions stimulate reflective consideration of the reader's own family and cultural history as well as to develop an awareness of one's own biases. Reflective questions can be identified by specially designed bullets (∞).
- ■ *Figures, Tables, and Boxes.* Throughout the book are photographs, illustrations, tables, and boxes that exemplify and expand on information referenced in the chapter.
- ■ *HEALTH Traditions Imagery.* These symbolic images are used to link the chapters. The images were selected to awaken you to the richness of a given heritage and the practices inherent within both modern and traditional cultures, as well as the beliefs surrounding health and HEALTH. (HEALTH, when written this way, is defined as the balance of the person, both within one's being—physical, mental, spiritual—and in the outside world—natural, familial and communal, metaphysical.)
- ■ *Keeping Up.* Selected resources that present information that is frequently published in a timely manner to keep you abreast of data, on such topics as poverty, income, immigration, and so forth, as the facts and figures change. This is an ongoing feature in this text.

■ Supplemental Resources

- ■ *Online Student Resources.* The student resources available for download at pearsonhighered.com/nursingresources include a wealth of supplemental material to accompany each chapter. The resources present chapter-related review questions, case studies, and exercises to provide additional information.
  - ■ **The CULTURALCARE Museum.** This museum contains a collection of the author's photographs and culturally significant images.
  - ■ **Bibliography.** An extensive bibliography is provided to suggest further reading and research.
- ■ *Instructor's Resource Center.* Available to instructors adopting this book are Lecture Note PowerPoints, an Instructor's Manual, and a complete test bank available for download from the Instructor's Resource Center, which can be accessed through the online catalog.

About the Author

Dr. Rachel E. Spector has been a student of culturally diverse HEALTH and ILLNESS beliefs and practices for over 40 years and has researched and taught courses on culture and HEALTHCARE for the same time span. Dr. Spector has had the opportunity to work in many different communities, including the American Indian and Hispanic communities in Boston, Massachusetts. Her studies have taken her to many places: most of the United States, Canada, and Mexico; several European countries, including Denmark, England, Greece, Finland, Iceland, Italy, France, Russia, Spain, and Switzerland; Cuba; Israel; Pakistan; and Australia and New Zealand. She was fortunate enough to collect traditional amulets and remedies from many of these diverse communities, visit shrines, and meet practitioners of traditional HEALTHCARE in several places. She was instrumental in the creation and presentation of the exhibit "Immigrant HEALTH Traditions" at the Ellis Island Immigration Museum, May 1994 through January 1995. She has exhibited HEALTH-related objects in several other settings. Recently, she served as a *Colaboradora Honorifica* (Honorary Collaborator) in the University of Alicante in Alicante, Spain, and Tamaulipas, Mexico. In 2006, she was a Lady Davis Fellow in the Henrietta Zold-Hadassah Hebrew University School of Nursing in Jerusalem, Israel. This text was translated into Spanish by Maria Munoz and published in Madrid by Prentice Hall as *Las Culturas de la SALUD* in 2003 and into Chinese in 2010. There have been two International Editions of the book. She is a Fellow in the American Academy of Nursing and a Scholar in the Transcultural Nursing Society. The American Nurses' Association–Massachusetts, the state organization of the American Nurses' Association, honored her as a "Living Legend" in 2007. In 2008, she received the Honorary Human Rights Award from the American Nurses Association. This award recognized her contributions and accomplishments that have been of national significance to human rights and have influenced healthcare and nursing practice.

Acknowledgments

I have had a 45-year adventure of studying the forces of culture, ethnicity, and religion and their profound influence on HEALTH, ILLNESS, and HEALING beliefs and practices. Many, many people have contributed generously to the knowledge I have acquired over this time as I have tried to serve as a voice for traditional people and the HEALTH, ILLNESS, and HEALING beliefs and practices derived from their given heritage. It has been a continuous struggle to ensure that this information be included not only in nursing education, but in the educational content of all helping professions—including medicine, the allied health professions, and social work.

For the past 15 years I have been teaching a course, Holistic Living, to students who are not nursing majors. The course explores HEALTH under the embracing umbrella of spirituality. I have learned a lot from the students. Not only have they been interested in learning about health/HEALTH, but also they have become empowered by learning about their cultural heritage. The questions "Who are you?" and "Why are you here?" are fundamental themes of this course. These questions have given students an opportunity to explore both their generational heritage and their intangible cultural heritage. They have opened doors to knowledge and experiences they had never expected to encounter. Given that they will be living and working in a society that is far more complex and multicultural than the one I began my adult life in, they heartily embrace the cultural aspects of this book and course.

I particularly wish to thank the following people for their guidance, professional support, and encouragement over the 40 years that this book, now in its ninth edition, has been an integral part of my life. They are people from many walks of life and have touched me in many ways. The people from Appleton-Century-Crofts, which became Appleton & Lange, then became Prentice Hall, and is now Pearson. They include Katrin Beacom, Erin Rafferty, and countless people involved in the production of this edition. My first encounter with publishing was with Leslie Boyer, an acquisition editor from Appleton-Century-Crofts, who simply said "write a book" in 1976. I had no idea what she was talking about or what she really meant and what this would set in motion! In 1976, when the first edition of this book was conceived, I never dreamt that this is where it would be in 2016. The experience of preparing this ninth edition has been a formidable one. Most of the new content has been gathered via the World Wide Web. In addition, for this edition I have worked closely with the developmental editor Addy McCulloch. Without her outstanding help and guidance, this book would not be here today. It is impossible to thank her for all she has contributed.

The many people who helped with advice and guidance to resources over the years include Dr. Gaurdia E, Bannister, Dr. Billye Brown, Jenny Chan, Dr. P. K. Chan, Joe Colorado, Miriam Cook, Elizabeth Cucchiaro, Norine Dresser, Dr. Jose Siles Gonzalez, Orlando Isaza, Henry and Pandora Law, Dr. S. Dale McLemore, Dr. Anita Noble, Dr. Carl Rutberg, Sister Mary Nicholas Vincelli, Dr. David Warner, Dr. Deborah Washington, and the late Elsie Basque, Louise Buchanan, Julian Castillo, Leonel J. Castillo, Dr. Marjory Gordon, Hawk Littlejohn, Father Richard McCabe, Drª. Carmen Chamizo Vega, and Irving K. Zola.

My students, over the many years that I have taught, have generously shared their experiences and insights. When the fall semester, 2015, ended, Elizabeth G. Arone, Alice I. Choi, Sydney L. Hoffman, and Jennifer M. Taylor helped by reviewing the new chapters for this edition. It was most useful to see their comments about the new work, and I deeply appreciate their efforts.

The reviewers for the manuscript added invaluable assistance. I hope they will be quite pleased when they read the completed book. I thank them for their diligence and attention to detail.

I wish to thank my friends and family, who have tolerated my distracted responses and absence at countless social functions, and the many people who have provided the numerous support services necessary for the completion of an undertaking such as this. My husband, Manny, has been the rock who has sustained and supported me through all these years—most of all, I can never thank him enough.

A lot has happened in my life since the first edition of this book was published in 1979. My family has shrunk with the deaths of my parents and in-laws, and it has greatly expanded with a new daughter, Hilary, and a new son, Perry, and five granddaughters—Julia, Emma, Naomi, Rose, and Miriam. The generations have gone, and come.

■ Reviewers

Teresa S. Burckhalter, MSN, RN, BC
University of South Carolina–Beaufort
Beaufort, SC

Margherite Matteis, PhD, RN, PMHCNS-BC
Regis College
Weston, MA

Kate Lewis Nolt, MPH, PhD
Motivation Intervention
Philadelphia, PA

Linda Sweigart, MSN, APRN
Ball State University
Muncie, IN

Unit I

Cultural Foundations

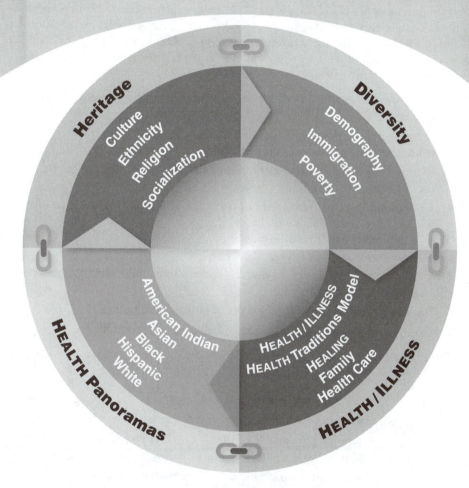

The *HERITAGECHAIN* (Figure U1-1) is the essential, distinct, and unifying theme of this book. It is a given that each of us is comprised of a genetic chain that is passed from generation to generation. We also possess an intangible cultural heritage (United Nations Educational, Scientific and Cultural Organization, n.d.) or sociocultural *HERITAGECHAIN* that includes traditional HEALTH beliefs and practices. These, too, are passed from generation to generation, but may have been lost or submerged in this modern era. The focus of this book will be the impact that the *HeritageChain* has on our HEALTH, ILLNESS, and HEALING beliefs and practices. The chapters represent major concepts; the *HeritageChain* links concept to concept. The concepts include cultural foundations, health domains, and HEALTH and ILLNESS panoramas. The theoretical links will be discussed in each chapter of this book.

Unit I creates the foundation for this book and is designed to help you become aware of the importance of developing knowledge in the topics of (1) cultural and linguistic competency; (2) *cultural* heritage and history—both your own and those of other people; (3) *diversity*—demographic, immigration, and economic; and (4) the customary concepts of *health* and *illness*. The chapters in Unit I will present an overview of relevant historical and contemporary theoretical content. You will:

1. Understand the critical need for the development of cultural and linguistic competency.
2. Identify and discuss the factors that contribute to heritage consistency—culture, ethnicity, religion, acculturation, and socialization.
3. Identify and discuss sociocultural events that may influence the life trajectory of a given person.
4. Understand diversity in the population of the United States by observing:
   - The Census estimates for 2015,
   - Immigration patterns and issues, and
   - Economic issues.
5. Understand health and illness and the sociocultural and historical phenomena that affect them.
6. Reexamine and redefine the concepts of health and illness.
7. Understand the multiple relationships between health and illness.

Before you read Unit I, please answer the following questions:

1. Do you speak a language other than English?
2. What is your sociocultural heritage?
3. What major sociocultural events have occurred in your lifetime?
4. What is the demographic profile of the community you grew up in? Has it changed; if so, how has it changed?
5. How would you acquire economic help if necessary?
6. How do you define *health*?
7. How do you define *illness*?
8. What do you do to maintain and protect your health?
9. What do you do when you experience a noticeable change in your health?
10. Do you diagnose your own health problems? If yes, how do you do so? If no, why not?
11. From whom do you seek healthcare?
12. What do you do to restore your health? Give examples.

CHAPTER 1

Building Cultural and Linguistic Competence

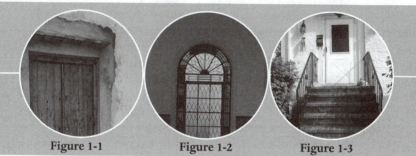

Figure 1-1 Figure 1-2 Figure 1-3

When there is a very dense cultural barrier, you do the best you can, and if something happens despite that, you have to be satisfied with little success instead of total successes. You have to give up total control....

—*Anne Fadiman (2001)*

■ Objectives

1. Discuss the critical need for cultural and linguistic competence.
2. Describe the National Standards for Culturally and Linguistically Appropriate Services in Health Care.
3. Describe institutional mandates regarding cultural and linguistic competence.
4. Articulate the attributes of CULTURALCOMPETENCY[1] and CULTURALCARE.

The opening images for this chapter depict the rationale for the building of CULTURALCOMPETENCY. Figure 1-1 is a "bolted fake door" in Vejer de la Frontera, Spain. It is a reminder of personal beliefs that shut out all other arguments and ways of understanding people. Figure 1-2 is a translucent door in Avila, Spain, where it is possible to look into a different reality and because

---

[1] When terms such as *HERITAGECHAIN*, CULTURALCOMPETENCY, and CULTURALCARE and others, such as HEALTH, ILLNESS, and HEALING, are written in all capital letters, it is done so to imply that they are referring to a holistic philosophy, rather than to a dualistic philosophy.

it is not locked, you can open it and recognize the views of others. Figure 1-3 represents the practical side—the steps to CULTURALCOMPETENCY. A more detailed discussion of each image follows in the forthcoming text.

In May 1988, Anne Fadiman, editor of *The American Scholar*, met the Lee family of Merced, California. Her subsequent book, *The Spirit Catches You and You Fall Down*, published in 1997, tells the compelling story of the Lees and their daughter, Lia, and their tragic encounter with the American healthcare delivery system. This book has now become a classic and is used by many healthcare educators and providers in situations where there is an effort to demonstrate the need for developing CULTURALCOMPETENCY.

When Lia was 3 months old, she was taken to the emergency room of the county hospital with epileptic seizures. The family was unable to communicate in English; the hospital staff did not include competent Hmong interpreters. From the parents' point of view, Lia was experiencing "the fleeing of her soul from her body and the soul had become lost." They knew these symptoms to be *quag dab peg*—"the spirit catches you and you fall down." The Hmong regarded this experience with ambivalence, yet they knew that it was serious and potentially dangerous, as it was epilepsy. It was also an illness that evokes a sense of both concern and pride.

The parents and the healthcare providers both wanted the best for Lia, yet a complex and dense trajectory of misunderstanding and misinterpreting was set in motion. The tragic cultural conflict lasted for several years and caused considerable pain to each party (Fadiman, 2001). This moving incident exemplifies the extreme events that can occur when two antithetical cultural belief systems collide within the overall environment of the healthcare delivery system. Each party comes to a healthcare event with a set notion of what ought to happen—and, unless each is able to understand the view of the other, complex difficulties can arise.

The catastrophic events of September 11, 2001; the wars in Iraq, Afghanistan, and Libya; the Islamic State and the increase in incidents of global terrorism, such as the 2015 massacre in Paris, France; the countless natural disasters such as Hurricane Katrina and the earthquakes in Haiti and Japan; and our ongoing preoccupation with domestic terrorist threats—and reality in San Bernardino, California—have pierced the consciousness of all Americans in general and healthcare providers in particular. Now, more than ever, providers *must* become informed about and sensitive to the culturally diverse subjective meanings of **health/HEALTH, illness/ILLNESS**, and **curing/HEALING** practices. Cultural diversity and pluralism are a core part of the social and economic engines that drive the country. Their impact has significant implications for healthcare delivery and policymaking throughout the United States.

In all clinical practice areas—from institutional settings, such as acute and long-term care settings, to community-based settings, such as nurse practitioners', physician assistants', and doctors' offices and clinics, schools and universities, public health, and occupational settings—one observes diversity every day. The undeniable need for culturally and linguistically competent healthcare services for diverse populations has attracted increased attention from healthcare providers and those who judge their quality and efficiency for many years.

Personal cultural background, heritage, and language have a considerable impact on both how patients access and respond to healthcare services and how the providers practice within the system. Cultural and linguistic competence suggests an ability of healthcare providers and healthcare organizations to understand and respond effectively to the cultural and linguistic needs brought to the healthcare experience. This is a phenomenon that recognizes the diversity that exists among the patients, physicians, nurses, and caregivers. This phenomenon is not limited to the changes in the patient population in that it also embraces the members of the workforce—including providers from other countries. Many of the people in the workforce are new immigrants and/or are from ethnocultural backgrounds that differ from that of the dominant culture.

In addition, health and illness can be interpreted and explained in terms of personal experience and expectations. We can define our own health or illness and determine what these states mean to us in our daily lives. We learn from our own cultural and ethnic backgrounds how to be healthy, how to recognize illness, and how to be ill. Furthermore, the meanings we attach to the notions of health and illness are related to the basic, culture-bound values by which we define a given experience and perception.

It is now *imperative,* according to the most recent policies of the Joint Commission of Hospital Accreditation and the Centers for Medicare & Medicaid Services, that *all* healthcare providers be "culturally competent." In this context, cultural competency implies that within the delivery of care, the healthcare provider understands and attends to the total context of the patient's situation; it is a complex combination of knowledge, attitudes, and skills, yet:

- How do you *really* inspire people to hear the content?
- How do you *motivate* providers to see the worldview and lived experience of the patient?
- How do you assist providers to *really* bear witness to the living conditions and lifeways of patients?
- How do you liberate providers from the burdens of prejudice, xenophobia, the "isms"—racism, ethnocentrism—and the "antis" such as anti-Semitism, anti-Catholicism, anti-Islamism, anti-immigrant, and so forth?
- How do you inspire philosophical changes from dualistic thinking to holistic thinking?

It can be argued that the development of CULTURALCOMPETENCY does not occur in a short encounter with programs on cultural diversity but that it takes time to develop the skills, knowledge, and attitudes to safely and satisfactorily become "CULTURALLYCOMPETENT" and to deliver CULTURALCARE. Indeed, the reality of becoming "CULTURALLYCOMPETENT" is a complex process—it is time consuming, difficult, frustrating, and extremely interesting. It is a philosophical change wherein the CULTURALLYCOMPETENT person is able to hear, understand, and respect the nonverbal and/or non-articulated needs and perspectives of a given patient.

CULTURALCOMPETENCY embraces the premise that all things are connected. Consider Figure U1-1, the HERITAGECHAIN. Each concept, or facet, discussed in this book—heritage, culture, ethnicity, religion, socialization, and identity—is a link connected to diversity, demographic change, population, immigration, and poverty. These links are connected to health/HEALTH, illness/ILLNESS, curing/HEALING, beliefs and practices, modern and traditional. All of these links are connected to the healthcare delivery system—the culture, costs, and politics of healthcare, the internal and external political issues, public health issues, and housing and other infrastructure issues. In order to fully understand a person's health/HEALTH beliefs and practices, each of these topics must be in the background of a provider's mind. Three assessment tools (see Appendix B) have been developed from the theoretical links that are delineated within the text:

1. Heritage Assessment
2. Ethnofamily Health Interview/Assessment
3. Ethnocultural Community Assessment

They will be further discussed in forthcoming chapters.

I have had the opportunity to live and teach in Spain and to explore many areas, including Cadiz and the surrounding small villages. There was a fake door within the walls of a small village, Vejer de la Frontera (Figure 1-1), that appeared to be bolted shut. The door was placed there during the early 14th century to fool the Barbary pirates. The people were able to vanquish them while they tried to pry the door open. It reminded me of the attempt to keep other ideas and people away and not open up to new and different ideas. Another door (Figure 1-2), found in Avila, Spain, was made of translucent glass. Here, the person has a choice—peer through the door and view the garden behind it, or open it and actually go into the garden for a finite walk. This reminded me of people who are able to understand the needs of others and return to their own life and heritage when work is completed. This polarity represents the challenges of "CULTURALCOMPETENCY."

The way to CULTURALCOMPETENCY is complex, but I have learned over the years that there are five steps, Figure 1-3, to master as you begin to achieve this goal:

1. *Personal heritage:* Who are *you*? What is *your* heritage? What are your health/HEALTH beliefs?
2. *Heritage of others—demographics:* Who is the other? Family? Community?
3. *Health and HEALTH beliefs and practices:* What the competing philosophies are.
4. *Healthcare culture and system:* What all the issues and problems are.
5. *Traditional HEALTHCARE systems:* The way HEALTH was for most, and the way HEALTH still is for many.

Once you have reached the sixth step, CULTURALCOMPETENCY, you are ready to open the door to CULTURALCARE.

Each link in the *HeritageChain* represents a discrete unit of study. The links represent the fundamental terms, or language, of the content. Table 1-1 lists many examples of the links, and these terms are used in the

Table 1-1   Selected CulturalCare Terms

Access	Acupuncture	Ageism	Alien
Allopathic philosophy	Amulet	Apparel	Assimilation
Bankes	Borders	Calendar	Care
Census	Citizen	CLAS	Community
Costs	Cultural conflict	CulturalCare	CulturalCompetency
Culturally appropriate	Culturally competent	Culturally sensitive	**Culture**
Curandera/o	Customs	Cycle of poverty	Demographic disparity
Demographic parity	**Demography**	Diagnosis	**Diversity**
Documentation	Education	*Empacho*	*Envidia*
Ethics	**Ethnicity**	Ethnicity	Ethnocentrism
Evil eye	**Family**	Financing	Food
Garments	Gender specific care	Green Card	Gris-gris
Habits	Halal	**Healing**	**Health**
Health	**Healthcare system**	Health disparities	**Health** Traditions
Healthy People 2020	Herbalist	Heritage	Heritage consistency
Heritage inconsistency	Heterosexism	Hex	Homeland security
Homeopathic philosophy	Homophobia	Iatrogenic	**Illness**
Illness	**Immigration**	Kosher	Language
Law	Legal Permanent Resident (LPR)	Life trajectory	*Limpia*
Linguistic competence	Literacy	Mal ojo	Manpower
Meridians	Migrant labor	*Milagros*	Modern
Modesty	Morbidity	Mortality	Naturalization
Office of Minority Health	*Orisha*	Osteopathy	*Partera*
Pasmo	Politics	**Poverty**	Poverty guidelines
Powwow	Procedures	*Promesa*	*Quag dab peg*
Racism	Reflexology	Refugee	**Religion**
Remedies	Sacred objects	Sacred places	Sacred practices
Sacred spaces	Sacred times	*Santera/o*	*Senoria*
Sexism	Silence	Silence	Singer
Socialization	Spell	Spirits	Spiritual
Spirituality	Title VI	Traditional	Undocumented person
Visitors	Voodoo	Vulnerability	Welfare
Worldview	Xenophobia	*Yin & Yang*	*Yoruba*

following chapters as appropriate and are defined in the Key Terms list in Appendix A. These selected terms and many more are the evolving language or jargon of CULTURALCARE.

Contrary to popular belief and practice, CULTURALCOMPETENCY is not a "condition" that is rapidly achieved. Rather, it is an ongoing process of growth and the development of knowledge that takes a considerable amount of time to ingest, digest, assimilate, circulate, and master. It is, for many, a philosophical change in that they develop the skills to understand where a person from a different cultural background than theirs is coming from.

This discussion now presents an overview of the significant content related to the ongoing development of the concepts of cultural and linguistic competency as they are described by several different organizations. Presently, there has been a proliferation of resources related to this content and a discussion of selected items is included here. Box 1-2, at the conclusion of the chapter, lists numerous resources.

■ National Standards for Culturally and Linguistically Appropriate Services in Health Care

In 1997, the Office of Minority Health undertook the development of national standards to provide a much-needed alternative to the patchwork that had been undertaken in the field of cultural diversity. It developed the National Standards for Culturally and Linguistically Appropriate Services (CLAS) in Health Care. These 15 standards, improved over time (Box 1-1), must be met by most healthcare-related agencies. The standards are based on an analytical review of key laws, regulations, contracts, and standards currently in use by federal and state agencies and other national organizations. The standards were developed with input from a national advisory committee of policymakers, healthcare providers, and researchers and were primarily directed at healthcare organizations. The current 15 enhanced standards are a comprehensive series of guidelines. They guide practices related to culturally and linguistically appropriate health services. The goal is to advance health equity along the healthcare continuum. The CLAS principles and activities must be integrated throughout an organization and implemented in partnership with the communities being served (https://www.thinkculturalhealth.hhs.gov/).

■ Cultural Competence

Cultural competence implies that professional healthcare must be developed to be culturally sensitive, culturally appropriate, and culturally competent. Culturally competent care is critical to meet the complex culture-bound healthcare needs of a given person, family, and community. It is the provision of healthcare across cultural boundaries and takes into account the context in which the patient lives, as well as the situations in which the patient's health problems arise.

Box 1-1

The National Standards for Culturally and Linguistically Appropriate Services in Health and Health Care (The National CLAS Standards)

Principal Standard

1. Provide effective, equitable, understandable, and respectful quality care and services that are responsive to diverse cultural health beliefs and practices, preferred languages, health literacy, and other communication needs.

Governance, Leadership and Workforce

2. Advance and sustain organizational governance and leadership that promotes CLAS and health equity through policy, practices, and allocated resources.
3. Recruit, promote, and support a culturally and linguistically diverse governance, leadership, and workforce that are responsive to the population in the service area.
4. Educate and train governance, leadership, and workforce in culturally and linguistically appropriate policies and practices on an ongoing basis.

Communication and Language Assistance

5. Offer language assistance to individuals who have limited English proficiency and/or other communication needs, at no cost to them, to facilitate timely access to all health care and services.
6. Inform all individuals of the availability of language assistance services clearly and in their preferred language, verbally and in writing.
7. Ensure the competence of individuals providing language assistance, recognizing that the use of untrained individuals and/or minors as interpreters should be avoided.
8. Provide easy-to-understand print and multimedia materials and signage in the languages commonly used by the populations in the service area.

Engagement, Continuous Improvement and Accountability

9. Establish culturally and linguistically appropriate goals, policies, and management accountability, and infuse them throughout the organization's planning and operations.
10. Conduct ongoing assessments of the organization's CLAS-related activities and integrate CLAS-related measures into assessment measurement and continuous quality improvement activities.
11. Collect and maintain accurate and reliable demographic data to monitor and evaluate the impact of CLAS on health equity and outcomes and to inform service delivery.
12. Conduct regular assessments of community health assets and needs and use the results to plan and implement services that respond to the cultural and linguistic diversity of populations in the service area.
13. Partner with the community to design, implement, and evaluate policies, practices, and services to ensure cultural and linguistic appropriateness.

(continued)

Box 1-1   *Continued*

14. Create conflict- and grievance-resolution processes that are culturally and linguistically appropriate to identify, prevent, and resolve conflicts or complaints.
15. Communicate the organization's progress in implementing and sustaining CLAS to all stakeholders, constituents, and the general public.

CLAS standards are non-regulatory and therefore do not have the force and effect of law. The standards are not mandatory, but they greatly assist healthcare providers and organizations in responding effectively to their patients' cultural and linguistic needs. Compliance with Title VI of the Civil Rights Act of 1964 is mandatory and requires healthcare providers and organizations that receive federal financial assistance to take reasonable steps to ensure Limited English Proficiency (LEP) persons have meaningful access to services.

CLAS standards use the term patients/consumers to refer to "individuals, including accompanying family members, guardians, or companions, seeking physical or mental healthcare services, or other health-related services" (p. 5 of the comprehensive final report; see http://minorityhealth.hhs.gov/templates/browse.aspx?lvl=2&lvlID=15).

Source: National Standards for Culturally and Linguistically Appropriate Services in Health Care, by U.S. Department of Health and Human Services, Office of Minority Health, ThinkHealth. Retrieved from https://www.thinkculturalhealth.hhs.gov/Content/clas.asp

- *Culturally competent.* Within the delivered care, the provider understands and attends to the total context of the patient's situation, and this is a complex combination of knowledge, attitudes, and skills.
- *Culturally appropriate.* The provider applies the underlying background knowledge that must be possessed to provide a patient with the best possible health/HEALTHcare.
- *Culturally sensitive.* The provider possesses some basic knowledge of and constructive attitudes toward the health/HEALTH traditions observed among the diverse cultural groups found in the setting in which he or she is practicing.

■ Linguistic Competence

Title VI of the Civil Rights Act of 1964 states, "No person in the United States shall, on ground of race, color, or national origin, be excluded from participation in, be denied the benefits of, or be subjected to discrimination under any program or activity receiving Federal financial assistance." To avoid discrimination based on national origin, Title VI and its implementing regulations require recipients of federal financial assistance to take reasonable steps to provide meaningful access to Limited English Proficiency (LEP) persons. Therefore, under the provisions of Title VI of the Civil Rights Act of 1964, when people with LEP seek healthcare in healthcare settings such as hospitals, nursing homes, clinics, daycare centers, and mental health centers, services cannot be denied to them. It is said that "language barriers have a deleterious effect on healthcare and patients are less likely to have a usual source of healthcare, and have an increased risk if non-adherence to medication regimens" (Flores, 2006, p. 230).

The United States is home to millions of people from many national origins. Currently, because there are growing concerns about racial, ethnic, and language disparities in health and healthcare and the need for healthcare systems to accommodate increasingly diverse patient populations, language access services (LAS) have become more and more a matter of national importance. This need has become increasingly pertinent given the continued growth in language diversity within the United States. English is the official language of the United States and, according to the 2011 American Community Survey estimates, it is spoken at home by 79.2% of the residents over 5 years old. In the same year, however, 9% of the population over 5 years old spoke "no English at all." In the total of over 37.5 million Spanish-speaking people over 5 years old, 62.9% spoke "no English at all." Of the people over the age of 5 speaking other Indo-European languages, most spoke English very well. However, there are a number of people from many of the Indo-European countries, such as Russia and Armenia, that speak no English. Of those who speak the Asian and Pacific Island languages, most speak English very well or well, but there are many who either speak English not well or not at all (Ryan, 2013, p. 1).

People who are limited in their ability to speak, read, write, and understand the English language experience countless language barriers that can result in limiting their access to critical public health, hospital, and other medical and social services to which they are legally entitled. Many health and social service programs who once provided information about their services in English only are now using interpreter services and information in the languages of the populations in their service area. Each patient must be carefully assessed to determine his or her language needs, and information must be delivered in a manner that is understandable by the patient. When a patient does not understand English, competent interpreters or language resources must be available.

■ Institutional Mandates

Since 2003, the Joint Commission has been actively pursuing a course that ensures that cultural and linguistic competency standards become a part of their accreditation requirements. Since this time, they have published several documents relevant to this topic, and in 2010 they published a monograph, *Advancing Effective Communication, Cultural Competence, and Patient and Family Centered Care: A Roadmap for Hospitals*. The monograph provides checklists to improve effective communication during the admission, assessment, treatment, end-of-life, and discharge and transfer stages of a given patient's hospitalization trajectory. They strongly state that:

> Every patient that enters the hospital has a unique set of needs—clinical symptoms that require medical attention and issues specific to the individual that can affect his or her care. (The Joint Commission, 2010, p. 1)

They implicitly recognize that when a given person moves through the hospitalization continuum, he or she requires not only medical and nursing intervention, but also care that addresses the spectrum of each person's demographic and personal characteristics. The Joint Commission has made many efforts to understand personal needs and then provide guidance to organizations to address those needs. They initially focused on studying language, culture, and health literacy needs, and presently (as of 2011), they are focusing on effective communication, cultural competence, and patient- and family-centered care.

The Joint Commission defines cultural competency as:

> the ability of health care providers and health care organizations to understand and respond effectively to the cultural and language needs brought by the patient to the health care encounter. (The Joint Commission, 2010, p. 91)

They further recognize that:

> cultural competence requires organizations and their personnel to: (1) value diversity; (2) assess themselves; (3) manage the dynamics of difference; (4) acquire and institutionalize cultural knowledge; and (5) adapt to diversity and the cultural contexts of individuals and communities served. (The Joint Commission, 2010, p. 91)

These principles apply to each segment of the institutional experience from admission to discharge or end of life, and for each facet, specific actions must be undertaken. These actions include informing patients of their rights, assessing communication needs, and involving the patient and family in care plans. Each segment is accompanied by a checklist for activities; for example, there is a checklist to Improve Effective Communication, Cultural Competence, and Patient- and Family-Centered Care during admission (The Joint Commission, 2010, p. 9).

■ CULTURALCARE

The term *CULTURALCARE* expresses all that is inherent in the development of healthcare delivery to meet the mandates of the CLAS standards and other cultural competency mandates. CULTURALCARE is holistic care. There are countless conflicts in the healthcare delivery arenas that are predicated on cultural misunderstandings. Although many of these misunderstandings are related to universal situations—such as verbal and nonverbal language misunderstandings, the conventions of courtesy and manners, the order in which conversations take place, how interactions are worded, and how the provider is perceived by the patient—many cultural misunderstandings are unique to the delivery of healthcare. The need to provide CULTURALCARE is essential, and providers must be able to assess and interpret a patient's health beliefs and practices and cultural and linguistic needs. CULTURALCARE alters the perspective of healthcare delivery as it enables the provider to understand, from a cultural perspective, the manifestations of the patient's cultural heritage and life trajectory. The provider must serve as a bridge in the healthcare setting between the given institution, the patient, and people who are from different cultural backgrounds.

In conclusion, cultural and linguistic competency must be understood to be the foundations of a new healthcare *philosophy*. It is comprised of countless facets—each of which is a topic for study. CULTURALCOMPETENCY is a philosophy that appreciates and values holistic perspectives rather than, or in addition to, dualistic—modern and technological—viewpoints. CULTURALCOMPETENCY is more than a "willingness"—it is a philosophy that *must* be part of an institution's and a professional's mission and goal statement. Within the philosophy of cultural competency, **HEALTH**, **ILLNESS**, and **HEALING** are understood holistically.

The development of CULTURALCOMPETENCY is an ongoing, lifelong endeavor. This is a topic that requires deep study, reflection, and time. The days when a "bagged lunch" with an hour's lecture or discussion have passed, and hours—even a lifetime—must be dedicated to the topics, and countless others, this book presents. Critical questions must be asked: "Are healthcare providers institutional advocates? Modern healthcare advocates? Or, patient advocates?"

Explore  MediaLink

Go to the Student Resource Site at pearsonhighered.com/nursingresources for chapter-related review questions, case studies, and activities. Contents of the CULTURALCARE Guide and CULTURALCARE Museum can also be found on the Student Resource Site. Click on Chapter 1 to select the activities for this chapter.

Box 1-2

Keeping Up

There are countless references, published weekly, monthly, annually, and periodically, that may be accessed to maintain currency in the domains of cultural and linguistic competency and with professional organizations concerned with this specialty area of practice. The following are selected suggestions:

American Association of Colleges of Nursing (AACN)

The AACN's Toolkit for Cultural Competent Education provides extensive resources including content and teaching-learning activities.

(continued)

Box 1-2   *Continued*

Health and Human Services (HHS) Data Council

The HHS Data Council coordinates all health and human services data collection and analysis activities of the Department of Health and Human Services, including integrated data collection strategy, coordination of health data standards and health and human services, and privacy policy activities.

Institute of Medicine

The Institute of Medicine (IOM) is a division of the National Academies of Sciences, Engineering, and Medicine. The Academies are private, nonprofit institutions that provide independent, objective analysis and advice to the nation and conduct other activities to solve complex problems and inform public policy decisions related to science, technology, and medicine. The IOM aids those in government and the private sector make informed health decisions predicated on reliable evidence.

Kaiser Family Foundation

Kaiser Fast Facts provides direct access to facts, data, and slides about the nation's healthcare system and programs, in an easy-to-use format.

The Kaiser Family Foundation has launched a new internet resource, State Health Facts Online, that offers comprehensive and current health information for all 50 states, the District of Columbia, and U.S. territories. State Health Facts Online offers health policy information on a broad range of issues such as managed care, health insurance coverage and the uninsured, Medicaid, Medicare, women's health, minority health, and data and slides about the nation's healthcare system and programs, in an easy-to-use format.

National Breast and Cervical Cancer Early Detection Program (NBCCEDP)

NBCCEDP provides access to critical breast and cervical cancer screening services for underserved women in the United States, the District of Columbia, 4 U.S. territories, and 13 American Indian/Alaska Native organizations.

Office of Minority Health (OMH)

The OMH was created in 1986 and is one of the most significant outcomes of the 1985 *Secretary's Task Force Report on Black and Minority Health*. Reauthorized by the Patient Protection and Affordable Care Act of 2010 (Pub. L. 111–148), the OMH is dedicated to improving the health of racial and ethnic minority populations through the development of health policies and programs that will help eliminate health disparities. In addition to the new standards, *National Standards for Culturally and Linguistically Appropriate Services in Health and Health Care: A Blueprint for Advancing and Sustaining CLAS Policy and Practice* are available on the OMH website. The OMH also offers an excellent resource, Think Cultural Health: Advancing Health Equity at Every Point of Contact.

Robert Wood Johnson

The Robert Wood Johnson Foundation has an online tool that ranks state counties by health status, taking into account clinical care, socioeconomic, and environmental factors.

The National Center for Health Statistics (NCHS)

The NCHS provides quick and easy access to the wide range of information and data available, including HHS surveys and data collection systems.

The Joint Commission

Since 2007, the Joint Commission has been working toward improving access to care for all patients at its accredited organizations, emphasizing better communication, cultural competence, and patient- and family-centered care.

The *Online Journal of Cultural Competence in Nursing and Healthcare*

This journal's first issue appeared online in January 2011. It is a free quarterly peer-reviewed publication that provides a forum for discussion of the issues, trends, theory, research, evidence-based, and best practices in the provision of culturally congruent and competent nursing and healthcare.

Transcultural Nursing Society

The Transcultural Nursing Society has developed a core curriculum in Transcultural Nursing; Douglas, M. K., Editor-in-Chief, and Pacquiao, D. F., Senior Editor. (2010). *Core Curriculum for Transcultural Nursing and Health Care* is available here.

The Transcultural Nursing Society has also developed Standards for Culturally Competent Nursing Care and they can be found in Douglas, M. K., Pierce, J. U., Rosenkoetter, M., et al. (2011). Standards of Practice for Culturally Competent Care. *Journal of Transcultural Nursing, 22*(4), 318.

University of Michigan Health System: The Cultural Competency Division

The Cultural Competency Division plays a vital role in implementing cultural competency in the UMHS and in promoting good community healthcare practices. This is an excellent website with links to numerous sites.

■ References

Civil Rights Act of 1964, Pub. L. No. 88–352, § 601, 78 Stat. 252 (42 U.S.C. 2000).

Fadiman, A. (2001). *The spirit catches you and you fall down.* New York, NY: Farrar, Straus, and Giroux.

Flores, G. (2006). Language barriers to health care in the United States. *New England Journal of Medicine, 355*(3), 229–231.

The Joint Commission. (2010). *Advancing effective communication, cultural competence, and patient- and family-centered care: A roadmap for hospitals.* Oakbrook Terrace, IL: The Joint Commission. Retrieved from http://www.jointcommission.org/

Ryan, C. (2013). *Language use in the United States: 2011.* American Community Survey Reports. U.S. Census Bureau. Retrieved from https://www.census.gov/prod/2013pubs/acs-22.pdf

United Nations Educational, Scientific and Cultural Organization. (n.d.). *What is intangible cultural heritage?* Retrieved from http://www.unesco.org/culture/ich/en/what-is-intangible-heritage-00003

CHAPTER 2 Cultural Heritage and History

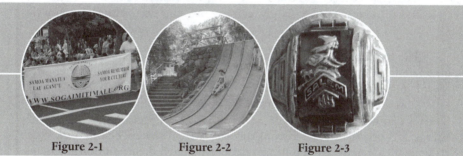

Figure 2-1   Figure 2-2   Figure 2-3

Samoans, remember your culture. — — — — — — — — — — — — — — — — — —

◼ Objectives

1. Explain the links on the *HERITAGECHAIN* that contribute to heritage consistency—culture, ethnicity, and religion.
2. Explain the links related to acculturation themes.
3. Discuss and give examples of cultural conflicts.
4. Explain the factors involved in the cultural phenomena affecting health and healthcare.

This link on the *HERITAGECHAIN* explores the concept of heritage—cultural, religious, and ethnic; acculturation themes, and cultural phenomena affecting health and healthcare. The banner (Figure 2-1) admonishes Samoans—"remember YOUR culture"—a searing message for each of us to hear. It is imperative for all of us to know our culture and heritage as we move forward to become CULTURALLYCOMPETENT. Figure 2-2 is a cement slide that was built into the side of a hill in a small playground. I played on it as a child, as did my mother, my children, and my grandchildren—a four-generation relic that evokes countless memories of childhood and child rearing. Figure 2-3 is my class ring, a cherished icon—I graduated from Salem (Massachusetts) High School.

As you begin to consider aspects of heritage consistency, first ask yourself:

ⓒ *Who are you?* What is *your* cultural, ethnic, and religious heritage? What are images of the places and icons of your generation and culture? How and where were you socialized to the roles and rules of your family, community, and occupation?

ⓒ *Who is the person next to you?* What is this person's cultural, ethnic, and religious heritage? How and where was this person socialized to the roles and rules of his or her family, community, and occupation? Are you this person's healthcare provider, instructor, colleague, or supervisor?

The foundation for CULTURALCOMPETENCY rests in the knowledge and understanding of heritage, not only your own, but also that of others with whom you are interacting.

This second chapter presents an overview of the salient and complex theoretical content related to one's heritage and its impact on health/HEALTH beliefs and practices. Two sets of theories are presented, the first of which analyzes the degree to which people have maintained their traditional heritage; the second, and opposite, set of theories relates to socialization and acculturation and the quasi-creation of a melting pot or some other common threads that are part of an American whole. It then becomes possible to analyze health beliefs by determining a person's ties to his or her traditional heritage, rather than to signs of acculturation. The assumption is that there is a relationship between people with strong identities—either with their heritage or the level at which they are acculturated into the American culture—and their health/HEALTH beliefs and practices. Hand in hand with the concept of ethnocultural heritage is that of a person's ethnocultural history; the journey a person has experienced predicated on the historical sociocultural events that have touched his or her life directly or indirectly.

■ Heritage Consistency

Heritage consistency is a concept developed by Estes and Zitzow (1980, p. 1) to describe "the degree to which one's lifestyle reflects his or her respective tribal culture." The theory has been expanded in an attempt to study the degree to which a person's lifestyle reflects his or her traditional culture, such as European, Asian, African, or Hispanic. The values indicating heritage consistency exist on a continuum, and a person can possess value characteristics of both a consistent heritage (traditional) and an inconsistent heritage (acculturated). The concept of heritage consistency includes a determination of one's cultural, ethnic, and religious background. Another way to consider the relationship between heritage and cultural, ethnic, and religious backgrounds is as a chain, with heritage forming the first link and the other factors—culture, religion, and ethnicity—being subsequent links (Figure 2-4).

It has been found over time that the greater a given person identifies with his or her traditional heritage—that is, his or her culture, ethnicity, and

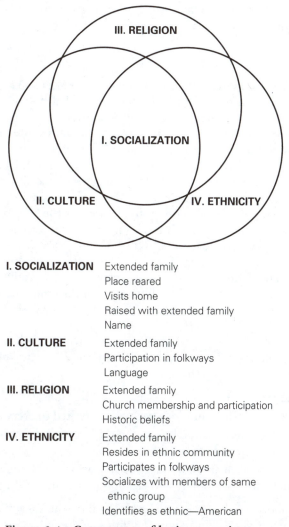

I. SOCIALIZATION   Extended family
                    Place reared
                    Visits home
                    Raised with extended family
                    Name

II. CULTURE   Extended family
                    Participation in folkways
                    Language

III. RELIGION   Extended family
                    Church membership and participation
                    Historic beliefs

IV. ETHNICITY   Extended family
                    Resides in ethnic community
                    Participates in folkways
                    Socializes with members of same
                      ethnic group
                    Identifies as ethnic—American

Figure 2-4   Components of heritage consistency.

religion—the greater the chance that the person's health and illness beliefs and practices may vary from those of the mainstream society and modern health-care providers. For example, Estes and Zitzow observed that when people who identified highly with their tribal culture were treated for alcoholism by a medicine man, the outcome was more favorable than with treatment in the modern culture. Other research found that people with a high level of heritage consistency frequented healthcare sources not used by modern providers. The Heritage Assessment Tool, another link on the chain of interrelated concepts and assessment tools that can be found in Appendix B, is a screening tool to assess for a person's immersion in their particular heritage. It is a useful tool in research development. A given respondent who answers affirmatively to a large number of factors on this tool may well be "heritage consistent"—that is, identify deeply with their traditional heritage.

Culture

The word *culture* showed 1,460,000,000 results on August 22, 2015, on the internet. There is no single definition of *culture*, and all too often definitions omit salient aspects of culture or are too general to have any real meaning. Of the countless ideas of the meaning of this term, some are of particular note. The classical definition by Fejos (1959, p. 43) describes culture as "the sum total of socially inherited characteristics of a human group that comprises everything which one generation can tell, convey, or hand down to the next; in other words, the nonphysically inherited traits we possess." Another way of understanding the concept of culture is to picture it as the luggage that each of us carries around for our lifetime. It is the sum of beliefs, practices, habits, likes, dislikes, norms, customs, rituals, and so forth that we learned from our families during the years of socialization. In turn, we transmit this cultural luggage to our children. The definition that is most relevant in the study of traditional HEALTH beliefs and practices is that culture is a "metacommunication system," wherein not only the spoken words have meaning but everything else does as well (Matsumoto, 1989, p. 14).

All facets of human behavior can be interpreted through the lens of culture, and everything can be related to and from this context. Culture has several characteristics, including that it is:

1. The medium of personhood and social relationships
2. A complex whole in which each part is related to every other part
3. Learned, and must be learned by each person in a family and social community, and
4. Dependent on an underlying social matrix, that includes knowledge, beliefs, art, law, morals, and customs (Bohannan, 1992, p. 13).

The symbols of culture—sound and acts—form the basis of all languages. Symbols are everywhere—in religion, politics, and gender; the meanings of which vary between and within cultural groups. There are countless cultural symbols relevant to traditional HEALTH and ILLNESS beliefs and practices and will be discussed in later chapters of this text.

Ethnicity

The word *ethnicity* showed 179,000,000 results on August 22, 2015, on the internet. A random exploration of selected sites did not provide information different from the classical information in the following discussion.

Cultural background is a fundamental component of one's ethnic background. Before we proceed with this discussion, though, we need to define some terms, so that we can move forward from the same point of reference. The classic reference defines *ethnic* as an adjective "relating to large groups of people classed according to common racial, national, tribal, religious, linguistic, or cultural origin or background" ("Ethnic," *Merriam-Webster Dictionary*, n.d.). O'Neil (2008) described *ethnicity* as selected cultural and sometimes physical characteristics used to classify people into groups or categories considered to be significantly different from others.

The term *ethnic* has for some time aroused strongly negative feelings and is often rejected by the general population. One can speculate that the upsurge in the use of the term stems from the recent interest of people in discovering their personal backgrounds, a fact used by some politicians who overtly court "the ethnics." Paradoxically, in a nation as large as the United States and comprising as many different peoples as it does—with the American Indians being the only true native population—we find ourselves still reluctant to speak of ethnicity and ethnic differences. This stance stems from the fact that most foreign groups that come to this land often shed the ways of the "old country" and quickly attempt to assimilate into the mainstream, or the so-called melting pot (Novak, 1973). Other terms related to *ethnic* include:

- *Ethnocentrism:* (1) belief in the superiority of one's own ethnic group; (2) overriding concern with race
- *Xenophobia:* a morbid fear of strangers
- *Xenophobe:* a person unduly fearful or contemptuous of strangers or foreigners, especially as reflected in his or her political or cultural views.

The behavioral manifestations of these phenomena occur in response to people's needs, especially when they are foreign born and must find a way to function (1) before they are assimilated into the mainstream and (2) in order to accept themselves. The people cluster together against the majority, who in turn may be discriminating against them.

Ethnicity is indicative of the following selected characteristics a group may share in some combination:

1. Geographic origin and migratory status
2. Race
3. Language and dialect
4. Religious faith or faiths
5. Ties that transcend kinship, neighborhood, and community boundaries
6. Traditions, values, and symbols
7. Literature, folklore, and music.

There are at least 106 ethnic groups and 567 federally recognized American Indian tribes and Alaska Natives (Bureau of Indian Affairs, 2016) in the United States that meet many of these criteria. People from every country in the world have immigrated to this country. Some nations, such as Germany, England, Italy, and Ireland, were heavily represented in early immigration times. People continue to immigrate to the United States, with the present influx coming from Mexico, Haiti, South and Central America, India, and China (U.S. Department of Homeland Security, 2014, pp. 12–13).

Religion

The third major component of heritage consistency is religion. The word *religion* showed 660,000,000 results on August 24, 2015, on the internet. One customary way to understand religion is that it is "the belief in a divine or superhuman power or powers to be obeyed and worshipped as the creator(s) and ruler(s) of the universe; it is a system of beliefs, practices, and ethical values" (Abramson, 1980, pp. 869–875). Another way is to see religion as "an organized system of beliefs, ceremonies, and rules used to worship a god or a group of gods" ("Religion," *Merriam-Webster Dictionary*, n.d.). The practice of religion is revealed in numerous cults, sects, denominations, and churches. Ethnicity and religion are clearly related, and one's religion quite often determines one's ethnic group. Religion gives a person a frame of reference and a perspective with which to organize information. Religious teachings help present a meaningful philosophy and system of practices within a system of social controls having specific values, norms, and ethics. These are related to health in that adherence to a religious code is conducive to spiritual harmony and health. Illness is sometimes seen as a punishment for the violation of religious codes and morals.

Religion plays a fundamental and vital role in the health beliefs and practices of many people. For example, the use of meditation; rules regarding immunization; rules regarding modesty and who can examine a given person; family relationships; the concept of hope with terminal illness; and childrearing. Specific examples of a religious tradition and its influence on health include:

1. The Jewish and Muslim faiths prohibit eating pig products.
2. The Catholic faith forbids abortion.
3. The Jehovah's Witness faith forbids blood transfusions.
4. The Mormon faith prohibits the use of caffeine and tobacco.

An additional way of understanding the relationship of religion to health is to conceptualize religion as the domain of life that deals with things of the spirit and matters of ultimate concern, a way to answer the questions "*Who am I?*" and "*Why am I here?*" In addition, religious affiliation and membership benefit health by promoting healthy behavior and lifestyles in the following ways:

1. Regular religious fellowship benefits health by offering support that buffers and affects stress and isolation.
2. Participation in worship and prayer benefits health through the physiological effects of positive emotions.
3. Religious beliefs benefit health by their similarity to health promoting beliefs and personality styles.
4. Simple faith benefits health by leading to thoughts of hope, optimism, and positive expectation.

5. Mystical experiences benefit health by activating a healing bioenergy or life force or altered state of consciousness.

6. Absent prayer for others is capable of healing by paranormal means or by divine intervention (Levin, 2001, p. 9).

Unlike some countries, the United States does not include a question about religion in its census and has not done so for over 55 years. Religious adherent statistics in the United States are obtained from surveys and organizational reporting. A 2006 survey by Putnam and Campbell found that Americans are a highly religious people. We have high rates of belonging, behaving, and believing, and when compared to other industrialized nations, the United States ranks 7th in the rate of weekly attendance at religious services. Jordan, Indonesia, and Brazil are ahead of us. They also found that Mormons, Black Protestants, and Evangelicals are the most religiously observant groups in America; and that the Deep South, Utah, and the Mississippi Valley are the most religious regions of the country (Putnam & Campbell, 2010, pp. 7–23).

One source of information on religious preference is the Pew Forum on Religion and Public Life (2015). The forum delivers timely, impartial information on issues at the intersection of religion and public affairs. In a 2014 study by the Pew Research Center, it was found that the Christian share of the American population was declining and that the number of American adults who do not identify with any organized religion was growing. Christians now comprise 70.6%; Jews, 1.9%; Buddhists, 0.7%; Muslims. 0.9%; Hindus, 0.7%; and Other World Religions, 0.3%. Individuals identifying as unaffiliated were 22.8% of the population studied (Pew Forum on Religion and Public Life, 2015, p. 2).

Examples of Heritage Consistency

The following are examples of each factor that is examined in determining a person's degree of Heritage:

1. The person's childhood development occurred in the person's country of origin or in an immigrant neighborhood in the United States of like ethnic group.

   The person was raised in a specific ethnic neighborhood, such as Italian, Black, Hispanic, or Jewish, in a given part of a city and was exposed to only the culture, language, foods, and customs of that group.

2. Extended family members encouraged participation in traditional religious and cultural activities.

   The parents sent the person to religious school, and most social activities were church-related.

3. The individual engages in frequent visits to the country of origin or returns to the "old neighborhood" in the United States.

   The desire to return to the old country or to the old neighborhood is prevalent in many people; however, many people, for various reasons, cannot return. The people who came here to escape religious persecution or whose families were killed during world wars or the Holocaust may not want to return to European homelands.

Other reasons people may not return to their native country include political conditions in the homeland and lack of relatives or friends in that land.

4. The individual's family home is within the ethnic community of which he or she is a member.

   As an adult, the person has elected to live with family in an ethnic neighborhood.

5. The individual participates in ethnic cultural events, such as religious festivals or national holidays, sometimes with singing, dancing, and costumes.

   The person holds membership in ethno- or religious-specific organizations and primarily participates in activities with the groups.

6. The individual was raised in an extended family setting.

   When the person was growing up, there may have been grandparents living in the same household, or aunts and uncles living in the same house or close by. The person's social frame of reference was the family.

7. The individual maintains regular contact with the extended family.

   The person maintains close ties with members of the same generation, the surviving members of the older generation, and members of the younger generation who are family members.

8. The individual's name has not been Americanized.

   The person has restored the family name to its European original if it had been changed by immigration authorities at the time the family immigrated or if the family changed the name at a later time in an attempt to assimilate more fully.

9. The individual was educated in a parochial (nonpublic) school with a religious or ethnic philosophy similar to the family's background.

   The person's education plays an enormous role in socialization, and the major purpose of education is to socialize a person into the dominant culture. Children learn English and the customs and norms of American life in the schools. In the parochial schools, they not only learn English but also are socialized in the culture and norms of the religious or ethnic group that is sponsoring the school.

10. The individual engages in social activities primarily with others of the same religious or ethnic background.

    The major portion of the person's personal time is spent with primary structural groups.

11. The individual has knowledge of the culture and language of origin.

    The person has been socialized in the traditional ways of the family and expresses this as a central theme of life.

12. The individual expresses pride in his or her heritage.

    The person may identify him- or herself as ethnic American and be supportive of ethnic activities to a great extent.

It is not possible to isolate the aspects of culture, religion, and ethnicity that shape a person's worldview. Each is part of the other, and all three are united within the person. When one writes of religion, one cannot eliminate culture or ethnicity, but descriptions and comparisons can be made. Understanding such differences can help enhance your understanding of the needs of patients and their families and the support systems that people may have or need.

■ Acculturation Themes

Several factors, also links on the chain, are relevant to the overall experience of acculturation. *Acculturation* is the broad term used to describe the process of adapting to and becoming absorbed into the dominant social culture. The overall process of acculturation into a new society is extremely difficult. Have you ever moved to a new community? Imagine moving to a new country and society where you are unable to communicate, do not know your way around, and do not know the "rules." The three facets to the process of overall acculturation are socialization, acculturation, and assimilation.

Socialization

Socialization is the process of being raised within a culture and acquiring the characteristics of that group. Education—be it preschool, elementary school, high school, college, or a healthcare provider program—is a form of socialization. For many people who have been socialized within the boundaries of a "traditional culture" or a non-Western culture, modern American culture becomes a second cultural identity. Those who immigrate here, legally or illegally, from non-Western or nonmodern countries may find socialization into the American culture, whether in schools or in society at large, to be an extremely difficult and painful process. They may experience biculturalism, which is a dual pattern of identification and one often of divided loyalty (LaFrombose, Coleman, & Gerton, 1993).

Understanding culturally determined health and illness beliefs and practices from different heritages requires moving away from linear models of process to more complex patterns of cultural beliefs and interrelationships.

Acculturation

While becoming a competent participant in the dominant culture, a member of the nondominant culture is always identified as a member of his or her original culture. The process of acculturation is involuntary, and a member of the nondominant cultural group is forced to learn the new culture to survive. *Acculturation* also refers to cultural or behavioral assimilation and may be defined as the changes of one's cultural patterns to those of the host society. In the United States, people assume that the usual course of acculturation takes three generations; hence, the adult grandchild of an immigrant is considered fully Americanized. It is with this population that the answers on the Heritage Assessment Tool may become more negative as family ties, spoken language at home, and other variables may be lost.

Assimilation

Acculturation also may be referred to as assimilation, the process by which an individual develops a new cultural identity. Assimilation means becoming in all ways like the members of the dominant culture. The process of assimilation encompasses various aspects, such as cultural or behavioral, marital, identification, and civic. The underlying assumption is that the person from a given cultural group loses this cultural identity to acquire the new one. In fact, this is not always possible, and the process may cause stress and anxiety (LaFrombose et al., 1993). Assimilation can be described as a collection of subprocesses: a process of inclusion through which a person gradually ceases to conform to any standard of life that differs from the dominant group standards and, at the same time, a process through which the person learns to conform to all the dominant group standards. The process of assimilation is considered complete when the foreigner is fully merged into the dominant cultural group (McLemore, 1980, p. 4).

The concepts of socialization, assimilation, and acculturation are complex and sensitive. The dominant society expects that all immigrants are in the process of acculturation and assimilation and that the worldview we share as healthcare practitioners is shared by our patients. Because we live in a pluralistic society, however, many variations of health beliefs and practices exist.

The debate still rages between those who believe that America is a melting pot and that all groups of immigrants must be acculturated and assimilated to an American norm, and those who dispute theories of acculturation and believe that the various groups maintain their own identities within the American whole. The concept of heritage consistency is one way of exploring whether people are maintaining their traditional heritage and of determining the depth of a person's traditional cultural heritage.

■ Cultural Conflicts

There are countless ways by which cultural conflicts occur. One is in the general way, a second is generational differences, and a third is within healthcare.

Cultural Conflicts

Hunter (1994) limited the classical discussion of "cultural conflicts" as events that occur when there is polarization between two groups and their differences are intensified by the way they are perceived. There may also be polarization between two people and between people and institutions. Hunter described the fields of conflict as found in family, education, media and the arts, law, and electoral politics. The struggles are centered on the control of the symbols of culture. This argument must be extended to include healthcare as a sixth field, and the conflict is between those who actively participate in traditional healthcare practices—that is, the practices of their given ethnocultural heritage—and those who are progressive and see the answers to contemporary health problems in the science and technology of the present.

When cultures clash, many misanthropic feelings, or "isms," can enter into a person's consciousness. Just as Hunter proclaimed that the "differences" must be confronted, so, too, must stereotypes, prejudices, and discrimination. It is impossible to describe traditional health and illness beliefs without a temptation to stereotype, but each person is an individual; therefore, just as levels of heritage consistency differ within and between ethnic groups, so do health beliefs and practices.

Prejudice—such as racism, sexism, homophobia, ageism, and xenophobia—occurs either because the person making the judgment does not understand the given person or his or her heritage, or because the person making the judgment generalizes an experience of one individual from a culture to all members of that group. Discrimination occurs when a person acts on prejudice and denies another person one or more of his or her fundamental rights.

Generational Differences

Generational differences have been described as deep and gut-level ways of experiencing and looking at the cultural events that surround us. The ethnocultural life trajectories of population cohorts have established a situation where generations in America today are poles apart. Given the technology explosion and other social changes, the differences between elders and the millennials can be staggering. For example, I was discussing Humphrey Bogart with a group of senior college students, and they had no frame of reference as to who he was and what he had accomplished. And yet, when they discuss many of the popular culture figures of today, I, too, often react in wonderment! The changes in the past several decades have created cultural barriers that openly or more subtly create misunderstandings, tensions, and often conflicts between family members, coworkers, and other individuals. Remember, the cycle of our lives is an ethnocultural journey, and many of the aspects of this journey are derived from the social, political, religious, and cultural contexts in which we grew up. Factors that imprint our lives are the characters and events that we interacted with between 10 and 19 years of age, more or less.

The following are examples of what life may have been and what it is for people from various generations:

- *The Silent Generation,* people born between 1938 and 1945, may well remember World War II and Hiroshima. Members of this generation believe in community service and tend to conform to societies' norms.
- *The Boomer Generation,* people born between 1946 and 1964, is now entering retirement times and remembers Elvis Presley, Marilyn Monroe, and Rosa Parks. "Boomers" work and play hard, vote if convenient, may live a distance from family, and are close with friends.
- *Generation X,* people born between 1965 and 1980, grew up during the Vietnam War, Kent State, and Watergate. Members of this generation tend to not actively participate in voting and to work hard if work does not interfere with good times.

■ *The Millennial Generation,* people born between 1977 and 1994, is the first generation to come of age in this new millennium. The older members well remember September 11, 2001, and the wars in Iraq and Afghanistan. Many millennials depend on smartphones, tablets, computers, and social media (Taylor & the Pew Research Center, 2014).

■ *Generation Z,* people born between 1995 and 2012, is characterized by independence and an eagerness to move into life. They prefer personal contact but are technologically proficient. They are connected to people all over the world because of social media and want to take an active role in their communities (Levit, 2005).

Another example of generational conflict between elders and the millennials is both within families, the workplace, and institutional settings where the people are cared for not only by providers who are immigrants, but also by those who are much younger and have limited knowledge as to what has been their life trajectory. The patient may also be an immigrant who experienced a much different life trajectory than others of the same age and the caregivers. Imagine your life today and what it may have been like to live without a computer, a cell phone, an iPod, or an iPad. Many people may see today's commonplace objects as "strangers" rather than "friends," and could be "digital immigrants," not "digital natives."

Commingling Variables

Six commingling variables relate to this overall situation of social and generational divisions as they, too, are potential sources of conflict:

1. *Decade of birth.* As mentioned above, people's life experiences vary greatly, depending on the events of the decades in which they were born and the cultural values and norms of the times. People who tend to be heritage consistent—that is, have a high level of identification and association with a traditional heritage—tend to be less caught up in the secular fads of the time and popular sociocultural events.

2. *Generation in the United States.* Worldviews differ greatly between the immigrant generation and subsequent generations, and between people who score high as heritage consistent and mainstream people who may score low on the heritage consistency assessment and have been born into families who have resided in the United States for multiple generations.

3. *Class and income.* Social class is how people are rated or may rate themselves as "upper, middle, lower, blue collar, or working poor" and is an important factor to consider. There are countless differences among people predicated on class, including such variables as education, living conditions, social status, occupation, income, access to and utilization of healthcare, and so forth. Between 1979 and 2013, women's earnings rose for most age groups. However,

women's earnings were 74% to 80% of the earnings of men (U.S. Bureau of Labor Statistics, 2013, p. 2).

4. *Language.* There are frequent misunderstandings, as discussed in Chapter 1, when people who do not understand English must help and care for or take direction from English speakers. There are also countless conflicts when people who are hard of hearing attempt to understand people with limited English-speaking skills, and many cultural and social misunderstandings can develop.

5. *Education.* Increasing percentages of students have completed high school, from 69% in 1980 to 85.3% in 2009. "Every child in America deserves a world-class education." With these words, President Obama signed *A Blueprint for Reform: The Reauthorization of the Elementary and Secondary Education Act* in March 2010. This blueprint challenged the nation to embrace education standards that would put America back on a path to global leadership in education. It provides incentives for states to adopt academic standards that prepare students to succeed in college and the workplace, and to create accountability systems that measure student growth toward meeting the goal that all children graduate and succeed in college. (U.S. Department of Education, 2010).

6. *Literacy.* The 2003 National Assessment of Adult Literacy is a nationally representative assessment of English literacy among American adults age 16 and older. Eleven million adults fell in the *Below Basic* rank; 7 million could not answer simple test questions, and 4 million could not take the test because of language barriers. Fifty-five percent of adults with *Below Basic* prose literacy did not graduate from high school, compared to 15% of adults in the general population (Baer, Kutner, Sabatini, & White, 2009).

■ Cultural Phenomena Affecting Health

The cultural phenomena identified by Giger and Davidhizar (1995) that vary among cultural groups and affect social interaction and/or healthcare are biological variations, communication, environmental control, social organization, space, and time orientation. The following discussion broadly defines these phenomena and provides examples of practical manners when they are faced.

Biological Variations

The several ways in which people from one cultural group differ biologically (i.e., physically and genetically) from members of other cultural groups constitute their biological variations; for example, body build and structure, including specific bone and structural differences between groups, such as the smaller stature of Asians, and skin color, including variations in tone, texture, healing abilities, and hair follicles.

It is important to know the variations in food intolerance as found in many people and in the amount of time that it may take a person to physically heal after surgery.

Communication

Communication differences present themselves in many ways, including language differences, verbal and nonverbal behaviors, and silence. Language differences are possibly the most important obstacle to providing multicultural healthcare because they affect all stages of the patient–caregiver relationship.

Proper manners dictate that you understand the correct greetings (e.g., if a form of touch such as a handshake is permissible), what gestures mean, and the interpretation of eye contact. People from most European cultures believe that if a person does not look them in the eye, the person is lying; however, many people from African and Asian heritages do not allow eye contact.

Environmental Control

Environmental control is the ability of members of a particular cultural group to plan activities that control nature or direct environmental factors. Included in this concept are the complex systems of traditional health and illness beliefs, the practice of folk medicine, and the use of traditional healers.

Be knowledgeable of the dietary practices of people and the health beliefs and practices they may adhere to.

Social Organization

The social environment in which people grow up and live plays an essential role in their cultural development and identification. Children learn their culture's responses to life events from the family and its ethnoreligious group. This socialization process is an inherent part of heritage—one's cultural, religious, and ethnic background.

Be sensitive to the celebration of religious holidays by those from backgrounds other than your own.

Space

Personal space refers to people's behaviors and attitudes toward the space around themselves. Territoriality is the behavior and attitude people exhibit about an area they have claimed and defend or react emotionally to when others encroach on it. Both personal space and territoriality are influenced by culture, and thus different ethnocultural groups have varying norms related to the use of space.

Be respectful of the distance people may choose when interacting and body language.

Time Orientation

The viewing of time in the present, past, or future varies among cultural groups. Certain cultures in the United States and Canada tend to be future-oriented. People who are future-oriented are concerned with long-range goals and with healthcare measures in the present to prevent the occurrence of illness in the future. Others are oriented more to the present than the future and may be late for appointments because they are less concerned about planning to be on time. This difference in time orientation may become important in healthcare measures such as long-term planning and explanations of medication schedules.

*Be aware of the meaning of **time** to a person and when their expectations are that you will be prompt. Avoid scheduling elective procedures and meetings during holidays (see Appendix C).*

The examples used in the text to illustrate cultural phenomena affecting health and health traditions in different cultures are not intended to be stereotypical. With careful listening, observing, and questioning, the provider should be able to sort out the traditional health and illness beliefs of a given person.

This chapter has presented an overview of the link on the *HERITAGECHAIN* that explores the concept of heritage—cultural, religious, and ethnic; acculturation themes; and cultural phenomena affecting health and healthcare. It has served as the foundation that delineates the multiple, interrelating phenomena that underlie the cultural conflict that occurs between healthcare providers and patients, many of whom have difficulty interacting with the healthcare providers and healthcare system. It has presented both classical and contemporary definitions and explanations relevant to the foundation of this conflict and sets the stage for further discussion.

Explore ⊙ MediaLink

Go to the Student Resource Site at pearsonhighered.com/nursingresources for chapter-related review questions, case studies, and activities. Contents of the CULTURALCARE Guide and CULTURALCARE Museum can also be found on the Student Resource Site. Click on Chapter 2 to select the activities for this chapter.

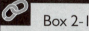 Box 2-1

Keeping Up

The following resources will be helpful in maintaining current information related to religious participation.

Department of Education
Pew Research Center

References

Abramson, H. J. (1980). Religion. In S. Thernstrom (Ed.), *Harvard encyclopedia of American ethnic groups*. Cambridge, MA: Harvard University Press.

Baer, J., Kutner, M., Sabatini, J., & White, S. (2009, February). *Basic reading skills and the literacy of America's least literate adults: Results from the 2003 National Assessment of Adult Literacy (NAAL) Supplemental Studies* (NCES 2009-481). Washington, DC: National Center for Education Statistics, Institute of Education Sciences, U.S. Department of Education. Retrieved from http://nces.ed.gov/pubs2009/2009481.pdf

Bohannan, P. (1992). *We, the alien: An introduction to cultural anthropology*. Prospect Heights, IL: Waveland Press.

Bureau of Indian Affairs. (2016). *What we do*. Retrieved from http://www.indianaffairs.gov/WhatWeDo/index.htm

Estes, G., & Zitzow, D. (1980, November). *Heritage consistency as a consideration in counseling Native Americans*. Paper presented at the National Indian Education Association Convention, Dallas, TX.

Ethnic. (n.d.). *Merriam-Webster Dictionary*. Retrieved from http://www.merriam-webster.com/interstitial-ad?next=%2Fdictionary%2Fethnic

Fejos, P. (1959). Man, magic, and medicine. In L. Goldston (Ed.), *Medicine and anthropology*. New York, NY: International University Press.

Giger, J. N., & Davidhizar, R. E. (Eds.). (1995). *Transcultural nursing assessment and intervention* (2nd ed.). St. Louis, MO: Mosby-Year Book.

Hunter, J. D. (1994). *Before the shooting begins: Searching for democracy in America's culture wars*. New York, NY: Free Press.

LaFrombose, T., Coleman, L. K., & Gerton, J. (1993). Psychological impact of biculturalism: Evidence and theory. *Psychological Bulletin, 114*(3), 395.

Levin, J. (2001). *God, faith, and health*. New York, NY: John Wiley & Sons.

Levit, A. (2015). Make way for Generation Z. *The New York Times*. Retrieved from http://www.nytimes.com/2015/03/29/jobs/make-way-for-generation-z.html

Matsumoto, M. (1989). *The unspoken way*. Tokyo, Japan: Kodahsha International.

McLemore, S. D. (1980). *Racial and ethnic relations in America*. Boston, MA: Allyn & Bacon.

Novak, M. (1973). How American are you if your grandparents came from Serbia in 1888? In S. Te Selle (Ed.), *The rediscovery of ethnicity: Its implications for culture and politics in America*. New York, NY: Harper & Row.

O'Neil, D. (2008). *Ethnicity and race: An introduction to the nature of social group differentiation and inequality*. San Marcos, CA: Palomar College. Retrieved from http://anthro.palomar.edu/ethnicity/Default.htm

Pew Forum on Religion and Public Life. (2015). *America's changing religious landscape*. Retrieved from http://religions.pewforum.org/

Putnam, R. D., & Campbell, D. E. (2010). *American grace: How religion divides and unites us*. New York, NY: Simon & Schuster.

Religion. (n.d.). *Merriam-Webster Dictionary*. http://www.merriam-webster.com/dictionary/religion. March 15, 2016.

Taylor, P., & the Pew Research Center. (2014). *The next America*. New York, NY: Public Affairs.

U.S. Bureau of Labor Statistics. (2013). *Highlights of Women in 2013*. Washington, DC: U.S. Department of Labor. Retrieved from http://www.bls.gov/opub/ted/2013/ted_20131203.htm

U.S. Department of Education. (2010). *A blueprint for reform: The reauthorization of the Elementary and Secondary Education Act*. Retrieved from http://www2 .ed.gov/policy/elsec/leg/blueprint/blueprint.pdf

U.S. Department of Homeland Security. (2014, August). *Yearbook of Immigration Statistics: 2013*. Washington, DC: U.S. Department of Homeland Security, Office of Immigration Statistics. Retrieved from http://www.dhs.gov/sites /default/files/publications/ois_yb_2013_0.pdf

CHAPTER

3 Diversity

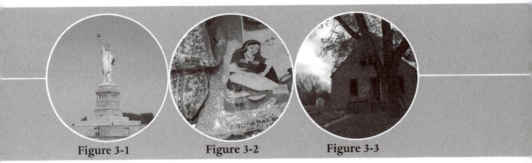

Figure 3-1   Figure 3-2   Figure 3-3

... Give me your tired, your poor,
Your huddled masses yearning to breathe free,
The wretched refuse of your teeming shore.
Send these, the homeless, tempest-tost to me,
I lift my lamp beside the golden door!

— *—Emma Lazarus,* The New *Colossus (1886)*

■ Objectives

1. Describe the total population characteristics of the United States as presented in Census 2010.
2. Compare the population characteristics of the United States in 2000, 2010, and 2014.
3. Discuss the changes in points of origin of recent and past immigrants.
4. Explain the meanings of terms related to immigration, such as *citizen, refugee, legal permanent resident, and naturalization.*
5. Discuss the concepts of poverty.
6. Analyze the cycle of poverty.

The next links on the *HERITAGECHAIN* explore the diversity in our nation, and the opening images for this chapter represent the demographic and socioeconomic diversity that exists in countless communities in this nation. The first figure, Figure 3-1, is that of the Statue of Liberty—a reminder that most of the people who live in the United States of America are the descendants of immigrants or are themselves immigrants. Figure 3-2 depicts a location where people are able to purchase food and other necessities from their homeland. Pictured here are lentils in an Indian grocery store in Waltham, Massachusetts. Figure 3-3 portrays the poverty in this land of plenty—a dark, lonely, abandoned home in a deteriorating neighborhood in an urban midwestern city. An infinite number of images could be placed in this chapter's opening.

∞ What comes to your mind when you think about the demographic diversity in your home community? What are your images of poverty and homelessness?

Diversity—namely, the population's characteristics, immigration, and poverty—will be described in this chapter. Healthcare providers are entangled in the revolutionary consequences of the enormous demographic, social, and cultural changes that have been occurring in the United States. Many of these changes are playing a dramatic role both in the delivery of healthcare to patients, their families, and communities, and in the workforce and environment in which the provider practices. Table 3-1 demonstrates the growth of

Table 3-1   Population by Hispanic or Latino Origin and by Race for the United States: 2000, 2010, and 2014 Estimates

Hispanic or Latino Origin and Race	2000	2010	2014 Estimates
Total population	281,421,906	308,745,538	318,857,056
	Percentage of Total Population		
Hispanic or Latino	12.5	16.3	17.3
Not Hispanic or Latino	87.5	83.7	82.7
White alone	69.1	63.7	61.9
Race			
One race	97.6	97.1	97.0
White	75.1	72.4	73.4
Black or African American	12.3	12.6	12.7
American Indian and Alaska Native	0.9	0.9	0.8
Asian	3.6	4.8	5.2
Native Hawaiian and other Pacific Islander	0.1	0.2	0.2
Some other race	5.5	6.2	4.7
Two or more races	2.4	2.9	3.0

Sources: "Overview of Race and Hispanic Origin: 2010" (p. 4), by K. R. Humes, N. A. Jones, and R. R. Ramirez, 2011, *2010 Census Briefs*. Retrieved from http://2010.census.gov/2010census/data/, June 26, 2011; and U.S. Census Bureau Factfinder. (2015). "Annual Estimates of the Resident Population by Sex, Single Year of Age, Race Alone or in Combination, and Hispanic Origin for the United States: April 1, 2010 to July 1, 2014," *2014 Population Estimates*, by U.S. Census Bureau Factfinder, 2015. Retrieved from http://factfinder.census.gov/faces/tableservices/jsf/pages/productview.xhtml?pid=PEP_2014_PEPALL5N&prodType=table.

the emerging majority—people of color—that constituted 30.9% of the population in 2000, grew to 36.3% in the 2010 census, and is estimated to be 38% for 2014 (Humes, Jones, & Ramirez, 2011, p. 6; U.S. Census Bureau, 2014 American Community Survey 1-Year Estimates). The comments and data presented in this chapter are designed to provide you with an impression of the demographic features, derived from Census 2000, 2010, and the American Community Survey of 2014, which provides the most recent data from the Census Bureau on recent immigration, labor, and economic backgrounds of the American population.

In order to understand the profound changes that are taking place in the healthcare system, both in the delivery of services and in the profile of the people who are receiving and delivering services, we must look at the changes in the American population. The White majority is aging and shrinking; the Black, Hispanic, Asian, and American Indian populations are young and growing. It is imperative for those who deliver healthcare to be understanding of and sensitive to cultural differences, and the effect of the differences on a person's health and illness beliefs and practices and healthcare needs.

■ Census 2010 and 2014 Estimates

Every census adapts to the decade in which it is conducted. One of the most important changes to Census 2010 was the revision of the questions that were asked regarding race and Hispanic origin. The federal government considers race and Hispanic origin to be two separate concepts, and the questions on race and Hispanic origin were asked of all people living in the United States. The changes were developed to reflect the country's growing diversity. The respondents were given the option of selecting one or more race categories to indicate their racial identities. A factor that presents confusion is that people were free to define themselves as belonging to many groups. However, the overwhelming majority of the population reported one race.

In 1997, the Office of Management and Budget established federal guidelines to collect and present data on race and Hispanic origin. Census 2010 adhered to the guidelines and added "some other race." Data on race has been collected since the first census in 1790. The present categories are as follows:

1. *White*—refers to a person having origins in any of the original peoples of Europe, the Middle East, or North Africa. It includes people who indicated their race(s) as "White" or reported entries such as Irish, German, Italian, Lebanese, Arab, Moroccan, or Caucasian.

2. *Black or African American*—refers to a person having origins in any of the Black racial groups of Africa. It includes people who indicated their race(s) as "Black, African American, or Negro" or reported entries such as African American, Kenyan, Nigerian, or Haitian.

3. *American Indian or Alaska Native*—refers to a person having origins in any of the original peoples of North and South America (including Central America) and who maintains tribal affiliation or

community attachment. This category includes people who indicated their race(s) as "American Indian or Alaska Native" or reported their enrolled or principal tribe, such as Navajo, Blackfeet, Inupiat, Yup'ik, Central American Indian groups, or South American Indian groups.

4. *Asian*—refers to a person having origins in any of the original peoples of the Far East, Southeast Asia, or the Indian subcontinent, including, for example, Cambodia, China, India, Japan, Korea, Malaysia, Pakistan, the Philippine Islands, Thailand, and Vietnam. It includes people who indicated their race(s) as "Asian" or reported entries such as "Asian Indian," "Chinese," "Filipino," "Korean," "Japanese," "Vietnamese," and "Other Asian," or provided other detailed Asian responses.

5. *Native Hawaiian or Other Pacific Islander*—refers to a person having origins in any of the original peoples of Hawaii, Guam, Samoa, or other Pacific islands. It includes people who indicated their race(s) as "Pacific Islander" or reported entries such as "Native Hawaiian," "Guamanian or Chamorro," "Samoan," and "Other Pacific Islander," or provided other detailed Pacific Islander responses.

6. *Some Other Race*—includes all other responses not included in the White, Black or African American, American Indian or Alaska Native, Asian, or Native Hawaiian or Other Pacific Islander race categories described above. Respondents reporting entries such as multiracial, mixed, interracial, or a Hispanic or Latino group (e.g., Mexican, Puerto Rican, Cuban, or Spanish) in response to the race question are included in this category.

7. *Hispanic or Latino*—refers to a person of Cuban, Mexican, Puerto Rican, South or Central American, or other Spanish culture or origin regardless of race (Humes et al., 2011, p. 2).

These terms of classification will be used throughout this chapter and the text. The census does not break down the population by gender except to ask if the respondent is male or female. It questions neither gender preference nor if a person is abled or disabled. This text will follow census categories and not directly include either the lesbian, gay, bisexual, and transgender (LBGT) community or disabled populations in its discussions.

The American Community Survey (ACS) is a critical element in the Census Bureau's decennial census program. It is a nationwide survey designed to provide communities an annual look at how they are changing and is the foremost source for detailed information about the American people and workforce (U.S. Census Bureau, 2015).

Total Population Characteristics

The 2010 census percentages are compared with the 2000 census percentages and the estimated percentages of 2014 in Table 3-1. The figures demonstrate both the growth of the American population in general and the growth of people of color specifically. It is important to note changes related to age classification. The age classification is based on the age of the person in complete years as of April 1, 2010, and January 1, 2014–December 31, 2015. The age was derived from the date of birth information requested on the census form and ACS surveys. It is critical to note the following points regarding age in 2010 and 2014:

- The median age of the population was 37.2 in 2010 and estimated to be 37.7 years in 2014 (Table 3-2).
- The population between the ages of 18 and 64 was estimated to be 62.9% of the population in 2010 and 62.5% of the population in 2014.
- The older working-age population, ages 45 to 64, was 26.4% of the population in 2010 and estimated to be 26.2% of the population in 2014.
- The 65 and over population was 13% of the population in 2010 and estimated to be 14.5% of the population in 2014 (U.S. Census Bureau, 2010, 2015).

■ Immigration

Immigrants and their descendants constitute most of the population of the United States, and Americans who are not themselves immigrants have ancestors who came to the United States from elsewhere. The only people considered native to this land are the American Indians, the Aleuts, and the Inuit (or Eskimos), for they migrated here thousands of years before the Europeans (Thernstrom, 1980, p. vii).

Immigrants come to the United States seeking religious and political freedom and economic opportunities. The life of the immigrant is fraught with

Table 3-2   Median Ages of the Population, 2000, 2010, and 2014 Estimates

Population Group	Median Age		
	2000 Census	2010 Census	2014 Estimates
American Indian alone	27.7 years	31.0 years	31.4
Asian alone	32.5 years	35.5 years	34.1
Black alone	30.0 years	32.5 years	31.6
Hispanic	25.8 years	27.2 years	27.6
White alone—not of Hispanic heritage	38.6 years	39.8 years	39.6
Native Hawaiian and other Pacific Islander	26.8 years	28.6 years	27.9
2 or more races	19.8 years	19.7 years	28.1
Total Population	35.3 years	36.5 years	37.6

Sources: U.S. Census Bureau, 2001. Retrieved from http://www.census.gov/popest/national/asrh/NC-EST2009-asrh .html; "American Community Survey," U.S. Census Bureau, 2010. Retrieved from http://factfinder2.census.gov/faces/ tableservices/jsf/pages/productview.xhtml?fpt=table; and "Selected Population Profile in the United States," U.S. Census Bureau. Retrieved from http://factfinder.census.gov/faces/tableservices/jsf/pages/productview .xhtml?pid=ACS_14_1YR_S0201&prodType=table.

difficulties—going from an "old" to a "new" way of life, learning a new language, and adapting to a new climate, new foods, and a new culture. Socialization of immigrants occurs in American public schools, and Americanization, according to Greeley (1978), is for some a process of "vast psychic repression," wherein one's language and other familiar trappings are shed. In part, the concept of the melting pot has been created in schools, where children learn English, reject family traditions, and attempt to take on the values of the dominant culture and "pass" as Americans (Novak, 1973). This difficult experience, as noted and described by Greeley and Novak in the 1970s, continues today.

A citizen of the United States is a native-born person, a foreign-born child of citizens, or a naturalized person who owes *allegiance* to the United States and who is entitled to its *protection*. The 14th Amendment to the Constitution of the United States, ratified in 1868, grants citizenship to all persons born in the United States. **Naturalization** refers to the process by which foreign born people ages 18 and over may become citizens of the United States. **Refugees** are persons who seek residence in the United States in order to avoid persecution in their country of origin. Persons granted refugee status applied for admission while outside the United States and are granted asylum either at a port of entry or at some point after their entry into the United States. Persecution or the fear of persecution must be based on the person's race, religion, nationality, membership in a particular social group, or political opinion. People with no nationality must generally be outside their country of last habitual residence to qualify as a refugee. Refugees are subject to ceilings by geographic area set annually by the president in consultation with Congress and are eligible to apply for **lawful permanent resident** (LPR) status after 1 year of continuous presence in the United States. LPR status legally accords the person the privilege of residing in the United States. Most lawful permanent residents (also known as "green card" recipients) are eligible to apply for naturalization within 5 years after obtaining LPR status. Nonimmigrant admissions refer to arrivals of persons who are authorized to stay in the United States for a limited period of time. Most nonimmigrants enter the United States as tourists or business travelers, but some come to work, study, or engage in cultural exchange programs. An undocumented person, who entered the United States without inspection, for example, would be strictly defined as an immigrant but is not a legal permanent resident.

Foreign citizens or nationals seeking U.S. citizenship must fulfill the requirements for naturalization established by Congress. Box 3-1 contains an example of the questions a person is asked when taking the examination for naturalization. Persons seeking citizenship in the United States may obtain a civics book to study about our government and some history. They are interviewed to determine English language competency and expected to meet other requirements (U.S. Department of Homeland Security, 2014).

In 2013, a total of 990,553 people became Legal Permanent Residents of the United States. Among the LPRs, Mexico (13.6%), China (6.9%), and India (6.6%) were the leading countries of birth. In 1970, the highest percentage of people came from Europe, whereas in 2010, people from Mexico, China,

Box 3-1

Sample Questions and Answers for the Naturalization Test

Questions
1. What is one responsibility that is only for U.S. citizens?
2. What is the supreme law of the land?
3. What do we call the first ten amendments to the Constitution?
4. How many amendments does the Constitution have?
5. Who makes federal laws?
6. What is the highest court in the United States?
7. How many justices are on the Supreme Court?
8. Under our Constitution, what powers belong to the states?
9. How old do citizens have to be to vote for president?
10. What did Susan B. Anthony do?

Answers
1. Serve on a jury, vote in a federal election
2. The Constitution
3. The Bill of Rights
4. Twenty-seven (27)
5. Congress, Senate and House (of Representatives), (U.S. or national) legislature
6. The Supreme Court
7. Nine (9)
8. Provide schooling and education, provide protection (police), provide safety (fire departments), give a driver's license, approve zoning and land use
9. Eighteen (18) and older
10. Fought for women's rights, fought for civil rights

Source: Learn About the United States: Quick Civics Lessons for the Naturalization Test 2011, U.S. Department of Homeland Security, 2011. Retrieved from http://www.uscis.gov/citizenship.

and India were the highest in percentage. In 2010, 619,913 people were naturalized. The largest percentage (39%) came from Asia (U.S. Department of Homeland Security, 2014).

Table 3-3 lists the primary metropolitan areas for Legal Permanent Residents in 2013, and Table 3-4 lists the top 5 states where Legal Permanent Residents reside. Table 3-5 shows the leading 5 countries of origin for Legal Permanent Residents flow by country of birth in 2013. Table 3-6 compares selected characteristics of the native and foreign-born populations in 2005.

As of 2015, there were estimated to be 12 million undocumented people living in the United States. It is extremely difficult to count the number of people who are hiding because they are not documented. It is widely recognized

Table 3-3   Five Leading Legal Permanent Resident Flow Metropolitan Areas of Residence: 2013

1. New York, northern New Jersey–Long Island	16.9%
2. Los Angeles–Long Beach–Santa Ana, California	8.1%
3. Miami–Fort Lauderdale–Pompano Beach, Florida	6.7%
4. Washington, DC–Arlington–Alexandria, Virginia–Maryland, West Virginia	4.0%
5. Chicago-Naperville-Joliet, Illinois, Indiana, Wisconsin	3.0%

Source: U.S. Legal Permanent Residents: 2013 (p. 3), by R. Monger and J. Yankay, 2014 (May), Washington, DC: Department of Homeland Security. Retrieved from http://www.dhs.gov/sites/default/files/publications/ois_lpr _fr_2013.pdf.

that the population is growing by about 275,000 people each year. California is the leading state of residence for undocumented people. Other states include Texas, New York, and Florida.

Although the United States is predominantly a country of immigrants (Box 3-2), there has been an effort by the government to tighten both

Table 3-4   Permanent Resident Flow by State of Residence: 2011 to 2013

1. California	19.4%
2. New York	13.5%
3. Florida	10.4%
4. Texas	9.4%
5. New Jersey	5.4%

Source: U.S. Legal Permanent Residents: 2013 (p. 4), by R. Monger and J. Yankay, 2014 (May), Washington, DC: Department of Homeland Security. Retrieved from http://www.dhs.gov/sites /default/files/publications/ois_lpr_fr_2013.pdf.

Table 3-5   Leading 5 Countries of Origin for Legal Permanent Resident Flow by Country of Birth: 2013

Country	Legal Permanent Residents (%)
1. Mexico	13.6
2. People's Republic of China	7.2
3. India	6.9
4. Philippines	5.5
5. Dominican Republic	4.2

Source: U.S. Legal Permanent Residents: 2013 (p. 4), by R. Monger and J. Yankay, 2014 (May), Washington, DC: Department of Homeland Security. Retrieved from http://www.dhs.gov /sites/default/files/publications/ois_lpr_fr_2013.pdf.

Table 3-6   Selected Characteristics of the Native and Foreign-Born Populations:
2014

Characteristic	Native Population	Foreign Born	Naturalized Citizens	Not a U.S. Citizen
Population	276.5 million	42.4 million	20 million	22.4 million
Median age	35.9 years	43.5 years	50.8 years	37.7 years
Asian	2.0%	26.2%	32.3%	20.8%
Hispanic	13.0%	46.7%	32.4%	57.5%
Population 25 years and older, less than high school	9.6%	29.9%	20.2%	39.7%
Speak language other than English	10.8%	84.2%	79.0%	88.8 %
Speak English less than well	1.8%	49.7%	38.4%	59.8%
Family poverty rates	10.1%	17.5%	10.4%	26.4%
Renting household unit	34.8%	49.3%	36.2%	67.1%
Vehicle unavailable	8.5%	12.9%	11.1%	15.1%
No telephone service	2.3%	2.6%	1.9%	3.5%

Source: "Selected Population Profile in the United States," U.S. Census Bureau, 2014. Retrieved from http://factfinder
.census.gov/faces/tableservices/jsf/pages/productview.xhtml?pid=ACS_14_1YR_S0201&prodType=table

Box 3-2

Highlights of Immigration History

The history of immigration has many noteworthy events, including:

- The passage of the Naturalization Act in 1790
- The potato famine in Ireland that resulted in a massive influx of Irish to the United States in 1846
- The extension of naturalization in 1870 to Africans
- The opening of the Statue of Liberty in 1886
- The opening of the Ellis Island Immigration Station in 1892
- The end of the Vietnam War and the implementation of the Indochinese refugee program in 1975
- The formation of the Department of Homeland Security in 2003
- The passage of the Secure Fence Act in 2006

Sources: The United States Immigration History Timeline, by E. Lefcowitz, 1990, New York, NY: Terra Firma Press, reprinted with permission; "Significant Historic Dates in U.S. Immigration," Rapid Immigration, 2012. Retrieved from http://www.rapidimmigration.com/1_eng_immigration
_history.html; U.S. Department of Homeland Security, 2010. Retrieved from http://www.dhs
.gov/index.shtm.

immigration and travel access to the United States since the terrorist attacks in September 2001. On July 22, 2002, the Justice Department announced that it would use criminal penalties against immigrants and foreign visitors who fail to notify the government of a change of address within 10 days. This requirement is not a new one, but it has not been strictly enforced. Enforcing the requirement impacts at least 11 million people and visitors who stay in the United States for more than 30 days (Davis & Furtado, 2002, p. A2). In addition, this will have an impact on the healthcare system and on providers of healthcare both directly and indirectly. For example, it will be more difficult for people to work here and to visit family members who are ill. In addition, the passage of Proposition 187 in California in November 1994, and earlier laws relating to bilingual education in Texas, demonstrates that many citizens are no longer willing to provide basic human services, such as healthcare and education, to new residents in general and to those who are undocumented specifically. Thus far, the implementation of these laws has been held up in the courts. Despite such efforts, however, it is evident that immigration to this country will continue. It is predicted that by the year 2020, immigration will be a major source of new people for the United States and will be responsible for whatever growth occurs in the United States after 2030. The United States will continue to attract about two thirds of the world's immigrants. The solutions for the problem of undocumented residents continues to cause political debate and, as of 2015, no realistic solutions have been proposed.

The need for strict enforcement of Title VI and the Culturally and Linguistically Appropriate Services (CLAS) standards becomes self-evident when you realize the high numbers of people who do not understand and speak English, as seen in Table 3-6.

■ Poverty

There are countless ways to answer the question "What is poverty?" Poverty may be viewed through numerous lenses, including anthropological, cultural, demographic, economical, educational, environmental, historical, medical, philosophical, policy, political, racial, sexual, sociological, and theological points of view. The consequences of poverty are ubiquitous. They include, but are not limited to, battering, bullying, child abuse, gaming, poor dental health and dental care, poor health and healthcare, poor nutrition, obesity, spousal abuse, substance abuse, and violence. Poverty may also be viewed in a "holistic" way. Here, the physical, mental, and spiritual aspects of poverty are self-evident. Examples include, but are not limited to:

■ *Physical*—substandard housing, no telephone or vehicle, limited access to healthcare

■ *Mental*—inadequate education, poor opportunity, limited access to mental health services

■ *Spiritual*—despair, the experience of being disparaged and disenfranchised.

In 2014, the official poverty rate was 14.8%, and 14.8 million people were in poverty. Poverty rates differ by age, gender, race, and ethnicity. For example, the rates of poverty in 2014 in demographic groups were:

- 26.2% for Blacks
- 12.0% for Asians
- 23.6% for Hispanics
- 10.1% for non-Hispanic Whites
- 21.1 % for children under 18
- 10.0% for adults over 65 (DeNavas-Walt & Proctor, p. 13).

The federal government has an extensive history of efforts to improve the conditions of people living with limited incomes and material resources. Since the 1850s, countless initiatives have been enacted to help citizens who are "poor." More than 80 federal programs (including six tax expenditures) provide aid to people with low incomes, based on the GAO's survey of relevant federal agencies. The largest program is Medicaid, which, along with the Supplemental Nutrition Assistance Program (SNAP), Supplemental Security Income (SSI), and the refundable portion of the Earned Income Tax Credit (EITC), comprised almost two thirds of the fiscal year 2013 federal obligations of $742 billion for antipoverty programs. Aid is most often targeted to groups of the low-income population, such as people with disabilities and workers with children (GAO, 2015). The association between socioeconomic status and the health status of a person or family may be explained in part by the reduced access to healthcare among people with lower socioeconomic status. Higher income is related to health because it does the following:

- Increases access to healthcare
- Enables the person or family to live in a better neighborhood
- Enables the person or family to afford better housing
- Enables the person or family to reside in locations not abutting known environmentally degraded locations (heavy industrial pollution or known hazardous waste sites), and
- Increases the opportunity to engage in health promoting behaviors.

Health also may affect income by restricting the type and amount of employment a person may seek or by preventing a person from working.

There has been an increase in earning inequality over the last 25 years. The income for all races rose, then dipped in this time period. For Blacks and Hispanics, income during this period was much lower than for Whites and Asians and for people from the Pacific Islands. Much of this change and inequality was due to technological changes that increased income to highly skilled labor. At the same time, less skilled workers saw their wages decrease or stagnate. The other factors responsible for this phenomenon include:

- Globalization of the economy
- Decline in the real minimum wage

- Decline in unionization
- Increase in immigration, and
- Increase in families headed by women (from 10% in 1970, to 18% in 1996, to 24.7% in 2000, and 30.5% in 2014); for foreign-born women with no husband present and children under 5, the percentage below the poverty level was 55.2%—households headed by women generally have lower incomes.

Cycle of Poverty

Poor production may be the situation that begins the cycle of poverty (Figure 3-4). This is the result of un- and underemployment and low wages. The available water supply may not be potable due to chemical or bacterial contamination. Nutritional deficits occur when the food supply is inadequate, with the person eating "junk foods" and not fresh fruits, vegetables, and proteins. The quality of the housing

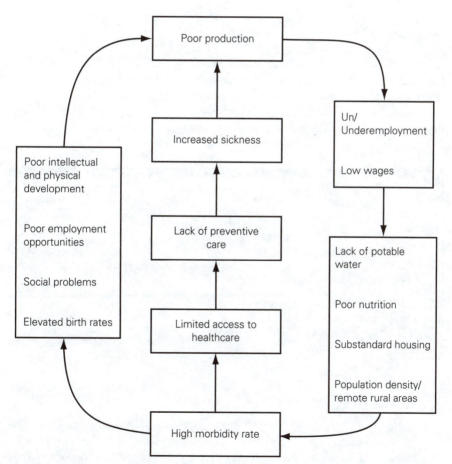

Figure 3-4 The cycle of poverty.

may be substandard, or the person may live in a densely populated or remote rural area. This contributes to a high morbidity rate, such as a high incidence of asthma or lead poisoning, high costs of healthcare needs, a lack of preventive care, and higher incidence of sickness. This leads to increased social problems such as substance abuse, child abuse, mental illness, violence, elevated birth rates, poor employment opportunities, and poor physical and mental growth and development. This is a cycle that has yet to be broken. Other barriers that are interrelated to this cycle are language and transportation issues. The issues of overcrowded housing, poor sanitation, inadequate nutrition, homelessness, and so forth that are part of the cycle of poverty have a profound and prolonged impact on the health status of people and in future generations.

This chapter has presented an overview of the major phenomena contributing to the profound diversity existing within the United States—demographic, immigration, and poverty. Additional issues will be explored in greater depth in the chapters relating to each of the major population groups identified in Census 2010.

Explore 🌐 MediaLink

Go to the Student Resource Site at pearsonhighered.com/nursingresources for chapter-related review questions, case studies, and activities. Contents of the CULTURALCARE Guide and CULTURALCARE Museum can also be found on the Student Resource Site. Click on Chapter 3 to select the activities for this chapter.

🔗 Box 3-3

Keeping Up

The following resources will be helpful in maintaining current information related to the demographics of your location, your state and the United States immigration issues and policies; and poverty:

U.S. Census Bureau
U.S. Department of Homeland Security
U.S. Government Accountability Office

■ References

Davis, F., & Furtado, C. (2002, July 22). INS to enforce change-of-address rule. *Boston Globe*, p. A2.

DeNavas-Walt, C., & Proctor, B. D. (2015). U.S. Census Bureau, Current Population Reports, P60-252, *Income and Poverty in the United States: 2014*,

Washington, DC: U.S. Government Printing Office. Retrieved from http://www.census.gov

Greeley, A. (1978). *Why can't they be like us? America's white ethnic groups.* New York, NY: E. P. Dutton.

Humes, K. R., Jones, N. A., & Ramirez, R. R. (2011, March). *Overview of race and Hispanic origin: 2010.* (2010 Census Briefs, p. 4). Retrieved from http://2010.census.gov/2010census/data/

Lefcowitz, E. (1990). *The United States immigration history timeline.* New York, NY: Terra Firma Press.

Monger, R., & Yankay, J. (2014). *U.S. Legal Permanent Residents: 2013* (p. 4). Washington, DC: Department of Homeland Security. Retrieved from http://www.dhs.gov/sites/default/files/publications/ois_lpr_fr_2013.pdf

Novak, M. (1973). How American are you if your grandparents came from Serbia in 1888? In S. Te Selle (Ed.), *The rediscovery of ethnicity: Its implications for culture and politics in America.* New York, NY: Harper & Row.

Rapid Immigration. (2012). *Significant historic dates in U.S. immigration.* Retrieved from http://www.rapidimmigration.com/1_eng_immigration_history.html

Thernstrom, S. (Ed.). (1980). *Harvard encyclopedia of American ethnic groups.* Cambridge, MA: Harvard University Press.

U.S. Census Bureau. (2001). Population Estimates. Retrieved from http://www.census.gov/popest/national/asrh/NC-EST2009-asrh.html

U.S. Census Bureau. (2010). *American Community Survey.* Retrieved from http://factfinder2.census.gov/faces/tableservices/jsf/pages/productview.xhtml?fpt=table

U.S. Census Bureau. (2014). Selected population profile in the United States. Retrieved from http://factfinder.census.gov/faces/tableservices/jsf/pages/productview.xhtml?pid=ACS_14_1YR_S0201&prodType=table

U.S. Census Bureau Factfinder. (2015). Annual estimates of the resident population by sex, single year of age, race alone or in combination, and Hispanic origin for the United States: April 1, 2010 to July 1, 2014. *2014 Population Estimates.* Retrieved from http://factfinder.census.gov/faces/tableservices/jsf/pages/productview.xhtml?pid=PEP_2014_PEPALL5N&prodType=table

U.S. Department of Homeland Security. (2011). *Learn about the United States: Quick civics lessons for the Naturalization Test 2011.* Retrieved from http://www.uscis.gov/citizenship

U.S. Department of Homeland Security. (2014). *2013 Yearbook of Immigration Statistics.* Washington, DC: U.S. Department of Homeland Security, Office of Immigration Statistics. Retrieved from https://www.dhs.gov/sites/default/files/publications/ois_yb_2013_0.pdf

U.S. Government Accountability Office (GAO). (2015). *Report to congressional requestors: Federal low-income programs: Multiple programs target diverse populations and needs.* Retrieved from http://gao.gov/assets/680/671779.pdf

CHAPTER
4 Health and Illness

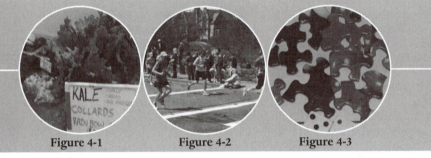

| Figure 4-1 | Figure 4-2 | Figure 4-3 |

All things are connected. Whatever befalls the earth befalls the children of the earth.

—Chief Seattle Suqwamish and Duwamish

◼ Objectives

1. Understand the subjective and objective determinants of health and illness.
2. Reexamine and redefine the concepts of health and illness.
3. Understand the multiple relationships between health and illness.
4. Associate the concepts of good and evil and light and dark with health and illness.
5. Describe significant components of *Healthy People 2020*.
6. Describe the concept of health disparities.
7. Compare the classic sick role models as described by Parsons, Alksen, and Suchman.
8. Understand the natural history of the health-illness trajectory.

The next links on the *HERITAGECHAIN* are health and illness. The opening images for this chapter represent facets of health and illness in various stages along the health/illness continuum. Figure 4-1 is suggestive of maintaining health and fresh, well-balanced food, especially fresh vegetables, that must be included in a healthy diet. One of the greatest signs of a healthy person is that of being able to accomplish demanding physical challenges; in Figure 4-2, marathon runners who are participating in a most demanding sport exemplify the notion of being fit and maintaining their overall health. Figure 4-3 represents board games and puzzles that require concentration and skill. There are countless images we can use to visualize comprehensive notions of health and illness.

∞ What do you do daily to maintain your health? Where do you go for help? What do you do when you experience a self-limiting ailment?

∞ How are ideas of health and illness reflected throughout the contemporary dominant culture in your family and home community? The community you work in? If you could pick three images relating to health and illness from your day-to-day experiences, what would they be?

■ Health

The answers to the question "What is health?" are not as readily articulated as you might assume. One response may be a flawless recitation of the World Health Organization (WHO) definition of *health* as a "state of complete physical, mental, and social well-being and not merely the absence of disease." This answer may be recited with great assurance—a challenge is neither expected nor welcomed, but may evoke an intense dispute in which the assumed right answer is completely torn apart. Answers such as "homeostasis," "kinetic energy in balance," "optimal functioning," and "freedom from pain" are open to discussion. Experienced healthcare providers may be unable to give a comprehensive, acceptable answer to such a seemingly simple question. It is difficult to give a definition that makes sense without the use of some form of medical jargon. It is also challenging to define *health* in terms that a layperson can understand. (We lack skill in understanding "health" from the layperson's perspective.) It is not unusual to hear healthcare providers define health in a negative manner—"the absence of disease."

When you google *health*, the response on the World Wide Web is about 3,140,000,000 results (0.32 sec) as of September 6, 2015. There are countless definitions for this term. Basic popular definitions include "the general condition of the body" or "the condition of being well or free from disease" ("Health," *Merriam-Webster Dictionary*, n.d.). As long ago as 1860, Florence Nightingale described health as "being well and using one's powers to the fullest extent." These definitions—varying in scope and context—are essentially those that the student practitioner and educator within the health professions agree convey the meaning of *health*; albeit, the most widely used and recognized definition is that of WHO. In analyzing these definitions, we are able to discern subtle variations in denotation. In fact, the connotation does not essentially change over time. If this occurs in the denotation of the word, what of the connotation? That is, are healthcare providers as familiar with implicit meanings as with more explicit ones? It may be argued that the connotation of health is most frequently seen as a two-dimensional phenomenon—body and mind—with the larger emphasis on the body.

The framework of both education and research in the health professions continues to rely on the more abstract definitions of the word *health*. When taken in a broader context, health can be regarded not only as the absence of disease, but also as a reward for "good behavior." In fact, a state of health is regarded by many people as the reward one receives for "good" behavior and illness as punishment for "bad" behavior. You may have heard something like "She is so good; no wonder she is so healthy" or a mother admonishing her child, "If you don't do such and such, you'll get sick." Situations and experiences may be avoided for the purpose of protecting and maintaining one's health. Conversely, some people seek out challenging, albeit dangerous, situations with the hope that they will experience the thrill of a challenge and still emerge in an intact state of health. Examples of such behavior include driving at high speeds, ongoing tobacco use, and not wearing seat belts.

Health can also be viewed as the freedom from and the absence of evil. In this context, health is analogous to day, which equals good and light. Conversely, illness is analogous to night, evil, and dark. Illness, to some, is seen as a punishment for being bad or doing evil deeds; it is the work of vindictive evil spirits. In the modern education of healthcare providers, these concepts of health and illness are rarely, if ever, discussed. However, if these concepts of health and illness are believed by some consumers of healthcare services, understanding these varying ideas is important for the provider. Each of us enters the healthcare community with our own culturally based concept of health. During the educational and socialization process in a healthcare provider profession—nursing, medicine, or social work—we are expected to shed these beliefs and adopt the standard definitions. In addition to shedding these old beliefs, we learn, if only by unspoken example, to view as deviant those who do not accept the prevailing, institutional connotation of the word *health*. In fact, you may agree, health tends to be defined as the absence of disease and not as a condition in its own right.

The following discussion illustrates the complex process necessary to enable providers to return to and appreciate our former interpretations of health, to understand the vast number of meanings of the word *health*, and to be aware of the difficulties that exist with definitions such as that of the World Health Organization.

How Do YOU Define Health?

You have been requested to describe the term *health* in your own words, and before you read further, jot down your definition of health. You may initially respond by reciting the WHO definition. What does this definition really mean? The following examples are representative of actual responses:

1. Physical and psychological well-being, *physical* meaning that there are no abnormal functions with the body—all systems are without those abnormal functions that would cause a problem physically—and *psychological* meaning that one's mind is capable of a clear and logical thinking process and association

2. Being able to use all of your body parts in the way that you want to—to have energy and enthusiasm
3. Being able to perform your normal activities, such as working, without discomfort and at an optimal level.

In the initial step of the unlocking process, it becomes clear that no single definition fully conveys what health really is.[1] We can all agree on the WHO definition, but when asked "What does that mean?" we are unable to clarify or to simplify that definition. As we begin to perceive a change in the connotation of the word, we may experience dismay, as that emotional response accompanies the breaking down of ideas. When this occurs, we begin to realize that as we were socialized into the healthcare provider culture by the educational process, our understanding of health changed, and we moved a great distance from our older cultural understanding of the term. The following list includes the definitions of *health* given by students at various levels of education and experience. The students ranged in age from 19-year-old college juniors to graduate students in both nursing and social work.

Beginning Students

■ A system involving all subsystems of one's body that constantly works on keeping one in good physical and mental condition

Senior Students

■ Ability to function in activities of daily living to optimal capacity without requiring medical attention
■ The state of physical, mental, and emotional well-being

Graduate Students

■ Ability to cope with stressors; absence of pain—mental and physical
■ State of optimal well-being, both physical and emotional
■ Not only the absence of disease but a state of balance or equilibrium of physical, emotional, and spiritual states of well-being.

It appears that the definition becomes more abstract and technical as the student advances in the educational program. The terms explaining health take on a more abstract and scientific character with each year of removal from the lay mode of thinking. Can these layers of jargon be removed, and can we help ourselves once again to view health in a more tangible manner?

In further probing this question, let us think back to the way we perceived health before our entrance into the educational program. I believe that

---

[1]The unlocking process includes those steps taken to help break down and understand the definitions of both terms—*health* and *illness*—in a living context. It consists of persistent questioning: What is health? No matter what the response, the question "What does that mean?" arises. Initially, this causes much confusion, but in classroom practice—as each term is written on the whiteboard and analyzed—the air clears and the process begins to make sense.

the farther back we can go in our memory of earlier concepts of health, the better. Again, the question "What is health?" is asked over and over. Initially, the responses continue to include such terms and phrases as "homeostasis," "freedom from disease," or "frame of mind." Slowly, and with considerable prodding, we are able to recall earlier perceptions of health. Once again, health becomes a personal, experiential concept, and the relation of health to being returns. The fragility and instability of this concept also are recognized as *health* gradually acquires meaning in relation to the term *being* and is seen in a positive light and not as "the absence of disease."

This process of unlocking a perception of a concept takes a considerable amount of time and patience. It also engenders dismay that briefly turns to anger and resentment. You may question why the definitions acquired and mastered in the learning process are now being challenged and torn apart. The feeling may be that of taking a giant step backward in a quest for new terminology and new knowledge.

With this unlocking process, however, we are able to perceive the concept of health in the way that a vast number of healthcare consumers may perceive it. The following illustrates the transition that the concept passed through in an unlocking process from the WHO definition to the realm of the healthcare consumer.

Initial Responses

- Feeling of well-being, no illness
- Complete physical, mental, and social well-being

Secondary Responses

- Frame of mind
- Ability to perform activities of daily living

Experiential Responses

- Health becomes tangible; the description is illustrated by using qualities that can be seen, felt, or touched.
- Shiny hair and warm, smooth, glossy skin
- Clear eyes and shiny teeth
- Being alert and happy
- Harmony between body and mind.

Even this itemized description does not completely answer the question "What is health?" The words are once again subjected to the question "What does that mean?" and once again the terms are stripped down, and a paradox begins to emerge. For example, *shiny hair* may, in fact, be present in an ill person or in a person whose hair has not been washed for a long time, and a healthy person may not always have clean, well-groomed, lustrous hair. It becomes clear that, no matter how much we go around in a circle in an attempt to define *health*, the terms and meanings attributed to the state can be challenged. As a result of this prolonged discussion, we never really come to an acceptable definition of *health*; yet, by going through the intense unlocking process, we are able, finally, to understand the ambiguity that surrounds the word. We are less likely to view as deviant the people whose beliefs and practices concerning their own health and healthcare differ from ours.

Health Maintenance and Protection

Health can be seen from many other viewpoints, and many areas of disagreement arise with respect to how *health* can be defined. The preparation of healthcare providers tends to organize their education from a perspective of illness. Rarely (or superficially) does it include an in-depth study of the concept of health. However, the emphasis in healthcare delivery has shifted from acute care to preventive care. The need for the provider of health services to comprehend this concept is therefore crucial and is exemplified in the desire of Surgeon General Dr. Vivek Murthy to establish "a culture of health" (Murthy, 2015). As this movement for preventive healthcare continues to grow, to become firmly entrenched, and to thrive, multiple issues must be constantly addressed in answering the question "What is health?" *Unless the provider is able to understand health from the viewpoint of the patient, a barrier of misunderstanding is perpetuated.* It is difficult to reexamine complex definitions dutifully memorized at an earlier time, yet an understanding of health from a patient's viewpoint is essential to the establishment of comprehensive primary healthcare services inclusive of health maintenance and protection services because, as has been discussed, the perception of health is a complex psychological process. There tends to be no established pattern in what individual people, families, or communities see as their health needs and how they go about practicing their own healthcare.

Health maintenance and protection or the prevention of illness are by no means new concepts. As long as human beings have existed, they have used a multitude of methods—ranging from magic and witchcraft to present-day immunization and lifestyle changes—in an ongoing effort to maintain good health and prevent debilitating illness and death. Logic suggests that in order to maintain health, we must prevent disease, and that is best accomplished by: complying with immunization schedules, enforced by school policies; eating balanced meals, including avoiding salt and cholesterol; exercising regularly; and seeing a healthcare provider once a year for a checkup. A provider's statement of good health is often required by a person seeking employment or life insurance. Furthermore, the annual physical examination has been advertised as the key to good health. A "clean bill of health" is considered essential for social, emotional, and even economic success. The general public has been conditioned to believe that health is guaranteed if a disease that may be developing is discovered early and treated with the ever-increasing varieties of modern medical technology. Although many people believe in and practice the annual physical and screening for early detection of a disease, there are some—both within and outside the healthcare professions—who do not subscribe to it.

Healthy People 2020

In 1979, the Surgeon General's Report, *Healthy People: The Surgeon General's Report on Health Promotion and Disease Prevention* was published. This seminal report was followed by *Healthy People 1990: Promoting Health/Preventing Disease: Objectives for the Nation*—a series of concrete objectives for addressing national public health issues. A decade later, this document was followed by *Healthy People 2000: National Health Promotion and Disease Prevention Objectives*. These early documents presented the initiative for a national strategy for significantly improving the health of the American people in the decades preceding 2000 and the decades to follow. The documents recognized that lifestyle and environmental factors are major determinants in disease prevention and health promotion. They provided strategies for significantly reducing preventable death and disability, for enhancing quality of life, and for reducing disparities in health status among various population groups within our society. *Healthy People 2000: National Health Promotion and Disease Prevention and Objectives* was a statement of national opportunities, and was followed by *Healthy People 2010* that was adjusted to continue in this trajectory; *Healthy People 2020*, released in early 2011, has been designed to continue this momentum.

The *Healthy People* series provides science-based, 10-year national objectives for improving the health of all Americans. Over the past decades, *Healthy People* has established benchmarks and monitored progress in order to:

1. Encourage collaborations in different areas and disciplines
2. Guide individuals toward making informed health decisions, and
3. Measure the impact of prevention activities.

The critical questions *Healthy People* addresses are:

1. What makes some people healthy and others unhealthy?
2. How can we create a society in which everyone has a chance to live long, healthy lives?

The vision statement of *Healthy People 2020* focuses on "the creation of a society in which all people live long and healthy lives" (Office of Disease Prevention and Health Promotion, 2015a). The overarching goals are to:

1. Attain high-quality, longer lives free of preventable disease, disability, injury, and premature death.
2. Achieve health equity, eliminate disparities, and improve the health of all groups.
3. Create social and physical environments that promote good health for all.
4. Promote quality of life, healthy development, and healthy behaviors across all life stages.

The elimination of health disparities has been one of the major goals of *Healthy People*. In *Healthy People 2000*, the goal was to reduce health disparities among

Americans. In *Healthy People 2010,* it was to eliminate, not just reduce, health disparities. In *Healthy People 2020,* the goal has expanded even further: to achieve health equity, eliminate disparities, and improve the health of all groups.

▥ *Health equity* is the "attainment of the highest level of health for all people. This requires valuing everyone equally."

▥ *Health disparity* is "a particular type of health difference that is closely linked with social, economic, and/or environmental disadvantage. The disparities adversely affect populations who have experienced greater obstacles to health based on their racial or ethnic group; religion; socioeconomic status; gender; age; mental health; cognitive, sensory, or physical disability; sexual orientation or gender identity; geographic location; or other characteristics historically linked to discrimination or exclusion."

Over the years, efforts to eliminate disparities and achieve health equity have focused primarily on diseases or illnesses and on healthcare services. However, the absence of disease does not automatically equate to good health.

In the next decade, *Healthy People* will assess health disparities in the U.S. population by tracking rates of illness, death, chronic conditions, behaviors, and other types of outcomes in relation to demographic factors including race and ethnicity, gender, sexual identity and orientation, disability status or special healthcare needs, and geographic location (rural and urban). Several goals have been developed for 2020, including the following two examples:

1. **Improve the health, safety, and well-being of lesbian, gay, bisexual, and transgender (LGBT) people.**

   LGBT people encompass all races and ethnicities, religions, and social classes. Sexual orientation and gender identity questions are not asked on most national or state surveys, making it difficult to estimate the number of LGBT people and their health needs. However, research suggests that LGBT people face health disparities linked to societal stigma, discrimination, and denial of their civil and human rights. Discrimination against LGBT persons has been associated with high rates of psychiatric disorders, substance abuse, and suicide. (Office of Disease Prevention and Health Promotion, 2015c)

2. **Improve health-related quality of life and well-being for all people.**

   Well-being considers the physical, mental, and social aspects of a person's life. **Physical well-being** *relates to vigor and vitality, feeling very healthy and full of energy.* **Mental well-being** *includes being satisfied with one's life; balancing positive and negative emotions; accepting one's self; finding purpose and meaning in one's life; seeking personal growth, autonomy, and competence; believing one's life and circumstances are under one's control; and generally experiencing optimism.* **Social well-being** *involves providing and receiving quality support from family, friends, and others. (Office of Disease Prevention and Health Promotion, 2015b; emphasis original)*

It is crucial to recognize that social determinants, which can also be viewed as "demographic disparities," have a profound impact on health outcomes of specific populations. This situation will be further illustrated in the forthcoming chapters. Chapters 9–12 contain numerous examples of the existing health and demographic disparities.

Health Beliefs

Health Beliefs, as described by Becker (1974), are useful for transitioning from a discussion of health to that of illness. They illustrate a layperson's perceptions of health and illness and/or those of healthcare providers as they illustrate the differences between lay and professional health beliefs and expectations. Forging a link between the two helps one better understand how people perceive themselves in relation to illness and what motivates them to seek medical help and then follow that advice. Three domains are identified:

1. *Perceived Susceptibility.* How susceptible to a certain condition do people consider themselves to be? For example, a woman whose family does not have a history of breast cancer is unlikely to consider herself susceptible to that disease. A woman whose mother and maternal aunt both died of breast cancer may well consider herself highly susceptible, however. In this case, the provider may concur with this perception of susceptibility on the basis of known risk factors.

2. *Perceived Seriousness.* The perception of the degree of a problem's seriousness varies from one person to another. It is in some measure related to the amount of difficulty the patient believes the condition will cause. From a background in pathophysiology, the provider knows—within a certain range—how serious a problem is and may withhold information from the patient. The provider may resort to euphemisms in explaining a problem. The patient may experience fear and dread by just hearing the name of a problem, such as cancer.

3. *Perceived Benefits: Taking Action.* What kinds of actions do people take when they feel susceptible, and what are the barriers that prevent them from taking action? If the condition is seen as serious, they may seek help from a doctor or some other significant person, or they may vacillate and delay seeking and using help. Many factors enter into the decision-making process. Several factors that may act as barriers to care are cost, availability, and the time that will be missed from work.

From the provider's viewpoint, there is a protocol governing who should be consulted when a problem occurs, when help should be sought during that problem's course, and what therapy should be prescribed. When the patient's belief about the causes of illness is "traditional" and the provider's is "modern," an inevitable conflict arises between the two viewpoints. This conflict is even more evident when the provider either is unaware of the patient's traditional beliefs or is aware of the manifestation of traditional beliefs and practices and devalues them.

In summary, this section has attempted to deal solely with the concept of health. The multiple denotations and connotations of the word have been explored. A method for helping you tune in to your health has been presented, a transitional discussion illustrating the plethora of issues to be raised later in the text has been included, an overview of *Healthy People 2020* has set the tone for the remainder of the text, and the Health Belief Model serves to provide a context for the discussion.

■ Illness

The next link on the chain is illness. It is a paradox that the world of illness is the one that is most familiar to the providers of healthcare. It is in this world that the provider feels most comfortable and useful. Many questions about illness need to be answered:

- What determines illness?
- How do you know when you are ill?
- What prompts you to seek help from the healthcare system?
- At what point does self-treatment seem no longer possible?
- Where do you go for help? And to whom?

We tend to regard illness as the absence of health, yet we demonstrated in the preceding discussion that *health* is at best an elusive term that defies a specific definition. Let us look at the present issue more closely. Is illness the opposite of health? Is it a permanent condition or a transient condition? How do you know if you are ill?

When you google *illness*, the response on the World Wide Web is well over 163,000,000 results in 0.36 sec (September 10, 2015). The basic dictionary definition for this term is "an unhealthy condition of body or mind: SICKNESS" ("Illness," *Merriam-Webster Dictionary*, n.d.). What is illness? A generalized response, such as "abnormal functioning of a body's system or systems," evolves into more specific assessments of what we observe and believe to be wrong. Illness is a sore throat, a headache, or a fever—the last one determined not necessarily by the measurement on a thermometer but by a flushed face; a warm-to-hot feeling of the forehead, back, and abdomen; and overall malaise. The diagnosis of intestinal obstruction is described as pain in the stomach (abdomen), a greater pain than that caused by "gas," accompanied by severely upset stomach, nausea, vomiting, and marked constipation.

Essentially, we are being pulled back in the popular direction and encouraged to use lay terms. We initially resist this because we want to employ professional jargon. (Why use lay terms when our knowledge is so much greater?) It is crucial that we be called to task for using jargon. We must learn to be constantly conscious of the way in which the laity perceive illness and healthcare.

Another factor emerges as the word *illness* is stripped down to its barest essentials. Many of the characteristics attributed to health occur in illness, too. You may receive a rude awakening when you realize that a person perceived as healthy by clinical assessment may then—by a given set of symptoms—defines him- or herself as ill (or vice versa). For example, in summertime, one may see a person with a red face and assume that she has a sunburn. The person may, in fact, have a fever. A person recently discharged from the hospital, pale and barely able to walk, may be judged ill. That individual may consider himself well, however, because he is much better than when he entered the hospital—now he is able to walk! Thus, perceptions are relative and, in this instance, the eyes of the beholder have been clouded by inadequate information. Unfortunately, at the provider's level of practice, we do not always ask the patient, "How do you view your state of health?" Rather, we determine the patient's state of health by objective and observational data.

As is the case with the concept of health, we learn in nursing or medical school how to determine what illness is and how people are expected to behave when they are ill. Once these terms are separated and examined, the models that healthcare providers have created tend to carry little weight. There is little agreement as to what, specifically, illness is, but we nonetheless have a high level of expectation as to what behavior should be demonstrated by both the patient and the provider when illness occurs. We discover that we have a vast amount of knowledge with respect to the acute illnesses and the services that ideally must be provided for the acutely ill person. When contradictions surface, however, it becomes apparent that our knowledge of the vast gray area is minimal—for example, whether someone is ill or becoming ill with what may later be an acute episode. Because of the ease with which we often identify cardinal symptoms, we find we are able to react to acute illness and may have negative attitudes toward those who do not seek help when the first symptom of an acute illness appears. The questions that then arise are "What is an acute illness, and how do we differentiate between it and some everyday indisposition that most people treat by themselves?" and "When do we draw the line and admit that the disorder is out of the realm of adequate self-treatment?"

These are certainly difficult questions to answer, especially when careful analysis shows that even the symptoms of an acute illness tend to vary from one person to another. In many acute illnesses, the symptoms are so severe that the person experiencing them has little choice but to seek immediate medical care. Such is the case with a severe myocardial infarction, but what about the person who experiences mild discomfort in the epigastric region? Such a symptom could lead the person to conclude he or she has indigestion and to self-medicate with baking soda, an antacid, milk, or Alka-Seltzer. A person who experiences mild pain in the left arm may delay seeking care, believing the pain will disappear. Obviously, this person may be as ill as the person who seeks help during the onset of symptoms but will, like most people, minimize these small aches because of not wanting to assume the sick role.

The Sick Role

The seminal work of Talcott Parsons (1966) helps explain the phenomenon of "the sick role." In our society, a person is expected to have the symptoms viewed as illness confirmed by a member of the healthcare profession. In other words, the sick role must first be legitimately conferred on this person by the keepers of this privilege. You cannot legitimize your own illness and have your own diagnosis accepted by society at large. There is a legitimate procedure for the definition and sanctioning of the adoption of the sick role, and it is fundamental for both the social system and the sick individual. Thus, illness is not only a "condition," but also a social role. Parsons describes four main components of the sick role:

1. *"The sick person is exempted from the performance of certain of his/her normal social obligations."* An example is a student or worker who has a severe sore throat and decides that he or she does not want to go to classes or work. For this person to be exempted from the day's activities, he or she must have this symptom validated by someone in the healthcare system, a provider who is either a physician or a nurse practitioner. The claim of illness must be legitimized or socially defined and validated by a sanctioned provider of healthcare services.

2. *"The sick person is also exempted from a certain type of responsibility for his/her own state."* For example, an ill person cannot be expected to control the situation or be spontaneously cured. The student or worker with the sore throat is expected to seek help and then to follow the advice of the attending physician or nurse in promoting recovery. The student or worker is not responsible for recovery except in a peripheral sense.

3. *"The legitimization of the sick role is, however, only partial."* When you are sick, you are in an undesirable state and should recover and leave this state as rapidly as possible. The student's or worker's sore throat is acceptable only for a while. Beyond a reasonable amount of time—as determined by the physician or nurse, peers, and the faculty or supervisors—legitimate absence from the classroom or work setting can no longer be claimed.

4. *"Being sick, except in the mildest of cases, is being in need of help."* Bona fide help, as defined by the majority of American society and other Western countries, is the exclusive realm of the physician or nurse practitioner. A person seeking the help of the provider now not only bears the sick role, but in addition takes on the role of patient. Patienthood carries with it a certain, prescribed set of responsibilities, some of which include compliance with a medical regimen, cooperation with the healthcare provider, and the following of orders without asking too many questions, all of which lead to the illness experience.

The Illness Experience

The experience of an illness is determined by what illness means to the sick person. Furthermore, *illness* refers to a specific status and role within a given society. Not only must illness be sanctioned by a physician or nurse practitioner for the sick person to assume the sick role, but it also must be sanctioned by the community or society structure of which the person is a member. Alksen,

Wellin, Suchman, & Patrick (n.d.) divide this experience into four stages, which are sufficiently general to apply to any society or culture.

The first stage, **onset**, is the time when the person experiences the first symptoms of a problem. This event can be slow and insidious or rapid and acute. When the onset is insidious, the patient may not be conscious of symptoms or may think that the discomfort will eventually go away. If, however, the onset is acute, the person is positive that illness has occurred and that immediate help must be sought. This stage is seen as the prelude to legitimization of illness. It is the time when the person with a sore throat in the preceding discussion may have experienced some fatigue, a raspy voice, or other vague symptoms.

In the second stage of the illness experience, **diagnosis**, the disease is identified or an effort is made to identify it. The person's role is now sanctioned, and the illness is socially recognized and identified. At this point, the healthcare providers make decisions pertaining to appropriate therapy. During the period of diagnosis, the person experiences another phenomenon: dealing with the unknown, which includes fearing what the diagnosis will be.

For many people, going through a medical workup is an unfamiliar experience. It is made doubly difficult because they are asked and expected to relate to strange people who are doing unfamiliar and often painful things to their bodies and minds. To the layperson, the environment of the hospital or the provider's office is both strange and unfamiliar, and it is natural to fear these qualities. Quite often, the ailing individual is faced with an unfamiliar diagnosis. Nonetheless, the person is expected to follow closely a prescribed treatment plan that usually is detailed by the healthcare providers but that, in all likelihood, may not accommodate a particular lifestyle. The situation is that of a horizontal-vertical relationship, the patient being figuratively and literally in the former position, the professional in the latter.

During the third stage, **patient status**, the person adjusts to the social aspects of being ill and gives in to the demands of his or her physical condition. The sick role becomes that of patienthood, and the person is expected to shift into this role as society determines it should be enacted. The person must make any necessary lifestyle alterations, become dependent on others in some circumstances for the basic needs of daily life, and adapt to the demands of the physical condition as well as to treatment limitations and expectations. The environment of the patient is highly structured. The boundaries of the patient's world are determined by the providers of the healthcare services, not by the patient. Herein lies the conflict.

Much has been written describing the environment of the hospital and the roles that people in such an institution play. As previously stated, the hospital is typically unfamiliar to the patient, who, nevertheless, is expected to conform to a predetermined set of rules and behaviors, many of which are unwritten and undefined for the patient—let alone by the patient.

The fourth stage—**recovery**—is generally characterized by the relinquishing of patient status and the assumption of prepatient roles and activities. There is often a change in the roles a person is able to play and the activities able to be performed once recovery takes place. Often, recovery is not complete. The person may be left with an undesirable or unexpected change in body image or in the ability to perform expected or routine activities. One example is a woman who enters the hospital with a small lump in her breast and who, after a surgery, may return home with only one breast or an incision where tissue in the afflicted breast has been removed. Another example is that of a man who is a laborer, who enters the hospital with a backache and returns home after a laminectomy. When he returns to work, he cannot resume his job as a loader. Obviously, an entire lifestyle must be altered to accommodate such newly imposed changes.

From the viewpoint of the provider, this person has recovered. His or her body no longer has the symptoms of the acute illness that made surgical treatment necessary. In the eyes of the former patient, illness persists because of the inability to perform as in the past. So many changes have been wrought that it should come as no surprise if the person seems perplexed and uncooperative. Here, too, there is certainly conflict between society's expectations and the person's expectation. Society releases the person from the sick role at a time when, subjectively, the person may not be ready to relinquish it.

Another method of dividing the illness experience into stages was developed by Edward A. Suchman (1965). He described the following five components:

1. *The symptom experience stage.* The person is physically and cognitively aware that something is wrong and responds emotionally.

2. *The assumption of the sick role stage.* The person seeks help and shares the problem with family and friends. After moving through the lay referral system, seeking advice, reassurance, and validation, the person is temporarily excused from such responsibilities as work, school, and other activities of daily living as the condition dictates.

3. *The medical care contact stage.* The person then seeks out the "scientific" rather than the "lay" diagnosis, wanting to know the following: Am I really sick? What is wrong with me? What does it mean? At this point, the sick person needs some knowledge of the healthcare system, what the system offers, and how it functions. This knowledge helps the person select resources and interpret the information received.

4. *The dependent-patient role stage.* The patient is now under the control of the healthcare providers and is expected to accept and comply with the prescribed treatments. The person may be quite ambivalent about this role, and certain factors (physical, administrative, social, or psychological) may create barriers that eventually will interfere with treatment and the willingness to comply.

5. *The recovery or rehabilitation stage.* The role of the patient is given up at the recovery stage, and the person resumes—as much as possible—his or her former roles.

The Natural History of the Health-Illness Continuum

Lastly, a way of explaining both health and illness is to explore the dynamics of the natural history of the health-illness continuum (Figure 4-4). Here, it is possible to follow the continuum or trajectory of a healthy state through an illness that a person may experience. This summarizes the social science approaches that have been discussed to answer our fundamental questions—"What is health?" and "What is illness?"—and begins to shift our focus to the responses and experiences people have both to and with states of health and illness. The focus now begins to move to the active role the person plays in shaping and experiencing the course of a state of health and a given illness. For example, the *seemingly healthy* person who develops an illness may experience the following continuum: healthy state, in which he or she is carrying on activities of daily living, actively participating in family life, work, other activities and so forth; an

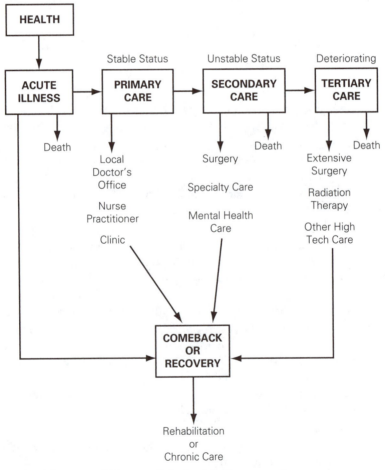

Figure 4-4   The natural history of the health-illness continuum.

illness, the symptoms of which may be acute, silent, or subtle in nature, occurs; the person may recover spontaneously or with treatment, or come back and resume his or her life in an expected manner or resume his or her earlier stable status; or, the illness episode may be more severe, and the person may become unstable or experience the illness as a chronic condition in which he or she may, over time, deteriorate; and at some point, death occurs. The person may die with the onset of the acute phase or later in the continuum. The acute phase most often is treated in the home or an acute care setting, and the early phases of comeback and rehabilitation occur in one of these settings. The management of the chronic phase, except for acute episodes, is performed at home or in an institution that is either a rehabilitation facility or a long-term care institution. The illness may profoundly affect the lives of the ill and his or her family in the scope of day-to-day living and hopes for the future.

As you can see, there have been countless explanatory words and models developed over time to define *health*, *illness*, and the experiences of each. Each of these theories is valid; each of them is time-tested; each is relevant as we go forward in time and space.

In summary, this chapter has presented an introductory overview of the modern culture's perception of health and illness through countless lenses. The writings of a number of preeminent theorists and sociologists have been examined in terms of applicability to healthcare. Box 4-1 suggests resources that provide timely information.

Explore MediaLink

Go to the Student Resource Site at pearsonhighered.com/nursingresources for chapter-related review questions, case studies, and activities. Contents of the CULTURALCARE Guide and CULTURALCARE Museum can also be found on the Student Resource Site. Click on Chapter 4 to select the activities for this chapter.

 Box 4-1

Keeping Up

Countless references that are published weekly, monthly, annually, and periodically may be accessed to maintain currency in the domains of health and illness. There is also a wealth of historical articles that can now be downloaded at either a nominal charge or no charge.

Google Scholar

Google Scholar is a search engine for literature related to countless topics, such as the Health Belief Model, sick role, the illness trajectory and/or the

(continued)

> **Box 4-1** *Continued*
>
> natural history of the health illness trajectory, and disparities. Many of the articles can be purchased from the publishers, and several articles may be downloaded at no charge as PDFs. It also links to dictionaries.
>
> **Healthy People 2020**
>
> Follow the progress of *Healthy People 2020*, review the history of *Healthy People 2000 and 2010*, and examine the evaluations that have been conducted on *Healthy People 2000 and 2010*.
>
> **Peer-Reviewed Resources**
>
> *The Centers for Disease Control, The National Center for Biotechnology Information* (PubMed), and the *National Institutes of Health* maintain a variety of Internet journal articles, data sources, and other resources for both patients and providers that are subject to peer review by medical professionals and generally considered reliable.
>
> **WebMD**
>
> WebMD is an informative resource as it provides health information in such topical areas as "Living Healthy," "Family and Pregnancy," and "Drugs and Supplements." It contains articles about countless health maladies, listings of physicians in most specialties, and current health-related news.

■ References

Alksen, L., Wellin, E., Suchman, E., & Patrick, S. (n.d.). *A conceptual framework for the analysis of cultural variations in the behavior of the ill*. Unpublished report (p. 2). New York, NY: New York City Department of Health.

Becker, M. H. (1974). *The health belief model and personal health behavior*. Thorofare, NJ: B. Slack.

Health. (n.d.). *Merriam-Webster Dictionary*. Retrieved from http://www.merriam-webster.com/dictionary/health

Illness. (n.d.). *Merriam-Webster Dictionary*. Retrieved from http://www.merriam-webster.com/dictionary/illness

Murthy, V. (2015, July 25). Not my job: Surgeon General Vivek Murthy gets quizzed on "General Hospital." NPR's *Wait, Wait, Don't Tell Me!* Retrieved from http://www.npr.org/2015/07/25/425887932/not-my-job-surgeon-general-vivek-murthy-gets-quizzed-on-general-hospital

Office of Disease Prevention and Health Promotion. (2015a). *Healthy People 2020*. Rockville, MD: U.S. Department of Health and Human Service. Retrieved from http://www.healthypeople.gov/sites/default/files/HP2020 Framework.pdf

Office of Disease Prevention and Health Promotion. (2015b). Health-related quality of life and well-being. *Healthy People 2020*. Rockville, MD: U.S. Department of Health and Human Service. Retrieved from http://www

.healthypeople.gov/2020/topics-objectives/topic/health-related-quality-of
-life-well-being

Office of Disease Prevention and Health Promotion. (2015c). Lesbian, gay,
bisexual, and transgender health. *Healthy People 2020*. Rockville, MD: U.S.
Department of Health and Human Service. Retrieved from http://www
.healthypeople.gov/2020/topics-objectives/topic/lesbian-gay-bisexual-and
-transgender-health

Parsons, T. (1966). Illness and the role of the physician: A sociological perspective.
In W. R. Scott & E. H. Volkart (Eds.), *Medical care: Readings in the sociology of
medical institutions* (p. 275). New York, NY: John Wiley & Sons.

Suchman, E. A. (1965, Fall). Stages of illness and medical care. *Journal of Health
and Human Behavior, 6*(3), 114.

Unit II

HEALTH Domains

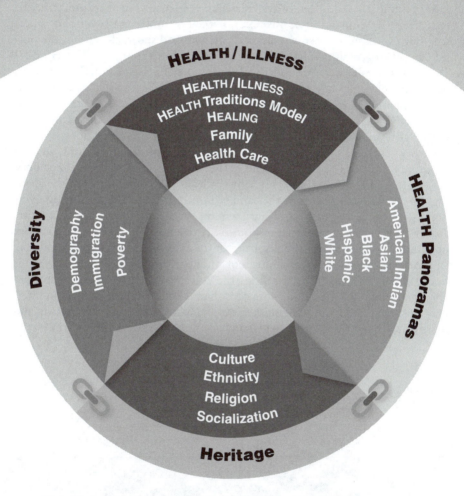

HEALTH / ILLNESS

HEALTH / ILLNESS
HEALTH Traditions Model
HEALING
Family
Health Care

HEALTH Panoramas

American Indian
Asian
Black
Hispanic
White

Diversity

Demography
Immigration
Poverty

Culture
Ethnicity
Religion
Socialization

Heritage

Unit II develops the "plot" of this book by providing background theoretical links on the *HERITAGECHAIN* for the dominant themes discussed in this unit. Chapter 5, "HEALTH Traditions," and Chapter 6, "HEALING Traditions," will explore the links of HEALTH and HEALING and the **traditional**[1] ways of maintaining, protecting, and restoring HEALTH, magico-religious traditions related to

HEALTH and HEALING, and HEALING practices. Chapter 7 will help you to explore your heritage and learn about the traditional HEALTH and HEALING beliefs and practices from your background.

■ Health

HEALTH and the countless ways by which it is maintained, protected, and restored is the foundation of this text. *HEALTH* connotes the **balance** of a person, both within one's being—physical, mental, and spiritual—and in the outside world—natural, familial and communal, and metaphysical. The HEALTH Traditions Model is a method for describing beliefs and practices used to **maintain** through daily HEALTH practices, such as diet, activities, and clothing; to **protect** through special HEALTH practices, such as food taboos, seasonal activities, and protective items worn, carried, or hung in the home or workplace; and/or to **restore** through special HEALTH practices, such as diet changes, rest, special clothing or objects, and **physical, mental**, and/or **spiritual** HEALTH. The accompanying image Figure UII-2, *salud*, is a metaphor for HEALTH in countless ways. Here, it is whole and emerging from the shadows of early morning. Just as the sand sculpture is fragile, disappearing overnight, so, too, is HEALTH. It brings to mind the reality that HEALTH is finite, and each of us has the internal responsibility to maintain, protect, and restore our HEALTH. The reciprocal holds true for the external familial, environmental, and societal forces—they, too, must look after and safeguard our HEALTH. This book, in part, is a mirror that reflects the countless ways by which people are able to maintain, protect, and/or restore their HEALTH. Just as there is an interplay between a sand sculpture and the natural forces that can create, harm, and destroy it, so, too, it is with HEALTH and the forces of the outside world.

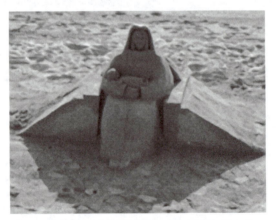

**Figure II-2   Sand Sculpture—Postiquet Beach,
Alicante, Spain.**

[1]Tradition is the handing down of statements, beliefs, legends, customs, and information, from generation to generation, especially by word of mouth or by practice.

ILLNESS is the imbalance of the person, both within one's being—physical, mental, and spiritual—and in the outside world—natural, familial and communal, and metaphysical. HEALING is the restoration of this balance. The relationships of the person to the outside world are reciprocal.

When these terms, HEALTH, ILLNESS, and HEALING, are used in small capitals in this book, it is to connote that they are being used holistically. When they are written in the general text font—health, illness, and healing—they are to be understood in the everyday way.

Chapter 8 presents an overview of the issues related to the modern, scientific, high-technology healthcare delivery system in general and will discuss why an analytical understanding of the modern allopathic philosophy relevant in this arena is a vital link in regard to the development of a holistic philosophy of HEALTH, HEALING, and CulturalCare.

The chapters in Unit II will present an overview of relevant historical and contemporary theoretical content that will help you to:

1. Describe traditional aspects of HEALTH.
2. Describe traditional HEALTHCARE philosophies and systems.
3. Discuss various forms of HEALING practices.
4. Trace your family's beliefs and practices in
   a. Health/HEALTH maintenance
   b. Health/HEALTH protection
   c. Health/HEALTH restoration, and
   d. Curing/HEALING.
5. Discuss the interrelationships of sociocultural, public health, and medical events that have produced the crises in today's modern healthcare system.
6. Trace the complex web of factors that:
   a. Contribute to the high cost of healthcare
   b. Discuss ways of paying for healthcare services, and
   c. Impede a person's passage through the healthcare system.
7. Describe common barriers to utilization of the healthcare system.
8. Compare the modern and traditional systems of health/HEALTHcare.

As you proceed through this unit, you will encounter several activities that link Unit I to Unit II and will help the content resonate and come alive. These are activities in which several people may participate and share their experiences.

1. Re-answer questions 5–12 from Unit I, thinking of HEALTH rather than health. (Remember, when HEALTH is in small capital letters, it is to designate it as a holistic phenomenon rather than dualistic, as is the everyday way it is defined.) They are the following questions:

   How do you define *HEALTH*?
   How do you define *ILLNESS*?
   What do you do to maintain your HEALTH?
   What do you do to protect your HEALTH?

What do you do when you experience a noticeable change in your HEALTH?

Do you diagnose your own HEALTH problems? If yes, how do you do so? If no, why not?

From whom do you seek HEALTHCARE?

What do you do to restore your HEALTH? Give examples.

2. To whom do you turn first when you are ILL? Where do you go next?

3. You have just moved to a new location. You do not know a single person in this community. How do you find health/HEALTH care resources?

4. Visit an emergency room in a large city hospital. Visit an emergency room in a small community hospital. Spend some time quietly observing what occurs in each setting.

   a. How long do patients wait to be seen?

   b. Are patients called by name—first name, surname—or number?

   c. Are relatives or friends allowed into the treatment room with the patient?

5. Determine the cost of a day of hospitalization in an acute care hospital in your community.

   a. How much does a room cost? How much is a day in the intensive care unit or coronary care unit? How much is time in the emergency room? How is a surgical procedure charged?

   b. How much is charged for diagnostic procedures, such as a computed tomography (CT) scan or an ultrasound? How much is charged for equipment, such as a simple intravenous (IV) setup?

   c. What do medications such as "clot busters," antibiotics, and cardiac medications cost?

   d. How many days, or hours, are women kept in the hospital after delivery of a child? Is the newborn baby sent home at the same time? If not, why not? What is the cost of a normal vaginal delivery or cesarean section and normal newborn care?

6. Visit a homeopathic pharmacy or a natural food store and examine the shelves that contain herbal remedies and information about complementary or integrative HEALTHCARE.

   a. What is the cost of a variety of herbal remedies used to maintain HEALTH or to prevent common ailments?

   b. What is the cost of a variety of herbal remedies used to treat common ailments?

   c. What is the range of costs for the books and other reading and instructional materials sold in the store?

7. What does your faith tradition teach you in terms of how to maintain, protect, and/or restore your HEALTH?

8. Attend a service in a house of worship with which you are not familiar. Inquire of the clergyperson what is taught or done within the faith tradition to maintain, protect, and/or restore HEALTH.

9. Visit a HEALER other than a physician or nurse practitioner in your community.

10. Attend a HEALING service.

11. Explore other methods of HEALING, such as massage, herbal therapy, or prayer.

12. Explore birth and birthing practices and traditions in both your heritage and others' than those derived from your own sociocultural heritage.

13. Explore end-of-life beliefs and practices and mourning traditions in both your own heritage and of people from other sociocultural heritages.

CHAPTER

5 HEALTH Traditions

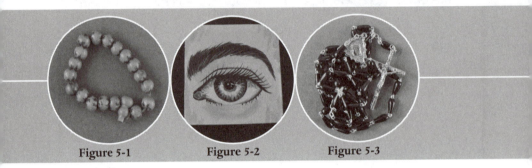

Figure 5-1   Figure 5-2   Figure 5-3

You can do nothing to bring the dead to life; but you can do much to save the living from death.

— *B. Frank School (1924)*

■ Objectives

1. Describe the interrelated components of the HEALTH Traditions Model.
   a. Give examples of the traditional ways people maintain their physical, mental, and spiritual HEALTH.
   b. Give examples of the traditional ways people protect their physical, mental, and spiritual HEALTH.
   c. Give examples of the traditional ways people restore their physical, mental, and spiritual HEALTH.
2. Describe the factors that constitute traditional epidemiology.
3. Give examples of the choices that people have in healthcare.
4. Give examples of the traditional HEALTHCARE philosophies and systems.
5. Describe examples of the information available from the National Center for Complementary and Integrative Health.

The next links on the *HERITAGECHAIN* are related to HEALTH. The three opening images in the chapter depict objects that are used to maintain protect and/ or restore physical, mental, and/or spiritual HEALTH. The items are symbolic of the HEALTH Traditions Model and its themes, which will be discussed later in the chapter. Figure 5-1 is a Buddhist *malas*, prayer bead bracelet. The beads are used to count mantras and prayer repetitions and also for meditation, for protection from negative energy, and to relieve stress. Figure 5-2 is an eye from Havana, Cuba. It may be hung in the home to protect the inhabitants from envy, jealousy, and/or malevolent forces. Figure 5-3 is of rosary beads, which are used in both spiritual HEALTH maintenance and/or restoration.

∞ Are there sacred objects that you and your family may have hung in your home, placed on your bed, or worn? If you could pick three items from your heritage that are used to maintain, protect, and/or restore your HEALTH, what would they be? Do you know where the items can be purchased? Do you continue to use sacred objects for your HEALTH?

Healthcare providers have the opportunity to observe the most incredible phenomenon of life: health/HEALTH and the recovery, in most cases, from illness/HEALTH. In today's society, the healer is primarily thought by many to be the physician, and the other members of the health team all play a significant role in the maintenance and protection of HEALTH and the detection and treatment of ILLNESS. However, human beings have existed, some sources suggest, for 2 million years. How, then, did the species *Homo sapiens* survive before the advent of scientific methods and modern technology? What did the people of other times do to maintain, protect, and restore their health/HEALTH? It is quite evident that numerous forms of health/HEALTH care and healing/HEALING existed long before the technological methodologies that we apply today.

In the natural course of any life, a person can expect to experience the following set of events: He or she becomes ill/ILL; the illness/ILLNESS may be acute, with concomitant symptoms or signs, such as pain, fever, nausea, bleeding, depression, anxiety, or despair. On the other hand, the illness/ILLNESS may be insidious, with a gradual progression and worsening of symptoms, which might encompass slow deterioration of movement or a profound intensification of pain or desperation. Or the person may not experience symptoms, seek care for a routine ailment, and discover he or she has a near fatal illness/ILLNESS.

If the illness/ILLNESS is mild, the person relies on self-treatment or, as is often the case, does nothing, and gradually the symptoms disappear. If the illness/ILLNESS is more severe or is of longer duration, the person may consult expert help from a healer—usually, in contemporary times, a physician or nurse practitioner.

The person recovers or expects to recover. As far back as historians and interested social scientists can trace in the history of humankind, this phenomenon of recovery has occurred. In fact, it made very little difference what mode of treatment was used; recovery was expected and usual. It is this occurrence of natural recovery that has given rise to all forms of therapies and healing/HEALING beliefs and practices that attempt to explain a phenomenon that is natural. That is, one may choose to rationalize the success of a healing/HEALING method by pointing to the patient's recovery. Over the generations, natural healing/HEALING has been attributed to all sorts of rituals, including trephining (puncturing the skull), cupping, magic, leeching, and bleeding. From medicine man to sorcerer, the arts of maintaining, protecting, restoring health/ HEALTH, and healing/HEALING have passed through succeeding generations. People knew the ailments of their time and devised treatments for them. In spite of ravaging plagues, disasters (both natural and those caused by humans), and pandemic and epidemic diseases, human beings as a species have survived!

This chapter explores the *HeritageChain's* links of HEALTH and ILLNESS and the HEALTH Traditions Model; the choices people have in terms of folk medicine, natural, or magico-religious medicine; complementary and integrative methods of health/HEALTH maintenance, protection, and/or restoration; and other schools of health/HEALTH care in contemporary American society. Just as the understanding of health and illness is fundamental in the socialization process into the healthcare professions, the understanding of HEALTH and ILLNESS within the traditional context is fundamental to the development of CULTURAL COMPETENCY and the skills necessary to deliver CULTURALCARE.

■ Health and Illness

In this section, the links of HEALTH and ILLNESS are going to be explored in greater depth. Once again, HEALTH is defined as "the balance of the person, both within one's being—physical, mental, and spiritual—and in the outside world—natural, communal, and metaphysical, is a complex, interrelated phenomenon." On the other hand, ILLNESS is "the imbalance of one's being—physical, mental, and spiritual—and in the outside world—natural, communal, and meta physical." When the terms HEALTH and ILLNESS are used in the remainder of this text, they denote the preceding definitions; small capitals are used to differentiate them from the terms *health* and *illness*, as defined in Chapter 4. *Health*/HEALTH and *illness*/ILLNESS are used in the text when there is an overlap between the terms.

The physical aspect of the person includes anatomical organs, such as the skin, skeleton, and muscles. It is our genetic inheritance, body chemistry, gender, age, and nutrition. The mind, mental, includes cognitive process, such as thoughts, memories, and knowledge. This includes emotional processes as feelings, defenses, and self-esteem. The spiritual facet includes both positive and negative learned spiritual practices and teachings, dreams, symbols, and stories; gifts and intuition; grace and protecting forces; and positive and negative metaphysical or innate forces. These facets are in constant flux and change over time, yet each is completely related to the others and related to the context of the person. The context includes the person's family, culture, work, community, history, and environment. There is also an overlap of the mental and spiritual facets of the person.

The person must be in a state of balance with the family, the community, and the forces of the natural world around him or her. This *balance* is what is perceived as HEALTH in a traditional sense and the way in which it is determined within most traditional cultures, as you will note in Chapters 9 through 13. ILLNESS, as stated, is the *imbalance* of one or all parts of a person (body, mind, and spirit); a person may be in a state of *imbalance* with the family, the community, or the forces of the natural world. The ways in which this *balance*, or harmony, is achieved, maintained, protected, or restored often differ from the prevailing scientific health philosophy of our modern societies. However, many of the traditional HEALTH-, ILLNESS-, and HEALING-related beliefs and practices exist today among people who know and live by the traditions of their own ethnocultural and/or religious heritage.

■ HEALTH Traditions Model

The HEALTH Traditions Model uses the concept of holistic HEALTH and explores what people do from a traditional perspective to maintain HEALTH, protect HEALTH or prevent ILLNESS, and restore HEALTH. HEALTH, in this traditional context, has nine interrelated facets, represented by:

1. Traditional methods of maintaining HEALTH—physical, mental, and spiritual
2. Traditional methods of protecting HEALTH—physical, mental, and spiritual
3. Traditional methods of restoring HEALTH—physical, mental, and spiritual.

The traditional methods of HEALTH maintenance, protection, and restoration require the knowledge and understanding of HEALTH-related resources from within a person's ethnocultural and religious heritage, and a reciprocal relationship exists between the person's needs and the available resources within the family and community to meet these needs. The methods may be used instead of or along with modern methods of healthcare. They are not alternative methods of healthcare because these methods are an integral part of a person's ethnocultural and religious heritage. Complementary and/or integrative healthcare is a system of healthcare that persons may elect to use that is generic and not necessarily a part of his or her personal heritage. The burgeoning system of complementary and integrative health approaches must not be confused with traditional HEALTH and ILLNESS beliefs and practices. In subsequent chapters of this book, traditional HEALTH and ILLNESS beliefs and practices are discussed, following (in part) the models (Figures 5-4 and 5-5). This model is two-dimensional in that it examines HEALTH as the internal perceptions of a person and addresses the ways by which a person can externally obtain the objects and/or substances necessary for his or her HEALTH. Tradition is the essential element in this model, and the model recognizes the fact that the role of tradition is fundamental. Given that the United States has been a melting pot, it has frequently weakened the traditions of immigrants during the processes of acculturation and assimilation, especially where health beliefs and practices are concerned. Many people relate that they "threw these practices away" when they came to the United States. Yet, for many people, modern medicine has not provided a compelling replacement. Examples of the barriers to modern healthcare are further explored in Chapter 8.

	PHYSICAL	MENTAL	SPIRITUAL
MAINTAIN HEALTH	Proper clothing Proper diet Exercise/Rest	Concentration Social and family support systems Hobbies	Religious worship Prayer Meditation
PROTECT HEALTH	Special foods and food combination Symbolic clothing	Avoid certain people who can cause illness Family activities	Religious customs Superstitions Wearing amulets and other symbolic objects to prevent the "Evil Eye" or defray other sources of harm
RESTORE HEALTH	Homeopathic remedies liniments Herbal teas Special foods Massage Acupuncture/ moxibustion	Relaxation Exorcism Curanderos and other traditional healers Nerve teas	Religious rituals—special prayers Meditation Traditional healings Exorcism

Figure 5-4   The nine interrelated facets of HEALTH (physical, mental, and spiritual) and personal methods of maintaining HEALTH, protecting HEALTH, and restoring HEALTH.

Traditional HEALTH Maintenance

The traditional ways of maintaining HEALTH are the active, everyday ways people go about living and attempting to stay well or HEALTHY—that is, ordinary functioning within their family, community, and society. These include such actions as wearing proper clothing—boots when it snows and sweaters when it is cold, long sleeves in the sun, and scarves to protect from drafts and dust. Many traditional ethnic or religious groups may also prescribe garments, such as special clothing or head coverings. Many "special objects," such as hats to protect the eyes and face, long skirts to keep the body clean, down comforters to keep warm, special shoes for work and comfort, glasses to improve vision, and canes to facilitate walking, are used to maintain HEALTH, and they can be found in many traditional homes.

    The food that is eaten and the methods for preparing it contribute to HEALTH. Here, too, one's ethnoreligious heritage plays a strong role in the determination of how foods are cooked, what combinations they may be eaten

	PHYSICAL	MENTAL	SPIRITUAL
MAINTAIN HEALTH	Availability of: Proper shelter, clothing, and food Safe air, water, soil	Availability of: Traditional sources of entertainment, concentration, and "rules" of the culture	Availability and promulgation of rules of ritual and religious worship Meditation
PROTECT HEALTH	Provision of the knowledge of necessary special foods and food combinations, the wearing of symbolic clothing, and avoidance of excessive heat or cold	Provision of the knowledge of what people and situations to avoid, family activities; Family activities	The teaching of: Religious customs Superstitions Wearing amulets and other symbolic objects to prevent the "Evil Eye" or how to defray other sources of harm
RESTORE HEALTH	Resources that provide Homeopathic remedies, liniments Herbal teas, Special foods, Massage, and other ways to restore the body's balance of hot and cold	Traditional healers with the knowledge to use such modalities as: relaxation exorcism, story-telling, and/or Nerve teas	The availability of healers who use magical and supernatural ways to restore health: including religious rituals, special prayers, meditation, traditional healings, and/or Exorcism

Figure 5-5   The nine interrelated facets of HEALTH (physical, mental, and spiritual) and personal methods of maintaining HEALTH, protecting HEALTH, and restoring HEALTH.

in, and what foods may be eaten. Foods are prepared in the home, and recipes from the family's tradition are followed. Traditional cooking methods do not use preservatives. Most foods are fresh and well prepared. Traditional diets are followed, and food taboos and restrictions are obeyed. Cleanliness of the self and the environment is vital. Hand washing and praying before and after meals are examples of necessary rituals.

Mental HEALTH in the traditional sense is maintained by concentrating and using the mind—reading and crafts are examples. There are countless games, books, music, art, and other expressions of identity that help in the maintenance of mental well-being. Hobbies also contribute to mental well-being.

The keys to maintaining HEALTH are, however, the family and social support systems. Spiritual HEALTH is maintained in the home with family closeness—prayer and celebrations. Rites of passage and kindred occasions are also family and community events. The strong identity with and connections to the "home" community are a great part of traditional life and the lifecycle, as well as factors that contribute to HEALTH and well-being.

■ Health Protection

The protection of HEALTH rests in the ability to understand the cause of a given ILLNESS or set of symptoms. Most of the traditional HEALTH and ILLNESS beliefs regarding the causation of ILLNESS differ from those of the modern epidemiological model. In modern epidemiology, we speak of viruses, bacteria, carcinogens, and other pathogens as the causative agents. In "traditional" epidemiology, factors such as the "evil eye," envy, hate, and/or jealousy may be the agents of ILLNESS.

Traditional Epidemiology

ILLNESS is most often attributed to the evil eye. When examining traditional epidemiology, the primary *link* to investigate is the "evil eye." Google the evil eye on the World Wide Web and you find that there have been about 17,200,000 results in 0.36 sec (September 15, 2015). It is essentially a belief that someone can project harm by gazing or staring at another's person or property. Researchers in evil eye beliefs assert that the belief in the evil eye is probably the oldest and most widespread of all superstitions, and it is found to exist in many parts of the world, such as southern Europe, the Middle East, and North Africa. It is thought by some to be merely a superstition, but what one person sees as superstition may well be seen by another person as religion. Immigrant populations carried various evil eye beliefs to the United States. The beliefs have persisted and may be quite strong among newer immigrants and heritage consistent peoples (Dundees, 1992; Maloney, 1976, p. vii; Radford, 2013).

The common beliefs in the evil eye assert that:

1. The power emanates from the eye (or mouth) and strikes the victim.
2. The injury, be it illness or other misfortune, is sudden.
3. The person who casts the evil eye may not be aware of having this power.
4. The afflicted person may or may not know the source of the evil eye.
5. The injury caused by the evil eye may be prevented or cured with rituals or symbols.
6. This belief helps explain sickness and misfortune (Dundees, 1992; Maloney, 1976, p. vii; Radford, 2013).

Various populations define the nature of the evil eye differently. The variables include how it is cast, who can cast it, who receives it, and the degree of power it has. In the Philippines, the evil is cast through the eye or mouth; in the Mediterranean, it is the avenging power of God; in Italy, it is a malevolent force, like a plague, and is warded off by wearing amulets.

In different parts of the world, various people cast it: in Mexico, by strangers; in Iran, by kinfolk; and in Greece, by witches. Its power varies, and in some places, such as the Mediterranean, it is seen as the "devil." In the Near East, it is seen as a deity, and among Slovak Americans, as a chronic but low grade phenomenon (Dundees, 1992; Maloney, 1976, p. xv; Radford, 2013).

Among Germans, the evil eye is known as *aberglobin* or *aberglaubisch*, and it causes preventable problems such as evil, harm, and illness/ILLNESS. Among the Polish, the evil eye is known as *szatan*, literally, "Satan." Some "evil spirits" are equated with the devil and can be warded off by praying to a patron saint or guardian angel. *Szatan* also is averted by prayer and repentance and the wearing of medals and scapulars. These serve as reminders of the "Blessed Mother and the Patrons in Heaven" and protect the wearer from harm. The evil eye is known in Yiddish as *kayn aynhoreh*. The expression *kineahora* is recited by Jews after a compliment or when a statement of luck is made to prevent the casting of an evil spell on another's health/HEALTH. Often, the speaker spits three times after uttering the word (Spector, 1983, pp. 126–127).

Agents of disease may also be "soul loss," "spirit possession," "spells," and "hexes." Here, prevention becomes a ritual of protecting oneself and one's children from these agents. Treatment requires the removal of these agents from the afflicted person (Zola, 1972, pp. 673–679).

ILLNESS also can be attributed to people who have the ability to make others ILL—for example, witches and practitioners of voodoo. The ailing person attempts to avoid these people to prevent ILLNESS and to identify them as part of the treatment. Other "agents" to be avoided are "envy," "hate," and "jealousy." A person may practice prevention by avoiding situations that could provoke the envy, hate, or jealousy of a friend, an acquaintance, or a neighbor. The evil eye belief contributes to this avoidance.

Another source of evil can be of human origin and occurs when a person is temporarily controlled by a soul not his or her own. In the Jewish tradition, this controlling spirit is known as *dybbuk*. The word comes from the Hebrew word meaning "cleaving" or "holding fast." A *dybbuk* is portrayed as a "wandering, disembodied soul which enters another person's body and holds fast" (Winkler, 1981, pp. 8–9).

Traditional practices used in the protection of HEALTH include, but are not limited to:

1. The use of protective objects—worn, carried, or hung in the home
2. The use of substances that are ingested in certain ways and amounts or eliminated from the diet, and substances worn or hung in the home
3. The practices of religion, such as the burning of candles, the rituals of redemption, and prayer.

Objects That Protect HEALTH

Amulets are sacred objects, such as charms, worn on a string or chain around the neck, wrist, or waist to protect the wearer from the evil eye or the evil spirits that could be transmitted from one person to another or have supernatural origins. For example, the *mano milagroso* (miraculous hand) (Figure 5-6) is worn by many people of Mexican origin for luck and the prevention of evil. A *mano negro* (black hand) (Figure 5-7) is placed on babies of Puerto Rican descent to ward off the evil eye. The *mano negro* is placed on the baby's wrist on a chain or pinned to the diaper or shirt and is worn throughout the early years of life.

Amulets may also be written documents on parchment scrolls, and these are hung in the home. Figure 5-8 is an example of a written amulet acquired in Jerusalem. It is hung in the home or workplace to protect the person, family, or business from the evil eye, famine, storms, diseases, and countless other dangers. Table 5-1 describes several practices found among selected ethnic groups to protect themselves from or to ward off the evil eye.

Bangles (Figure 5-9) are worn by people originating from the West Indies. The silver bracelets are open to "let out evil," yet closed to prevent evil from entering the body. They are worn from infancy, and as the person grows, they are replaced with larger bracelets. The bracelets tend to tarnish and leave a black ring on the skin when a person is becoming ILL. When this occurs, the person knows it is important to rest, to improve the diet, and to take other needed precautions. Many people believe they are extremely vulnerable to evil, even to death, when the bracelets are removed. Some people wear numerous bangles. When they move an arm, the bracelets tinkle. It is believed that this sound frightens away the evil spirit. Healthcare providers should realize that, when the bracelets are removed, the person experiences a great deal of anxiety.

In addition to amulets, there are talismans. A talisman is believed to possess extraordinary powers and may be worn on a rope around the waist or carried in a pocket or purse. The talisman illustrated in Figure 5-10 is a marionette,

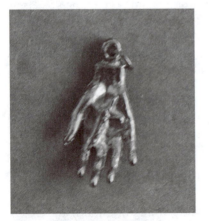

Figure 5-6   Mano milagroso.

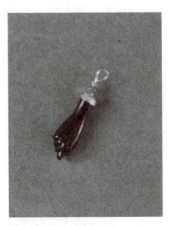

Figure 5-7   Mano negro.

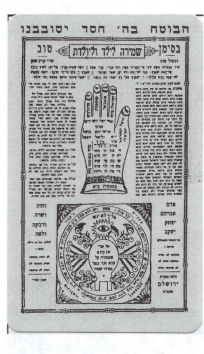

Figure 5-8   The Jerusalem amulet. This amulet serves as protection from pestilence, fire, bad wounds and infection, the evil eye, bad decrees and decisions, curses, witchcraft, and from everything bad; to heal nervous illness, weakness of body organs, children's diseases, and all kinds of suffering from pain; as a talisman for livelihood for success, fertility, honesty, and honor; and for charity, love, mercy, goodness, and grace. It also has the following admonition: "Know before whom you stand—the King of Kings, The Holy One, Blessed be He."

Table 5-1   Practices to Ward Off the Evil Eye

Origin	Practices
Eastern European Jews	Red ribbon woven into clothes or attached to crib
Greece	Blue "eye" bead, crucifix, charms
	Phylacto—a baptismal charm placed on a baby
	Cloves of garlic pinned to shirt
Guatemala	Small red bag containing herbs placed on baby or crib
India	Red string worn on the wrist
India/Pakistan Hindus or Muslims	Copper plates with magic drawings rolled in them
	Slips of paper with verses from the Qur'an
	Black or red string around a baby's wrist
Iran	Child covered with amulets—agate, blue beads
	Children left filthy and never washed to protect them from the evil eye
Italians	Red ribbon worn on clothing
	The *corno* (horn) worn on a necklace
Mexico	Amulet or seed wrapped with red yarn
Philippines	Charms, amulets, medals
Puerto Rico	*Mano negro*

(continued)

Table 5-1   *Continued*

Origin	Practices
Scotland	Red thread knotted into clothing
	Fragment of Bible worn on body
Sephardic Jews	Blue ribbon or blue bead worn
South Asia	Knotted hair or fragment of Qur'an worn on body
Tunisia	Amulets pinned on clothing consisting of tiny figures or writings from the Qur'an
	Charms of the fish symbol—widely used to ward off evil

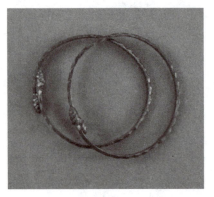

Figure 5-9   Bangles.

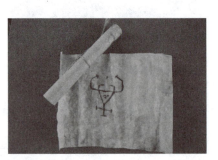

Figure 5-10   Talisman.

and it protects the wearer from evil. It is recommended that people who wear amulets or carry a talisman should be allowed to do so in healthcare institutions. The person who uses an amulet determines and interprets the meaning of the object.

Substances That Protect HEALTH

The second practice uses diet to protect HEALTH and consists of many different observances. People from many ethnic backgrounds eat raw garlic or onions (Figure 5-11) in an effort to prevent ILLNESS. Garlic or onions also may be worn on the body or hung in the Italian, Greek, or Native American home. The ginseng root is the most famous of Chinese medicines. It has universal medicinal applications and is used preventively to "build the blood," especially after childbirth. Tradition states that the more the root looks like a man, the more effective it is. Ginseng is also native to the United States and is used in this country as a restorative tonic (Figure 5-12).

Diet regimens also are used to protect HEALTH. It is believed that the body is kept in balance, or harmony, by the type of food one eats.

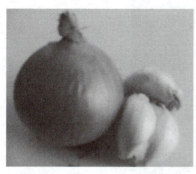

Figure 5-11   Onion and garlic.

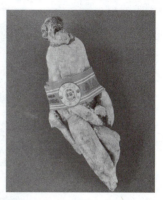

Figure 5-12   Ginseng root.

Traditionalists have strong beliefs about diet and foods and their relationship to the protection of HEALTH. The rules of the kosher diet practiced among Jewish people mandate the elimination of pig products and shellfish. Only fish with scales and fins are allowed, and only certain cuts of meat from animals with a cleft hoof and that chew cud can be consumed. Examples of this kind of animal are cattle and sheep. Many of the dietary practices, such as the avoidance of pig products, are also adhered to by Muslims, and the meats must be *halal*, sanctioned by Islamic law. Jews also believe that milk and meat must never be mixed and eaten at the same meal.

In traditional Chinese homes, a balance must be maintained between foods that are *yin* or *yang*. These are eaten in specified proportions. In Hispanic homes, foods must be balanced as to "hot" and "cold." These foods, too, must be eaten in the proper amounts, at certain times, and in certain combinations. There are also foods that are consumed at certain times of the week or year and not during other times.

Spiritual Practices That Protect HEALTH

A third traditional approach toward HEALTH protection centers, in part, on religion. The words *spirituality* and *religion* are frequently used synonymously, but they are not the same. *Spirituality* connotes the way we orient ourselves toward the Divine, the way we make meaning out of our lives, the recognition of the presence of Spirit (breath) within us, a cultivation of a lifestyle consistent with this presence, and a perspective to foster purpose, meaning, and direction to life. It may find expression through religion, or religion may be a tool for finding one's spirit (Hopkins, Woods, Kelley, Bentley, & Murphy, 1995, p. 11).

Religion is embedded in the life of many heritage-consistent traditional people in countless ways. For example, the religion's calendar gives order to people's lives by defining holidays in their season. A religion has sacred objects, spaces, and times; stipulates practices, such as dietary and wardrobe; teaches the rituals surrounding conception, pregnancy, birth, and the child's early

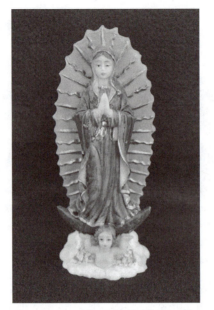

Figure 5-13   The Virgin of Guadalupe.

life; and instructs how to bring babies into the world, what the first words a newborn should hear, and how to care for and remember the dead. It may also, in many cases, instruct how to protect ourselves from the envy of others and/or the evil eye (Leontis, 2009, p. 32). It strongly affects the way people choose to protect HEALTH, and it plays a strong role in the rituals associated with HEALTH protection. It dictates social, moral, and dietary practices that are designed to keep a person in balance. Many people believe that ILLNESS and evil are prevented by strict adherence to religious codes, morals, and practices. They view ILLNESS as a punishment for breaking a religious code. For example, I once interviewed a woman who believed she had cancer because God was punishing her for spending the money her mother gave her to put in the church collection when she was a child. An example of a protective religious figure is the Virgin of Guadalupe (Figure 5-13), the patron saint of Mexico, who is pictured on medals that people wear or in pictures or icons hung in the home. She is believed to protect the person and home from evil and harm, and she serves as a figure of hope.

Religion and HEALTH

Religion helps to provide the believer with an ability to understand and interpret the events of the environment and life. Box 5-1 illustrates selected situations where religion and HEALTH intersect. Not every religious tradition speaks to each situation. Most often, these situations are not overtly linked to HEALTH, but if thought through, one can see their relationship.

Box 5-1

Selected Examples of Situations Where Religion and Health Intersect

Physical
- **Agriculture**—practices related to the planting, harvesting, and distributing of produce and meats
- **Blood**—admonitions regarding the acceptance of blood transfusions
- **Childbirth**—numerous rituals and rites surrounding immediate birth
- **Conception**—prohibitions against birth control and abortion
- **Death**—the immediate care of the body after death
- **Dietary practices**—food prohibitions
- **Dying**—care of the person in the final moments of life
- **Exercise practices**—physical daily care of the body
- **Garments**—special cloths and sacred clothes that must be worn at all times or for special occasions
- **Medications**—admonitions to take prescribed medications
- **Nature**—respect for the sustainability of the earth and natural resources—stewardship
- **Pregnancy**—countless rules to be followed
- **Specific maintenance and prevention practices**—cleanliness—hand washing

Mental
- **Child rearing**—how, when, and what children must be taught regarding rules of the given faith tradition
- **Face**—how the essential part of the person must be safeguarded, and that one must not compromise a person's face[2]
- **Familial relationships**—encouragement of close family bonds and respect for the elderly
- **Readings**—sacred readings developed to calm a person
- **Sense of self and self in world**—answers to the questions: "Who am I?" and "Why am I here?"
- **Time**—weekly and seasonal festivals and holidays to set the rhythm of the year and keep person in balance

Spiritual
- **Amulets and talismans**—sacred objects that may be worn, carried, or hung in the home
- **Beginning of life**—sacred ceremonies—baptism, circumcision, naming
- **Death**—rituals for funeral, burial, mourning, memorial services
- **Dying**—confession, prayers
- **End-of-life care**—use of resuscitation and extreme care versus not using
- **Forgiveness**—final words with family members and friends

[2]Face in this context refers to a person's sense of self and pride—saving face.

(continued)

Box 5-1   *Continued*

- **Pilgrimages**—visiting holy places such as shrines—sacred spaces
- **Prayer times**—times of day when prayers are recited
- **Prayer ways**—direction one faces, position of prayer, sacred garments that must be worn

---

HEALTH Restoration

HEALTH restoration in the physical sense can be accomplished by the use of countless traditional remedies, such as herbal teas, liniments, special foods and food combinations, massage, and other activities.

The restoration of HEALTH in the mental domain may be accomplished by the use of various techniques, such as performing exorcism, calling on traditional healers, using teas or massage, and seeking family and community support.

The restoration of HEALTH in the spiritual sense can be accomplished by healing rituals; religious healing rituals; or the use of symbols and prayer, meditation, special prayers, and exorcism. This will be further discussed in Chapter 6.

■ Healthcare Choices

There are countless ways to describe and label health/HEALTH care beliefs, practices, and systems. "Healthcare" may be labeled as "modern," "conventional," "traditional," "alternative," "complementary," "allopathic," "homeopathic," "folk," "integrative," and so forth. The use of the word *traditional* to describe "modern healthcare" is, by definition, a misnomer. *Traditional* connotes a tradition, such as the handing down of statements, beliefs, legends, customs, and information from generation to generation—"The passing down of elements of a culture from generation to generation, especially by oral communication: *cultural practices that are preserved by tradition*"; or "a mode of thought or behavior followed by a people continuously from generation to generation; a custom or usage" ("Tradition," *American Heritage Dictionary of the English Language,* 2011). The use of *traditional* to connote modern healthcare is a misnomer, as modern, allopathic, healthcare is a new science and has been passed down in writing for a relatively short amount of time, rather than orally over many generations.

There are also many reasons people may choose to use HEALTHCARE systems other than modern healthcare. These include, but are not limited to, access issues, such as poverty, language, availability, and lack of insurance, and preference for familiar and personal care. *Traditional* here connotes HEALTHCARE beliefs and practices observed among peoples who steadfastly maintain their heritage and observe HEALTHCARE practices derived from their ethnocultural or religious heritage.

As stated earlier, in nearly every situation when a person becomes ill, there is an expectation for the restoration of health/HEALTH, and the person usually recovers. As far back as historians and interested social scientists can trace in the extended history of humankind, the phenomenon of recovery has occurred. It made little difference what mode of treatment was used; health/HEALTH restoration was usual and expected. Established cultural norms have been attributed to the recovery from illness, and over time the successful methods for treating various maladies were preserved and passed down to each new generation within a traditional ethnocultural community. It is the occurrence of natural recovery that has given rise to all forms of therapeutic treatments, and the attempts to explain a phenomenon that is natural. Over the generations, natural recovery has been attributed to all sorts of rituals, including cupping, magic, leeching, and bleeding. Today, the people who are members of many different native, immigrant, and traditional cultural communities in the United States— American Indian, Black, Asian, European, and Hispanic—may continue to utilize the practices found within their tradition.

■ Folk Medicine

Folk medicine today is related to other types of medicine that are practiced in our society. It has coexisted, with increasing tensions, alongside modern medicine and was derived from academic medicine of earlier generations. There is ample evidence that the folk practices of ancient times have been abandoned only in part by modern healthcare belief systems, for many of these beliefs and practices continue to be observed today. Many may be practiced in secret, underground. Today's popular medicine is, in a sense, commercial folk medicine. Yoder (1972) describes two varieties of folk medicine:

1. Natural folk medicine—or rational folk medicine—is one of humans' earliest uses of the natural environment and utilizes herbs, plants, minerals, and animal substances to prevent and treat illnesses.
2. Magico-religious folk medicine—or occult folk medicine—is the use of charms, holy words, and holy actions to prevent and cure illnesses/ILLNESSES.

Natural Folk Medicine

Natural folk medicine has been widely practiced in the United States and throughout the world. In general, this form of prevention and treatment is found in old fashioned remedies and household medicines. These remedies have been passed down for generations, and many are in common use today. Much folk medicine is herbal, and the customs and rituals related to the use of the herbs vary among ethnic groups. Specific knowledge and usages are addressed throughout this text. Commonly, across cultures, the herbs are found in nature and are used by humans as a source of therapy, although how these medicines are gathered and specific modes of use vary from group to group and place to place. In general, folk medical traditions prescribed the time of year in which the herb was to be picked; how it was to be dried; how it was to be prepared; the method, amount, and frequency of taking; and so forth.

Natural Remedies

The use of natural products, such as wild herbs and berries, accessible to healers developed into today's science of pharmacology. Early humankind had a wealth of knowledge about the medicinal properties of the plants, trees, and fungi in their environment. They knew how to prepare concoctions from the bark and roots of trees and from berries and wildflowers. Countless herbal preparations that were used many generations ago are in popular use today. Examples include purple foxglove, which contains the cardiotonic digitalis and was used for centuries to slow the heart rate; and feverfew, used to treat headaches.

Magico-Religious Folk Medicine

The magico-religious form of folk medicine has existed for as long as humans have sought to maintain, protect, and/or restore their HEALTH. It has now, in this modern age of science and technology, come to be labeled by some as "superstition," "old fashioned nonsense," or "foolishness," yet for believers it may go so far on the continuum as to take the form of religious practices related to HEALTH maintenance, protection, restoration, and healing. Chapter 6 addresses these belief systems in greater detail.

■ Healthcare Philosophies

Two distinctly different health/HEALTH care philosophies determine the scope of health/HEALTH beliefs and practices: dualistic and holistic. Each of these philosophies espouses effective methods of maintaining, protecting, and restoring health/HEALTH, and the "battles for dominance" between the allopathic and homeopathic philosophies have been hard fought in this country over the past century. One manifestation of these struggles is an emerging preference for homeopathic or holistic, complementary, integrative, or alternative medicine among people from all walks of life.

The dominant healthcare system in the United States is predicated on the allopathic (dualistic) philosophy. The word *allopathy* has two roots. One comes from the Greek meaning "other than disease" because medications are often prescribed on a basis that has no consistent or logical relationship to the symptoms. The second root of *allopathy* is derived from the German meaning "all therapies." Allopathy is a "system of medicine that embraces all methods of proven, that is, empirical science and scientific methodology is used to prove the value in the treatment of diseases" (Weil, 1983, p. 17). After 1855, the American Medical Association (AMA) adopted the "all therapies" definition of *allopathy* and has exclusively determined who can practice medicine in the United States. For example, in the 1860s the AMA refused to admit women doctors to medical societies, practiced segregation, and demanded the purging of homeopaths. Allopaths continue to show little or limited tolerance or respect for other providers of healthcare, such as homeopaths, osteopaths, and chiropractors, and for such traditional healers as lay midwives, herbalists, and American Indian medicine men and women. The allopathic healthcare system, the modern healthcare system, is further discussed in Chapter 8.

The Homeopathic (Holistic) Philosophy is the other healthcare philosophy in the United States. Developed between 1790 and 1810 by Samuel C. Hahnemann in Germany, homeopathic medicine is extremely popular in much of Europe and other parts of the world. It is becoming, once again, more popular in the United States.

Homeopathy, or homoeopathy, comes from the Greek words *homoios* ("similar") and *pathos* ("suffering"). In the practice of homeopathy, the person, not the disease, is treated. This system has not been "tolerated" by the allopaths, yet it continues to thrive and is used by countless people. It espouses a holistic philosophy—that is, it sees health as a balance of the physical, mental, and spiritual whole. Homeopathic care encompasses a wide range of healthcare practices and is often referred to as "complementary medicine" or "alternative medicine." Complementary, alternative, unconventional, or unorthodox therapies are medical practices that do not conform to the scientific standards set by the allopathic medical community; they are not taught widely in the medical and nursing communities and are not generally available in the allopathic healthcare system, including the hospital settings. These include such therapies as acupuncture, massage therapy, and chiropractic medicine. Presently, this situation is changing, and the use of services such as acupuncture is more widespread in modern healthcare settings.

Table 5-3 demonstrates the health/HEALTH care choices, or pathways a person may follow when an illness occurs. The allopathic system comprises the conventional or familiar services within the dominant healthcare culture—acute care, chronic care, communtiy/public healthcare, psychiatric/mental health, rehabilitation, and so forth.

Two types of care in the holistic system are classified as complementary. These break down again into two categories, either alternative or integrative, and traditional or ethnocultural. Modern or allopathic therapies were discussed in Chapter 4. Alternative, or integrative, therapies are those that are *not* a part of one's ethnocultural or religious heritage, interventions neither taught widely in medical schools nor generally available in U.S. hospitals and other healthcare settings; traditional therapies are those that are part of one's traditional ethnocultural or religious heritage. In other words, a European American electing to use acupuncture as a method of treatment is seeking alternative treatment; a Chinese American using this treatment modality is using traditional medicine derived from his or her heritage.

Table 5-2   Selected Examples of Health/HEALTH Care Choices

Healthcare (Dualistic – mind/body)	Allopathic (Conventional)	Acute care Chronic care Community/public health Psychiatric/mental health Rehabilitation
HEALTHCARE (Holistic – mind/body/spirit)	Alternative (Integrative)	Aromatherapy Biofeedback Hypnotherapy Macrobiotics Massage therapy Reflexology
	Traditional (Ethnocultural)	Ayurveda *Curanderismo* *Qi gong* Reiki *Santeria* Voodoo

The following are selected examples of alternative/integrative care:

1. *Aromatherapy*—an ancient science, presently popular, that uses essential plant oils to produce strong physical and emotional effects in the body

2. *Biofeedback*—the use of an electronic machine to measure skin temperatures; the patient controls responses that are usually involuntary

3. *Hypnotherapy*—the use of hypnosis to stimulate emotions and involuntary responses such as blood pressure

4. *Macrobiotics*—a diet and lifestyle from the Far East and adapted for the United States by Michio Kushi; the principles of this vegetarian diet consists of balancing yin and yang energies of food

5. *Massage therapy*—use of manipulative techniques to relieve pain and return energy to the body, now popular among many groups, both modern and traditional

6. *Reflexology*—the natural science dealing with the reflex points in the hands and feet that correspond to every organ in the body. The goal is to clear the energy pathways and the flow of energy through the body.

The following are selected examples of traditional or ethnocultural HEALTHCARE systems:

1. *Ayurvedic.* This 4,000-year-old method of healing originated in India and is the most ancient existing medical system that uses diet, natural therapies, and herbs. Its chief aim is longevity and quality of life. It formed the foundation of Chinese medicine.

2. *Curanderismo.* This traditional Hispanic (Mexican) system of HEALTHCARE originated in Spain and is derived, in part from traditional practices of indigenous Indian and Spanish HEALTH practices.

3. *Qi gong.* This form of Chinese traditional medicine combines movement, meditation, and regulation of breathing to enhance the flow of qi (the vital energy), to improve circulation and enhance the immune system.

4. *Reiki.* This Japanese form of therapy is based on the belief that when spiritual energy is channeled through a practitioner, the patient's spirit is healed, and this in turn heals the physical body.

5. *Santeria.* A form of traditional HEALTHCARE observed among the practitioners of Santeria, this is a syncretic religion that comprises both African and Catholic beliefs. This religion is found practiced among Puerto Ricans and Dominicans.

6. *Voodoo.* This form of traditional HEALTHCARE is observed among the practitioners of Voodoo, a religion that combines Christian and African Yoruba religious beliefs.

Homeopathic Schools

The period from 1870 through 1930 was when the allopathic healthcare model as we know it today was established. During the time that the roots of this system of healthcare were becoming firmly established, the ideas of the eclectic and other schools of medical thought were also prevalent. The following are examples of healthcare systems that developed in this time:

1. *Homeopathic medicine.* As stated earlier in this chapter, homeopathic medicine was developed between 1790 and 1810 by Samuel C. Hahnemann in Germany. In the practice of homeopathy, the person, not the disease, is treated. The practitioner treats a person by using minute doses of plant, mineral, or animal substances. The medicines are selected using the principle of the "law of similars." A substance that is used to treat a specific set of symptoms is the same substance that, if given to a healthy person, would cause the symptoms. The medicines are administered in extremely small doses. These medicines are said to provide a gentle but powerful stimulus to the person's own defense system, helping the person recover. An increasing group of homeopaths exist in the United States, and there are larger practices in India, Great Britain, France, Greece, Germany, Brazil, Argentina, and Mexico (Homeopathic Educational Services, n.d.).

2. *Osteopathic medicine.* Dr. A. T. Still developed osteopathy in 1874 in Kirksville, Missouri. It was a uniquely American branch of medicine and a distinct form of medical practice as it was the art of curing without the use of surgery or drugs. Today, osteopathic medicine offers the benefits of allopathic medicine, including prescription medications, surgery, and the use of technology to

diagnose disease and treat injuries. It also attempts to discover and correct all mechanical disorders in the human body. Osteopathy is the knowledge of the structure, relation, and function of each part of the human body applied to the adjustment or correction of whatever interferes with the body's harmonious operation. Today, U.S. osteopathic physicians (DOs) are fully licensed, patient-centered medical doctors. They, like medical doctors, have completed 4 years of medical school, 1 year of internship, and generally a further residency in a specialty area. They take the same course work as do medical doctors, often use the same textbooks, and often take the same licensing examinations. The lines of distinction between the medical doctor and the osteopath arise because the osteopath, in addition to using modern scientific forms of medical diagnosis and treatment, uses manipulation of the bones, muscles, and joints as therapy. Osteopaths also employ structural diagnosis and take into account the relationship between body structure and organic functioning when they determine a diagnosis. The osteopathic doctor has the same legal power to treat patients as a medical doctor (AACOM, 2015).

3. *Chiropractic.* Chiropractic is a healthcare profession that focuses on the relationship between the body's structure—mainly the spine—and its functioning. It is a controversial form of healing that has been in existence for over a century. It, too, adheres to a disease theory and a method of therapy that differ from allopathy. It was developed as a form of healing in 1895 in Davenport, Iowa, by a storekeeper named Daniel David Palmer, also known as a "magnetic healer." Palmer's theory underlying the practice of chiropractic was that an interference with the normal transmission of "mental impulses" between the brain and the body organs produced diseases. The interference is caused by misalignment, or subluxation, of the vertebrae of the spine, which decreases the flow of "vital energy" from the brain through the nerves and spinal cord to all parts of the body. The treatment consists of manipulation to eradicate the subluxation (American Chiropractic Association, 2015).

4. *Christian Science.* The religious philosophy of scientism lies outside allopathic and most homeopathic philosophies and delivery systems. Christian Science, as a system of spiritual healing, was first explained in 1875 in Mary Baker Eddy's book *Science and Health with Key to the Scriptures* (Eddy, 1875). Eddy introduced the term *Christian Science* to designate the scientific system of divine healing. Eddy's revelation consists of two parts:

- The discovery of this divine science of mind healing, through a spiritual sense of the Scriptures, and
- The proof, by present demonstration, that the so called miracles of Jesus did not specially belong to a dispensation now ended, but

that they illustrated "an ever-operative divine principle" (Eddy, 1875, p. 123, lines 16–27).

Eddy's own early research and experiments in homeopathy, allopathy, and diet preceded her discoveries about spiritual healing. Ultimately, she found that "a mental method produces permanent health" (Eddy, 1875, p. 79, lines 8–9).

Christian Scientists are free to choose the method of healthcare they feel is most effective. Their choice is not compelled by a church. Individuals and families make their own decisions. Christian Scientists, like others, grapple with the moral, social, and cultural implications of modern medical approaches and technological developments—including gene therapy, cloning, and artificial life-support systems. They are free to make their own choices on important social health matters, such as abortion, birth control, blood transfusions, and organ donations. Christian Scientists turn to the Bible and the pages of *Science and Health* for answers to humanity's deepest questions (K. Graunke, (personal interview, January 8, 2003).

National Center for Complementary and Integrative Health

This agency was initially established as the National Center for Complementary and Alternative Medicine (NCCAM) at the National Institutes of Health in 1998. As of December 2014, it became the National Center for Complimentary and Integrative Health (NCCIH). NCCIH is the federal government's lead agency for scientific research on complementary and integrative health approaches. Its mission is to define, through rigorous scientific investigation, the usefulness and safety of complementary and integrative health approaches and the role they play in improving health and healthcare. The goals of this agency are:

1. Advance the science and practice of symptom management.
2. Develop effective, practical, personalized strategies for promoting health and well-being.
3. Enable better evidence-based decision making regarding complementary and integrative health approaches and their integration into healthcare and health promotion (NCCIH, 2015).

NCCIH describes the different approaches to healthcare that are outside the realm of conventional medicine as either complementary or alternative. When a nonmainstream practice is used together with conventional medicine, it is considered "complementary." When a nonmainstream practice is used in place of conventional medicine, it is considered "alternative." The agency generally uses the term "complementary health approaches" when discussing practices and products of nonmainstream origin. They use "integrative health" when they talk about incorporating complementary approaches into mainstream healthcare. Most complementary health approaches fall into one of two subgroups—natural products, or mind and body practices. Topics from acai to zinc are, will be, or were subjects for research by the agency. An example of an alternative therapy is using a special diet or medication to treat cancer instead of undergoing the surgery, radiation, or chemotherapy recommended by a conventional doctor.

The National Institutes of Health has found that about a third of Americans seek help for their health in a place that is outside their doctor's office. Fish oil, probiotics, melatonin, deep breathing, chiropractors, and yoga are among some of the alternatives Americans use to feel better. Most Americans who use these approaches do so as a complement to conventional care. Only about 5% of Americans use only alternative medicine solely (Christensen, 2015).

In addition, the 2012 National Health Interview Survey (NHIS), which included a comprehensive survey on the use of complementary health approaches by Americans, found that 17.7% of American adults had used a dietary supplement other than vitamins and minerals in the past (NCCIH, 2015). Furthermore, according to statistics released in July 2009 from a nationwide government survey, U.S. adults spent $33.9 billion out of pocket on visits to complementary and alternative medicine (CAM) practitioners and purchases of CAM products, classes, and materials (Nahin, Barnes, Stussman, & Bloom, 2009).

The use of complimentary and integrative therapies has grown rapidly. As early as 1998, Astin reported that three theories had been offered to explain why people seek this care:

1. *Dissatisfaction.* Patients are not satisfied with allopathic care because it is seen as ineffective, it produces adverse effects, or it is impersonal, too costly, or too technological.

2. *Need for personal control.* The providers of alternative therapies are less authoritarian and more empowering, as they offer the patient the opportunity to have autonomy and control in their healthcare decisions.

3. *Philosophical congruence.* The alternative methods of therapy are compatible with the patients' values, worldview, spiritual philosophy, or beliefs regarding the nature and meaning of *health*/HEALTH and *illness*/ILLNESS. These therapies are now frequently used by patients with cancer, arthritis, chronic back or other pain, stress-related problems, AIDS, gastrointestinal problems, and anxiety.

It is difficult to sort out which aspects of complementary and traditional medicine have merit and which are hoaxes. From the viewpoint of the patient, if he or she has faith in the efficacy of an herb, a diet, a pill, or a healer, it is not a hoax. From the viewpoint of the medical establishment, jealous of its territorial claim, the same herb, diet, pill, or healer is indeed a hoax if it is "scientifically" ineffective and prevents the person from using the method of treatment the physician healer or other healthcare provider believes is effective. The tensions between allopathic and homeopathic philosophies have been going on since the late 19th century.

This chapter has explored the *HERITAGECHAIN*'s links of HEALTH and ILLNESS and the HEALTH Traditions Model; the choices people have in terms of folk medicine, natural, or magico-religious medicine; complementary and integrative methods of health/HEALTH maintenance, protection, and/or restoration; and other schools of health/HEALTH care in contemporary American society. In this chapter, we have explored traditional ways of maintaining, protecting, and restoring HEALTH; the choices available to patients; and health/HEALTH care philosophies.

Explore  MediaLink

Go to the Student Resource Site at pearsonhighered.com/nursingresources for chapter-related review questions, case studies, and activities. Contents of the CULTURALCARE Guide and CULTURALCARE Museum can also be found on the Student Resource Site. Click on Chapter 5 to select the activities for this chapter.

Box 5-2

Keeping Up

Countless references may be accessed to maintain currency in the domain of health. Suggested resources include, but are not limited to:

Homeopathic Educational Services
National Center for Complementary and Integrative Health
American Association for Osteopathic Medicine
American Association for Chiropractic Medicine

■ References

American Association of Colleges of Osteopathic Medicine (AACOM). (2015). *The difference between U.S.-trained osteopathic physicians and osteopaths trained abroad.* Retrieved from http://www.aacom.org/home

American Chiropractic Association. (2015). *What is chiropractic?* Retrieved from http://www.acatoday.org/Patients/Why-Choose-Chiropractic/What-is-Chiropractic

Astin, J. A. (1998, May 20). Why patients use alternative medicine: Results of a national study. *Journal of the American Medical Association, 279*(19), 1548–1553.

Christensen, J. (2015). A third of Americans use alternative medicine. *CNN.* Retrieved from http://www.cnn.com/2015/02/11/health/feat-alternative-medicine-study/

Dundees, A. (1992). *The evil eye: A casebook.* Madison: University of Wisconsin Press.

Eddy, M. B. (1875). *Science and health with key to the scriptures.* Boston, MA: Christian Science Publishing.

Homeopathic Educational Services. (n.d.). Retrieved from http://www.homeopathic.com/

Hopkins, E., Woods, L., Kelley, R., Bentley, K., & Murphy, J. (1995). *Working with groups on spiritual themes.* Duluth, MN: Whole Person Associates.

Leontis, A. (2009). *Culture and customs of Greece.* Westport, CT: Greenwood Press.

Maloney, C. (Ed.). (1976). *The evil eye.* New York, NY: Columbia University Press.

Nahin, R. L., Barnes, P. M., Stussman, B. J., & Bloom, B. (2009). *Costs of complementary and alternative medicine (CAM) and frequency of visits to CAM practitioners: United States, 2007* (National Health Statistics Reports, No. 18). Hyattsville, MD: National Center for Health Statistics. Retrieved from https://nccih.nih.gov/research/statistics/costs

National Center for Complementary and Integrative Health (NCCIH). (2015). *Complementary, alternative, or integrative health: What's in a name?* U.S. Department of Health and Human Services, National Institutes of Health. Retrieved from https://nccih.nih.gov/health/integrative-health

Radford, B. (2013). The evil eye: Meaning of the curse and protection against it. *Livescience.* Retrieved from http://www.livescience.com/40633-evil-eye.html

Spector, R. E. (1983). *A description of the impact of Medicare on health—illness beliefs and practices of white ethnic senior citizens in central Texas* (Doctoral dissertation, pp. 126–127). University of Texas at Austin School of Nursing. University Microfilms International, Ann Arbor, MI.

Weil, A. (1983). *Health and healing.* Boston, MA: Houghton Mifflin.

Winkler, G. (1981). *Dybbuk.* New York, NY: Judaica Press.

Yoder, D. (1972). Folk medicine. In R. H. Dorson (Ed.), *Folklore and folklife* (pp. 191–193). Chicago, IL: University of Chicago Press.

Zola, I. K. (1972). The concept of trouble and sources of medical assistance to whom one can turn with what. *Social Science and Medicine, 6,* 673–679.

CHAPTER

6   HEALING Traditions

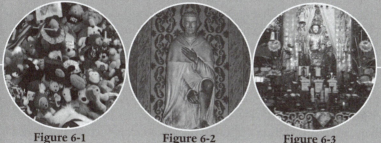

Figure 6-1   Figure 6-2   Figure 6-3

■ Objectives

1. Identify practices that were part of ancient forms of HEALING.
2. Distinguish the relationship between faith traditions and HEALING.
3. Identify selected saints related to HEALTH problems.
4. Discuss the various destinations and purposes of popular piety and spiritual journeys.
5. Discuss the relationship of HEALING to today's health/HEALTH beliefs and practices.
6. Describe various forms of HEALING.
7. Differentiate rituals of birth and death among people of selected faith traditions.

The *HeritageChain* link of HEALING evokes countless images and experiences. The opening images for this chapter represent secular and sacred shrines where people may visit to seek HEALTH or HEALING. Figure 6-1 is the Memorial Shrine at the site of the "Marathon Bombing" in Boston, Massachusetts, on April 15, 2013, where 3 people were killed and 260 wounded. Figure 6-2 is the statue of St. Peregrine, the patron saint for cancer sufferers in the Serra Chapel of the Mission Church in San Juan Capistrano, California. Figure 6-3 is a Buddhist Shrine in Honolulu, Hawaii, where people visit to pray for HEALTH and HEALING.

Consider your own experiences and background:

∞ Are you having difficulties in your life that you would like to change? Are you seeking answers to questions that you cannot easily answer? Do you know about the HEALING traditions within your ethnoreligious heritage or the places you may visit to find the help you need?

∞ What are the HEALING practices within your family and ethnocultural heritage? What are the shrines, or sacred places, that are a part of your tradition or that you have visited? In the minds of countless people, shrines such as the ones in the chapter opener are an invaluable resource. If you could pick three images from your heritage that are related to HEALING, what would they be?

What is HEALING? What is the connotation of this word from a magico-religious or traditional perspective? What compels people to travel to shrines in the United States or in other parts of the world? Could it be that people who experience the need to seek consolation and solutions for overpowering events for which they cannot find rational answers turn to sources such as holy shrines? The phenomenon of seeking HEALING is observed worldwide, and every religion and ethnic group offers substantive beliefs and practices in this genre. Are these examples of magic or of faith in a form of HEALTHCARE that is obtained from sources other than those that are conventional medicine? This chapter explores these questions by introducing a wide range of magico-religious and religious beliefs and practices regarding HEALING. It also discusses the traditions cross-culturally related to lifecycle crises—birth and death—as these phenomena are closely linked to the beliefs and practices inherent in HEALING.

■ HEALING

The professional history of nursing was born with Florence Nightingale's knowledge (1860) that "nature heals." In more recent times, numerous texts have been written to help nurses assist patients in upgrading their lives in a holistic sense and in HEALING the person—body, mind, and spirit. Krieger (1979) developed a method for teaching nurses how to use their hands to heal. Historically, Wallace (1979) described methods of helping nurses diagnose and deliver spiritual care. She points out that the word *spiritual* is often used synonymously with *religion*, but that the terms are not the same. If they are used synonymously as a basis for the healthcare and nursing assessment of needs, some of the patient's deepest needs may be glossed over. *Spiritual care* implies a much broader grasp of the search for meanings that goes on within every human life. In addition to answers to these questions from nursing raised in the introduction to this chapter, one is able to explore the concept from the classical and historical viewpoints of anthropology, sociology, psychology, and religion.

From the established literature of anthropology and sociology come classical texts that describe rituals, customs, beliefs, and practices that surround healing. Shaw (1975, p. 121) contends that, "for as long as man has practiced the art of magic, he has sought to find personal immortality through healing practices." Buxton (1973) describes traditional beliefs and indigenous HEALING rituals in Mandari and relates the source of these rituals with how humans view themselves in relation to God and Earth. In this culture, the healer experiences a religious calling to become a healer. HEALING is linked to beliefs in evil and the removal of evil from the sick person. Naegele (1970, p. 18) describes healing in our society as a form of "professional practice." He asserts, however, that "healing is not wholly a professional monopoly and that there are several forms of nonprofessional healing such as the 'specialized alternatives.'" These include Christian Science and the marginally professional activities of varying legitimacy, folk medicine, and quackery. Naegele (1970) states: "To understand modern society is to understand the tension between traditional patterns and self-conscious rational calculations devoted to the mastery of everyday life."

Literature from the field of psychology abounds with references to HEALING. Shames and Sterin (1978) describe the use of self-hypnosis to HEAL, and Progoff (1959), a depth psychologist, describes depth as the "dimension of wholeness in man." He has written extensively on how one's discovery of the inner self can be used for both HEALING and creation.

Krippner and Villaldo (1976, p. viii) contend that there is a "basic conflict between HEALING and technology" and that "the reality of miracles, of HEALING of any significant entity that could be called God is not thought to be compatible with the reality of science." They further contend that HEALINGS are psychosomatic in origin and useful only in the sense of the placebo effect.

The literature linking religion to HEALING is bountiful. The primary source is the Bible (both the Old and New Testaments) and prayers. Bishop (1967, p. 45) and MacNutt (1974) discuss miracles and their relationship to HEALING. Both authors concur that miracles must be considered in context, in relation to the time, place, and situation in which they occur. They further describe faith and its relationship to HEALING. As Bishop states, "something goes on in the process of faith healing," and HEALING "is the exception rather than the rule" (1967, p. 45). HEALING through faith generally is not accepted as a matter of plain fact, but it is an event to rejoice over.

Ford (1971, p. 6) describes HEALING of the spirit and methods of spiritual HEALING. He describes suffering in 3 dimensions: body, mind, and spirit. He fully describes telotherapy—spiritual HEALING—which is both a means and an invitation. His argument is that full HEALING takes place only when there is agape love—divine love—and no estrangement from God. Russell (1937, p. 221) and Cramer (1923, p. 11) assert that HEALING is the work of God alone. Russell asserts that "God's will normally expresses itself in HEALTH," and Cramer focuses on the unity of human beings with God and claims that permanent HEALTH is truth, that HEALING is the gift of Jesus, and that it is a spiritual gift.

Other ways of examining HEALING are found in the writings of Harner (1988), where he contends that the important aspect of shamanism (HEALING) is that it "provides us with an ancient means of solving everyday problems." Other authors, such as Chopra (1989), Fox (2000), and Moorjani (2012), focus on the personal and pragmatic elements of HEALING. Dossey (1993) focuses on the power of prayer in HEALING situations.

■ Ancient Forms of HEALING

ILLNESS was considered to be a crisis, and the people of ancient times developed elaborate systems of HEALING. The cause of an ILLNESS was attributed to the forces of evil, which originated either within or outside the body. Early forms of HEALING dealt with the removal of evil. Once a method of treatment was found effective, it was passed down through the generations in slightly altered forms.

If the source of sickness-causing evil was within the body, treatment involved drawing the evil out of the body. This may have been accomplished through the use of purgatives, which caused either vomiting or diarrhea, or by bloodletting, which involved "bleeding" the patient or "sucking out" blood. (The barbers of medieval Europe did not originate this practice; bleeding was done in ancient times.) Leeching was another method used to remove corrupt humors from the body.

If the source of the evil was outside the body, there were a number of ways to deal with it. One source of external evil was witchcraft. In a community, there were often many people or a single person who was "different" from the other people. Quite often, when an unexplainable or untreatable illness occurred, these people were seen as the causative agents. In such a belief system, successful treatment depended on the identification and punishment of the person believed responsible for the disease. The practice of scapegoating is in part derived from this belief. It was believed that if the "guilty" person was punished or removed from the community, the disease would be cured. In some communities, the HEALERS themselves were seen as witches and the possessors of evil skills. How easy it was for ancient humankind to turn things around and blame the person with the skills to treat the disease for causing the disease!

Various rituals were involved in the treatment of ILL people. Often, the sick person was isolated from the rest of the family and community. In addition, it was customary to chant special prayers and incantations on the patient's behalf. Sacrifices and dances often were performed in an effort to HEAL the ILLS. Often, the rituals of the HEALER involved reciting incantations in a language foreign to the ears of the general population ("speaking in tongues") and using practices that were strange to the observers. Given these strong beliefs, at times the HEALERS themselves were ostracized by the population.

Another cause of ILLNESS was believed to be the envy of people within the community. The best method of preventing such an ILLNESS was to avoid causing the envy of one's friends and neighbors. The treatment was to do away with whatever was provoking the envy—even though the act might have prevented a person from accomplishing a "mission in life," and the fear of being "responsible" might have been psychologically damaging.

Today, we tend to view the HEALING beliefs and methods of ancient people as "primitive"; yet to fully appreciate their efficacy, we need only make the simple observation that many forms of these methods exist today and have aided the survival of humankind.

■ Religion and HEALING

Religion plays a fundamental role in one's perception of HEALTH and ILLNESS. Just as culture and ethnicity are strong determinants in an individual's interpretation of the environment and the events within the environment, so, too, is religion. In fact, it is often difficult to distinguish between those aspects of a person's belief system arising from a religious background, and those that stem from an ethnic and cultural heritage. Some people may share an ethnicity yet be of different religions; a group of people can share a religion yet have a variety of ethnic and cultural backgrounds. It is never safe to assume that all individuals of a given ethnic group practice or believe in the same religion. The point was embarrassingly driven home when I once asked a Mexican American woman if she would like me to call the priest for her while her young son was awaiting critical surgery. The woman became angry with me. I could not understand why until I learned that she was Methodist and not Catholic. I had made an assumption, and I was wrong. She later told me that not all Chicanos are Catholic. After many years of hearing people make this assumption, she had learned to react with anger.

Religion strongly affects the way people interpret and respond to the signs and symptoms of ILLNESS. Religion and the piety of a person determine not only the role that faith plays in the process of recovery, but also in many instances the response to a given treatment and to the HEALING process. Each of these threads—religion, ethnicity, and culture—is woven into the fabric of each person's response to treatment and HEALING.

There are far too many religious beliefs and practices related to HEALING to include in this chapter. An introductory discussion of religious HEALING beliefs from the Judeo-Christian background, however, is possible.

The Old Testament does not focus on HEALING to the extent the New Testament does. God is seen to have total power over life and death and is the HEALER of all human woes. God is the giver of all good things and of all misfortune, including sickness. Sickness represented a break between God and humans. In Exodus 15:26, God is proclaimed the supreme HEALER ("I will put none of the diseases upon you which I put upon the Egyptians; for I am the Lord, your healer."). In a passage from Deuteronomy 32:39, it is stated "I kill, and I make alive. I have wounded and I heal." The Jewish person may believe that the "HEALING of illness comes from God through the mediation of His 'messenger,' the doctor." The person who is ill may combine hope for a cure with faith in God and faith in the doctor (Ausubel, 1964, pp. 192–195). A prayer is recited for HEALING each Sabbath and other times throughout the week, and people are invited to submit or speak the names of people for whom they are petitioning for a restoration of their HEALTH.

The HEALING practices of the Roman Catholic tradition include a variety of beliefs and numerous practices of both a preventive and a HEALING nature. For example, St. Blaise, an Armenian bishop who died in AD 316 as a martyr, is revered as the preventer of sore throats. The blessing of the throats on his feast day (February 3) derives from the tradition that he miraculously saved the life of a boy by removing a fishbone he had swallowed, and he is the patron saint of throat illnesses (Matz, 2000). Other saints concerned with aspects of ILLNESS include the following: St. Odilia, blindness; St. Vitus, cholera; St. Raymond Nonnatus, pregnancy; St. Lucy, eye diseases; and St. Dymphna, mental illness. These, and countless other saints, are the subject of prayers, and their medals may be worn, images hung in the home, and/or prayer cards carried by believers (Catholic Saints Online, 2015).

Many more saints could be included. I refer you to other sources for information, and I also recommend that you ask patients for information. I was caring for a young woman with terminal colon cancer. We began a conversation about St. Peregrine. She shared with me her belief in this saint, showed me a medal that she had carried with her, and expressed that she was comforted by sharing this information.

Spiritual Journeys

There are countless places in the United States and in this world where people make spiritual journeys, pilgrimages, or show popular piety for the purpose of petitioning or giving thanks for favors. These shrines are related to magico-religious folk medicine and the use of charms, holy words, and holy actions. For example, at many shrines, petitioners leave objects, written petitions, or money, and/or light candles. Shrines range from small memorials—such as shrines that are created at the sites where fatal incidences or accidents have occurred (see Figure 6-1)—to large, famous shrines where people who are part of a given religious tradition, or a follower of a given HEALER may go to pray or petition at the site. In the United States, and throughout the world, people make pilgrimages to a number of shrines in search of special favors and HEALING. Shrines are not limited to any one faith tradition, and they can be secular as well as religious. Over the years, I have visited many sacred shrines and have learned that they are indeed extraordinary places. The essentials that each of the shrines has in common are a feeling of peacefulness and serenity to the visitor; a calm, soothing atmosphere; and a place where petitions and/or objects are left when petitions for help with a specific problem or HEALING are made; or prayers have been answered, and people leave objects in gratitude. Most, but not all, have a source of water as part of the milieu, and it is a part of the tradition to take home water from the shrine.

The following are examples of selected shrines located in the United States:

■ The Callery pear tree was found alive in the rubble of the World Trade Center in 2001; it is now a secular shrine. The tree was replanted in the 9/11 Memorial Park and is visited by countless people seeking to pay their respects. In this image, the lower branches are covered with "clouties," an ancient Celtic traditional way of praying and making an offering for HEALING (Figure 6-4). The National September 11 Memorial Museum opened at the World Trade Center as a tribute to the victims and survivors of this event.

- The Tomb of Menachem Mendel Schneerson in Queens, New York, is a holy shrine where Jewish people from around the world gather to leave petitions and seek HEALING. People have reported HEALINGS when they visit his tomb (Figure 6-5).
- Chimayo, New Mexico, is the home of the Shrine of our Lord of Esquipulas. The shrine was built between 1814 and 1816 and is visited by thousands of people each year. The shrine has been called the "Lourdes of America," and countless HEALINGS have been reported in this location (Figure 6-6). There is a hole in the floor of the shrine, and it is believed that eating the dirt from this hole will cure many illnesses.

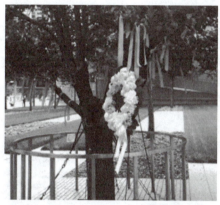

Figure 6-4   Callery pear tree, New York City.

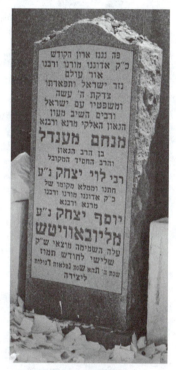

Figure 6-5   The tomb of Menachem Mendel Schneerson in Queens, New York.

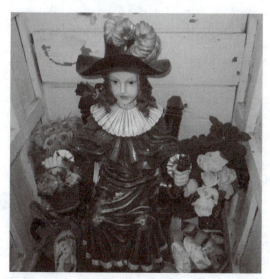

Figure 6-6   Chimayo—Shrine of our Lord of Esquipulas.

The dirt may also be mixed with water and the mud rubbed on the body (*Welcome to El Santuario de Chimayo*, 2010).

Three of the most revered and known shrines worldwide are located in France, Spain, and Portugal:

■ Lourdes, in France, is believed to be a site where the Virgin Mary visited Bernadette Soubirous. In 1858, she observed a vision of St. Mary in a grotto. The Virgin was reported to have visited her several times. There have been 67 accepted miracle cures at this site, and countless—over 5 million a year—pilgrims go there. Petitions may also be placed on line (Lourdes, France, n.d.).

■ Another famous shrine is found on a high, saw-toothed mountain near Barcelona, Spain. It is the Shrine of our Lady of Montserrat. Pilgrims have visited this site since the 13th century to venerate the miraculous statue of the Black Madonna, and many miracles have been reported here (Abadia de Montserrat, 2015).

■ Fatima is located in a small village in central Portugal, a short distance from Lisbon. It is a site of a shrine dedicated to the Virgin Mary. In 1917, three peasant children reported a vision of a woman who identified herself as the "Lady of the Rosary." The first national pilgrimage to the site occurred in 1927. Countless miraculous have been reported at this site. Prayers and petitions may be placed on line (Santuario de Fatima, 2015).

You need only visit these remarkable HEALING places and bear witness to the display of faith to begin to understand their important contributions in the complex areas of HEALING and faith.

There are numerous variations as to what a person's religion allows or disallows when they are receiving healthcare. The following are examples of the richly diverse beliefs of people from several religious backgrounds with respect to health/HEALTH, healing/HEALING, and other events related to healthcare delivery:

■ **Buddhists** are allowed to receive an abortion if necessary, practice birth control, receive transfusions as necessary, and donate organs. Buddhists have no restrictions on medications and HEALING beliefs and practices.

■ **Christians** have many different HEALTH-related practices and may allow abortion, artificial insemination, birth control, blood and blood products, most medications, and organ donations. However, Roman Catholics are prohibited from having an abortion and must use only natural methods of birth control.

■ **Hindus** have no policy regarding abortion, accept all types of birth control, blood and blood products, medications, and organ donations; traditional HEALING beliefs and practices may be followed.

■ **Jehovah's Witnesses** forbid abortion, artificial insemination, blood and blood products, faith healing, organ donation, and sterilization.

- *Judaism* permits therapeutic abortions and artificial insemination for most branches; has strict dietary laws, including not mixing milk and prohibiting consumption of meat and pork products and shellfish; has no restrictions on medications except pork-based insulin; and permits most surgical procedures.
- *Mormons* forbid abortions, do not use birth control, believe that the power of God can bring HEALING, employ the laying on of hands for HEALING, and have no restrictions regarding medications and most surgical procedures.
- *Muslims* do not accept abortion; forbid pork and alcohol; do not allow euthanasia; have no restrictions on blood and blood products; and allow most surgical procedures (Andrews & Hanson, 1995; Beliefnet, 2015).

Remember, these are examples, and you are urged not to generalize from this information when relating to a patient and family. It is important to show respect, sensitivity, and understanding of the different perspectives that may exist and to be able to convey to the patient and family your desire to understand their faith-based viewpoints on health and healthcare.

■ HEALING and Today's Beliefs

It is not an accident or a coincidence that today, more so than in recent years, we are not only curious, but vitally concerned about the ways of HEALING that our ancestors employed. Some critics of the healthcare system choose to condemn the system, with more vociferous critics, such as the visionary work of Illich (1975), citing its failure to create a utopia for humankind. It is obvious to those who embrace a more moderate viewpoint that diseases continue to occur and that they outflank our ability to cure or prevent them. Many people are seeking the services of people with knowledge in the arts of HEALING and folk medicine. Many patients may elect, at some point in their lives, more specifically during an ILLNESS, to use modalities outside the medical establishment. It is important to understand the various modalities of HEALING and HEALERS.

Types of HEALING

A review of HEALING and spiritual literature reveals that there are four types of HEALING:

- *Spiritual HEALING.* When a person is experiencing an illness of the spirit, spiritual HEALING applies. The cause of suffering is personal sin. The treatment method is repentance, which is followed by a natural healing process.
- *Inner HEALING.* When a person is suffering from an emotional (mental) illness, inner HEALING is used. The root of the problem may lie in the person's conscious or unconscious mind. The treatment method is

to heal the person's memory. The HEALING process is delicate and sensitive and takes considerable time and effort.

■ *Physical HEALING.* When a person is suffering from a disease or has been involved in an accident that resulted in some form of bodily damage, physical HEALING is appropriate. Laying on of hands and speaking in tongues usually accompany physical HEALING. The person is prayed over by both the leader and members of a prayer group.

■ *Deliverance or exorcism.* When the body and mind are victims of evil from the outside, exorcism is used. In order to effect treatment, the person must be delivered, or exorcised, from the evil. The ongoing popularity of films such as *The Exorcist* gives testimony to the return of these beliefs. Incidentally, the priest who has lectured in my classes stated that he does not, as yet, lend credence to exorcisms; however, he was guarded enough not to discount it, either.

The people who HEAL, both in the past and in the present, often have been those who received the gift of HEALING from a "divine" source. Many receive this gift in a vision and have been unable to explain to others how they know what to do. Other HEALERS learned their skills from one of their parents or other family members. Most of the HEALERS with acquired skills are women, who subsequently pass on their knowledge to their daughters. People who use herbs and other preparations to remove the evil from the sick person's body are known as *herbalists*. Other HEALERS include bone setters and midwives, and although early humankind did not separate ILLNESS of the body from those of the mind and spirit, some HEALERS were more adept at solving mental and spiritual problems.

There are numerous HEALERS in the general population, some of whom are legitimate and some of whom are not. They range from housewives and priests to *Romani* and witches. Many people seek their services. There are numerous technical differences between the scope of practice of a modern healthcare practitioner and that of a traditional HEALER (Table 6-1). I have visited with several traditional HEALERS. One man I visited was a *Santero*, a traditional HEALER from Puerto Rico. He enjoyed a reputation as a person who can "bring comfort to those most in need." I had an appointment for an interview but, when I arrived, he informed me that if I wanted to learn about his practice, I had to "sit." I did. He examined me by asking questions (history); examining my head and hands (palpation and observation); and casting cowrie shells (in-depth examination). He then told me a story, asked me to interpret it, and then, based on my interpretation, told me how to treat my "problem." I visited another *Santero* in Los Angeles in 2008 and was treated for a knee problem. He massaged my knee with a dark liquid, recited several incantations, and then I was wrapped in a large white sheet, placed in the center of his patio for a *limpia* (cleansing), and a circle was made around me with alcohol and was then lit on fire (Figure 6-7). I appreciated the treatment, and my knee has been better for a long time!

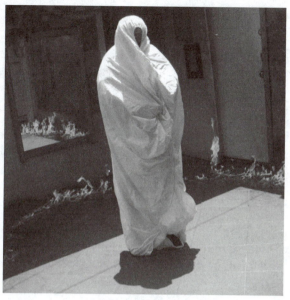

Figure 6-7   Ring of fire.

Table 6-1   Comparisons: Traditional Holistic HEALER Versus Modern Allopathic Healthcare Provider

Traditional Holistic HEALER	Modern Healthcare Provider
1. Maintains informal, friendly, affective relationship with the entire family	1. Businesslike, formal relationship; deals only with the patient but may involve family members
2. Comes to the house, day or night	2. Patient must go to the physician's office or clinic, and only during the day; may have to wait for hours to be seen; home visits are rarely, if ever, made
3. For diagnosis, consults with head of house, creates a mood of awe, talks to all family members, is not authoritarian, has social rapport, builds expectation of cure	3. Rest of family usually is ignored; deals solely with the ill person and may deal only with the sick part of the person; authoritarian manner creates fear
4. Generally less expensive than the physician	4. More expensive than the HEALER
5. Has ties to the "world of the sacred"; has rapport with the symbolic, spiritual, creative, or holy force	5. Secular; pays little attention to the religious beliefs or meaning of an illness
6. Shares the worldview of the patient—that is, speaks the same language, lives in the same neighborhood, or lives in some similar socioeconomic conditions; may know the same people; understands the lifestyle of the patient.	6. Generally does not share the worldview of the patient—that is, may not speak the same language, live in the same neighborhood, or understand the socioeconomic conditions; may not understand the lifestyle of the patient.

■ Ancient Rituals Related to the Lifecycle

Today, just as it did in antiquity, religion also plays a role in the rites surrounding both birth and death. Many of the rituals that we observe at the time of birth and death have their origins in the practices of ancient human beings. Close your eyes for a few moments and picture yourself living thousands and thousands of years ago. There is no electricity, no running water, no bathroom, and no plumbing. The nights are dark and cold. The only signs of the passage of time are the changing seasons and the apparent movement of the various planets and stars through the heavens. You are prey to all the elements, as well as to animals and the unknown. How do you survive? What sort of rituals and practices assist you in maintaining your equilibrium within this often hostile environment? It is from these living conditions that many of today's practices sprang.

There are two heritage links or critical moments that occur in the life of every human being: birth and death. When you examine the historical rites that were connected to birth and death, you see how many of them are relevant to our lives today. Many of the rites continue to be practiced in this modern era.

Birth Rituals

In the minds of early human beings, the number of evil spirits far exceeded the number of good spirits, and a great deal of energy and time was devoted to thwarting these spirits. They could be defeated by the use of gifts or rituals, or, when the evil spirits had to be removed from a person's body, with redemptive sacrifices. Once these evil spirits were expelled, they were prevented from returning by various magical ceremonies and rites. When a ceremony and an incantation were found to be effective, they were passed on through the generations. It has been suggested and supported by scholars that, from this original beginning, today's organized religions came into being. Many of the early rites have survived in changed forms, and we continue to practice them.

The power of the evil spirits was believed to endure for a certain length of time. The 3rd, 7th, and 40th days were the crucial days in the early life of a child and the new mother. Hence, it was on these days, or on the 8th day, that most of the rituals were observed. It was believed that, during this period, the newborn and the mother were at the greatest risk from the power of supernatural beings and thus in a taboo state. "The concept underlying taboo is that all things created by or emanating from a supernatural being are his, or are at least in his power" (Morgenstern, 1966, p. 31). The person was freed from this taboo by certain rituals, depending on the practices of a given community. When the various rites were completed and the 40 days were over, both the mother and child were believed to be redeemed from evil. The ceremonies that freed the person had a double character: They were partly magic and partly religious.

I have deliberately chosen to present the early practices of Semitic peoples because their beliefs and practices evolved into the Judaic, Christian, and Islamic religions of today. Because the newborn baby and mother were considered vulnerable to the threats of evil spirits, many rituals were developed to protect them. For example, in some communities, the mother and child were separated from the rest of the community for a certain length of time, usually 40 days. Various people performed precautionary measures, such as rubbing the baby with different oils or garlic, swaddling the baby, and lighting candles. In other communities, the baby and the mother were watched closely for a certain length of time, usually 7 days. During this time span, they were believed to be intensely susceptible to the effects of evil—hence, close guarding was in order (Morgenstern, 1966, pp. 22–30).

The birth of a male child was considered more significant than that of a female, and many rites were practiced in observance of this event. One ritual sacrifice was cutting off a lock of the child's hair and then sprinkling his forehead with sheep's blood. This ritual was performed on the 8th day of life and may be practiced today among Muslims. In other Semitic countries, when a child was named, a sheep was sacrificed and asked to give protection to the infant. Depending on regional or tribal differences, the mother might be given parts of the sheep. It was believed that if this sacrificial ritual was not performed on the 7th or 8th day of life, the child would die. The sheep's skin was saved, dried, and placed in the child's bed for 3 or 4 years as protection from evil spirits (Morgenstern, 1966, p. 87).

The practice of cutting a lock of a child's hair and the sacrifice of an animal served as a ceremony of redemption. The child could also be redeemed from the taboo state by giving silver—the weight of which equaled the weight of the hair—to the poor. Although not universally practiced, these rites are still observed in some form in some communities of the Muslim world (Lee, 2015).

Circumcision is closely related to the ceremony of cutting the child's hair and offering it as a sacrifice. Some authorities hold that the practice originated as a rite of puberty: a body mutilation performed to attract the opposite sex. (Circumcision was practiced by many peoples throughout the ancient world.) Other sources attribute circumcision to the concept of the sanctity of the male organ and claim that it was derived from the practice of ancestor worship. The Jews of ancient Israel, as today, practiced circumcision on the 8th day of life. The Muslims circumcise their sons on the 7th day in the tradition that Mohammed established. The rite of circumcision was accompanied by festivals of varying durations. Some families feasted for as long as a week.

The ceremony of baptism is also rooted in the past. It, too, symbolically expels the evil spirits, removes the taboo, and is redemptive. It is practiced mainly among members of the Christian faith, but the Yezidis and other non-Christian sects also perform the rite. Water was believed to possess magical powers and was used to cleanse the body from both physical and spiritual maladies, which included evil possession and other impurities. Usually, the child was baptized on the 40th day of life. In some communities, however, the child was baptized on the 8th day. The 40th (or 8th) day was chosen because it was believed that, given performance of the particular ritual, this day marked the end of the evil spirits' influence (Morgenstern, 1966).

Today, baptism is practiced by most Christians, but the timing and the procedure that is followed varies. For example, people who belong to the

Eastern Orthodox, Episcopalian, Roman Catholic, Russian Orthodox, and Unitarian faiths baptize infants; and members of the Church of Christ, Mormons, Methodists, and Pentecostals baptize children when older. The method used varies from sprinkling to immersion to full immersion.

Some rituals also involved the new mother. For example, not only was she (along with her infant) removed from her household and community for 40 days, but in many communities she had to practice ritual bathing before she could return to her husband, family, and community. Again, these practices were not universal, and they varied in scope and intensity from people to people.

Extensions of Birth Rituals to Today's Practices

Early human beings, in their quest for survival, strove to appease and prevent the evil spirits from interfering with their lives. Their beliefs seem simple and naive, yet the rituals that began in those years have evolved into those that exist today. Attacks of the evil spirits were warded off with the use of amulets, charms, and the like. People recited prayers and incantations. Because survival was predicated on people's ability to appease evil spirits, the prescribed rituals were performed with great care and respect. This accounts in part for the longevity of many of these practices through the ages. For example, circumcision and baptism still exist, even when the belief that they are being performed to release the child from a state of being taboo may not continue to be held. It is interesting also that adherence to a certain timetable is maintained. For example, as stated, the Jewish religion mandates that the ritual of circumcision be performed on the 8th day of life as commanded by Jewish law in the Bible.

The practice of closely guarding the new mother and baby through the initial hours after birth is certainly not foreign to us. The mother is closely watched for hemorrhage and signs of infection; the infant initially is watched for signs of choking or respiratory distress. This form of observation is very intense. Could factors such as these have been what our ancestors watched for? If early human beings believed that evil spirits caused the frequent complications that surrounded the birth of a baby, it stands to reason that they would seek to control or prevent these complications by adhering to astute observation, isolation, and rituals of redemption. In fact, in our present time, it is not unusual to observe women using ancient practices to facilitate pregnancy; ensure a safe pregnancy, labor, and delivery; and employ traditional ways of protecting both herself and her newborn child.

The care of the newborn baby also varies among people migrating here from different nations. In the West (Western Europe and other nations, such as Brazil, Cuba, Haiti, Ireland, and the Philippines, where the predominant populations are Christian), the father may attend the delivery, midwives may be used, breastfeeding is common, and BCG (Bacillus Calmette-Guérin) vaccine is used routinely to prevent tuberculosis. Regarding migrants from countries such as Afghanistan, Albania, Bangladesh, Egypt, Indonesia, Iraq, Pakistan, and Syria where the predominant faith is Islam, families may choose to have a traditional birth attendant and/or here prefer to have a female doctor deliver the baby when a midwife is not available. All Muslim fathers recite an *adhan* in the infant's right ear so that it is the first words the child hears. The *adhan* most often used is "there is no deity but God, and Muhammad is the messenger of God" (Lee, 2015). The babies are breastfed for 2 years, and the babies born in the country of origin are given BCG at birth.[1] In Eastern countries such as Cambodia, China, India, Japan, Korea, Laos, and Vietnam, where the majority populations are either Hindu or Buddhist, objects may be placed in the home to prevent evil spirits, the babies are breastfed and given BCG at birth or shortly thereafter. The United States does not administer BCG.

Death Rituals

It was believed that the work of evil spirits and the duration of their evil—whether it was 7 or 40 days—surrounded the person, family, and community at the time of and after death. Rites evolved to protect both dying and dead persons and the remaining family from these evil spirits. The dying person was cared for in specific ways (ritual washing), and the grave was prepared in set ways. For example, in many traditions, food and water are stored in the coffin for the journey after death. Further, rituals were performed to protect the deceased's survivors from the harm believed to be rendered by the deceased's ghost. It was believed that this ghost could return from the grave and, if not carefully appeased, harm surviving relatives (Morgenstern, 1966, pp. 117–160).

Countless ethnocultural and religious differences can be found in the ways we observe dying, announce death, and mourning. I have collected the terms for announcing a death for several years by randomly reading the local newspapers' death notices in several cities. It is interesting to observe the regional differences in expressions. In some cities, deaths are merely listed by the person's name; in other places, the event of death is followed by "expired," "suddenly," or "unexpected"; and some names are followed by comments such as "sunrise ... sunset" and "departed this life." The following are further examples of the ways a death may be announced:

> Boston, Massachusetts—"left this world entirely too early"
> New York, New York—"found her way over the rainbow"
> St. Albans, West Virginia—"ushered into his heavenly home"
> Los Angeles, California—"passed away"
> San Antonio, Texas—"entered into the arms of his Lord"
> Houston, Texas—"went to be with her heavenly father," and
> Honolulu, Hawaii—"went to the next room."

Just as the care of the newborn baby varies among people migrating here from different nations, so too does the care of the dying and dead. In the West (Western Europe and other nations, where the predominant populations are

---

[1]Bacillus Calmette-Guérin (BCG) vaccine is used routinely outside the United States to prevent tuberculosis.

Christians), there are such practices as isolating the dying person and withholding the truth; however, the person is not left alone, and the desire to die at home is vital. The family and friends stay with the body through the night, and burial is generally in 24 hours. White clothing representing death may be worn in nations such as Haiti, whereas black is worn in other nations, such as Greece. The watching or "waking" of the dead originates from keeping a vigil to keep evil spirits away from the deceased and is now a religious ritual among Catholics (U.S. Conference of Catholic Bishops, 2015).

Migrants from countries where the predominant faith is Islam follow the Muslim rites. The body generally remains in the home and is cared for, washed, and wrapped in a white cloth by family members. The Mullah is often in attendance, and friends and family visit. The person is buried in 24 hours and a ceremony is held 2 days after burial, followed by a meal. In Eastern countries where the majority population is either Hindu or Buddhist, many people may prefer quality rather than quantity of life, and the dying person may be helped to recall past good deeds. Non-Hindus are not allowed to touch the body, and the family cares for it. Mourning beliefs and practices vary widely depending on the religious and national origins of the family. The following are a limited number of examples:

- Buddhists may not allow pregnant women to attend funerals to prevent bad luck for the baby.
- Christians may show reserved grieving in public, and for others grief may be demonstrative. In many traditions the widow may wear dark mourning clothes for the rest of her life, and in other nations, white may be worn.
- Hindus believe in reincarnation and practice cremation.
- Jews bury the person as a soon as possible; and this is followed by a 7-day mourning period.
- Muslims may hold a ceremony 2 days after burial, followed by a meal.

Expressions of death and death rituals are also found in objects. Figures 6-8, 6-9, and 6-10 depict several objects that may be used.

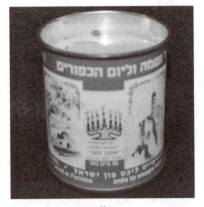

Figure 6-8   Candle.

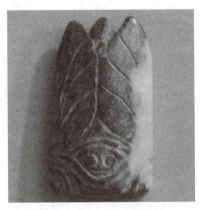

Figure 6-9   Jade stone.

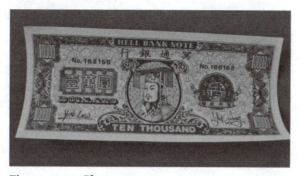

Figure 6-10   Ghost money.

- Candles (Figure 6-8) are used by many people after a death as a way of lighting the way for the soul of the deceased.
- Jade stone (Figure 6-9), from China, is placed in orifices of the body to block the entrance of evil spirits after death.
- Ghost money, from China (Figure 6-10), is burned to send payments to a deceased person and to ensure his or her well-being in the afterlife.

Intersections of HEALTH, HEALING, and RELIGION

There are several areas in which there is an intersection of HEALTH, HEALING, and RELIGION. The following are examples of additional spiritual/religious factors that link with the myriad of facets that have been described earlier in this chapter and in Chapter 5. One's religious affiliation may be seen as providing many links in a complex chain of life events. Religious affiliation frequently provides a background for a person regarding HEALTHY behavior and contributes to HEALTH. Participation in religious practices provides social support, and this in turn brings HEALTH. In addition, religious worship may create positive emotions; this, too, contributes to HEALTH. Table 6-2 illustrates several of these intersections, which must be known by healthcare providers.

This chapter has been no more than an overview of the topics introduced. The amount of relevant knowledge could fill many books. The issues raised here are those that have special meaning to the practice of nursing, medicine, and healthcare delivery. We must be aware (1) of what people are thinking that may differ from our own thoughts and (2) that sources of help exist outside the modern medical community. As the beliefs of ethnic communities are explored in later chapters, the text discussions will attempt to delineate who are specifically recognized and used as HEALERS by the members of the communities, and will describe some of the forms of treatment used by each community.

Table 6-2 **Areas of Intersection Between the Provision of Healthcare and HEALTH, HEALING, and RELIGION**

Communication	Spirituality and religion begin in silence; however, the need for adequate interpreters has been addressed, but it is also imperative to have available to people the members and leaders of their faith community who can reach out and interpret what is happening in regard to a health crisis at a deeper and spiritual level for the patient and family.
Gender	Understand the "rules" for gender care; in many faith traditions—for example, among Orthodox Jews and Muslims—care must be gender-specific, and people may be forbidden to be touched by someone of the opposite gender.
Manners	Religious and elderly people may be extremely sensitive as to the manner in which they are addressed—never call a person by their given name unless given permission to do so.
Modesty	Religious and elderly people may be extremely modest, and modesty *must* be safeguarded at all times.
Diet	Many food taboos are predicated by one's religion, and consideration must be given to see that improper foods are not served to patients.
Objects	Sacred objects, such as amulets and statues, must be allowed in the patient's space, and all precautions must be observed to safeguard them; when a person wears an amulet, every effort must be made to protect this amulet and permit the patient to wear it.
Social organization	Spirituality or a religious background contributes many positive factors to the healthcare situation; collaboration with the leaders of a faith community can result in strongly positive outcomes for a patient and family.
Space	Space must be defined and allocated for the patient's and family's private use.
Time	Healthcare providers must be knowledgeable about sacred time—for example, what day the patient and family observe as a day of rest—Friday for Muslims, Friday sunset until Saturday sunset for Jews, Saturday for Seventh-day Adventists, and Sunday for Christians; calendars must be posted that note holidays for all the faith traditions of people served within a given institution, and meetings should not be held on these dates; Appendix C contains a list of religious holidays that do not occur on the same date each year; clergy within the faith tradition *must* be contacted to provide the dates for the holidays on a yearly basis; major meetings should not be scheduled on holidays.

Explore 🌐 MediaLink

Go to the Student Resource Site at pearsonhighered.com/nursingresources for chapter-related review questions, case studies, and activities. Contents of the CULTURALCARE Guide and CULTURALCARE Museum can also be found on the Student Resource Site. Click on Chapter 6 to select the activities for this chapter.

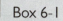

Box 6-1

Keeping Up

There are countless organizations and references that may be accessed to maintain relevant information in the domains of healing and spirituality.

American Holistic Nurses Association

A professional nursing specialty organization, the association promotes nursing education in all aspects of holistic caring and healing.

National Center for Cultural Competence

This center at Georgetown University offers current resources in the Biopsychosocial-Spiritual Model, Spirituality of Children, Spiritual Pain and Distress, and the Assessment of Spirituality and Religion.

Spiritual Competency Resource Center

Approved by the California Board of Behavioral Sciences, Continuing Education, the center offers resources and courses in topics such as Forgiveness, Mindfulness, Spirituality Oriented Interventions, and Self-Compassion.

■ References

Abadia de Montserrat. (2015). Retrieved from http://www.abadiamontserrat .net/(S(nd0kxpyyvci2b3vh5tw2temn))/Default.aspx

Andrews, M. M., & Hanson, P. A. (1995). Religion, culture, and nursing. In J. S. Boyle & M. M. Andrews (Eds.), *Transcultural concepts in nursing care* (2nd ed., pp. 371–406). Philadelphia, PA: J. B. Lippincott.

Ausubel, N. (1964). *The book of Jewish knowledge.* New York, NY: Crown.

Beliefnet. (2015). *Transition rituals.* Retrieved from http://www.beliefnet.com /Wellness/Health/Health-Support/Grief-and-Loss/2001/05/Transition -Rituals.aspx?p=1

Bishop, G. (1967). *Faith healing: God or fraud?* Los Angeles, CA: Sherbourne.

Buxton, J. (1973). *Religion and healing in Mandari.* Oxford, England: Clarendon.

Catholic Saints Online. (2015). Retrieved from http://www.catholic.org/saints

Chopra, D. (1989) *Quantum healing: Exploring the frontiers of mind/body medicine.* New York, NY: Bantam Books.

Cramer, E. (1923). *Divine science and healing.* Denver, CO: Colorado College of Divine Science.

Dossey, L. (1993). *Healing words.* San Francisco, CA: HarperCollins.

Ford, P. S. (1971). *The healing trinity: Prescriptions for body, mind, and spirit.* New York, NY: Harper & Row.

Fox, M. (2000). *One river, many wells.* New York, NY: Putnam.

Harner, M. (1988). Shaman's path. In Doore, G. (Ed.), *What is a Shaman?* (pp. 7-16). New York, NY: Random House.

Illich, I. (1975). *Medical nemesis: The expropriation of health.* London, England: Marion Bogars.

Krieger, D. (1979). *The therapeutic touch.* Englewood Cliffs, NJ: Prentice Hall.

Krippner, S., & Villaldo, A. (1976). *The realms of healing.* Millbrae, CA: Celestial Arts.

Lee, M. (2015). Muslim customs and traditions relating to childbirth. *Synonym.* Retrieved from http://classroom.synonym.com/muslim-customs-traditions -relating-childbirth-5240.html

Lourdes, France. (n.d.). *Numerous links to information and history of the site.* Retrieved from http://en.lourdes-france.org

MacNutt, F. (1974). *Healing,* New York, NY: Ave Maria Press.

Matz. T. (2000). St. Blaise. *Catholic Online.* Retrieved from http://www.catholic .org/saints/saint.php?saint_id=28

Moorjani, A. (2012). *Dying to be me: My journey from cancer, to near death, to true healing.* Carlsbad, CA: Hay House (self-publishing).

Morgenstern, J. (1966). *Rites of birth, marriage, death and kindred occasions among the Semites.* Chicago, IL: Quadrangle Books.

Naegele, K. (1970). *Health and healing.* San Francisco, CA: Jossey-Bass.

Nightingale, F. (1860, 1946). *Notes on nursing—What it is, what it is not* (A facsimile of the first edition published by D. Appleton and Co.). New York, NY: Appleton-Century.

Progoff, I. (1959). *Depth psychology and modern man.* New York, NY: McGraw-Hill.

Russell, A. J. (1937). *Healing in his wings.* London, England: Methuen.

Santuario de Fatima. (2015). Retrieved from http://www.fatima.pt/pt/

Shames, R., & Sterin, C. (1978). *Healing with mind power.* Emmaus, PA: Rodale Press.

Shaw, W. (1975). *Aspects of Malaysian magic.* Kuala Lumpur, Malaysia: Nazibum Negara.

U.S. Conference of Catholic Bishops. (2015). *An overview of Catholic funeral rites.* Retrieved from http://www.usccb.org/prayer-and-worship/bereavement -and-funerals/overview-of-catholic-funeral-rites.cfm

Welcome to El Santuario de Chimayo. (2010). Author. Retrieved from http://www .elsantuariodechimayo.us/Pilgrim/Santuario.html#l

Wallace, G. (1979, November). Spiritual care—A reality in nursing education and practice. *The Nurses Lamp, 5*(2), 1–4.

7 Familial HEALTH Traditions

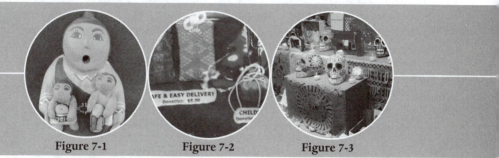

| Figure 7-1 | Figure 7-2 | Figure 7-3 |

As modern medicine becomes more impersonal, people are recalling with some wistfulness old country cures administered by parents and grandparents over the generations.

—*F. Kennet (1976)*

■ Objectives

1. Trace your family's heritage.
2. Describe your and your family's beliefs and practices in:
   a. Health/HEALTH maintenance
   b. Health/HEALTH protection
   c. Health/HEALTH restoration, and
   d. Curing/HEALING.
3. Compare and contrast the difference and similarities between you and your peers in respect to beliefs and practices in:
   a. Health/HEALTH maintenance
   b. Health/HEALTH protection
   c. Health/HEALTH restoration, and
   d. Curing/HEALING.

This link on the *HeritageChain* investigates the health/HEALTH traditions that may be a part of a family's heritage. A baby is born—a new life begins. The child may go home with birth parents, foster parents, or adoptive parents and to a nuclear, an extended, same gender, or a single-parent family with parents who have lived in this country for many generations or are immigrants, who are heritage consistent or heritage inconsistent. The family may use objects and remedies that were used in earlier generations or elect to use today's remedies for the maintenance, protection, and restoration of the family's health/HEALTH. The opening images portray a story of the passage of familial lore from the beginning of life to the end of life. Figure 7-1 is a mother, or grandmother, who may be telling the children their family stories. Figure 7-2 is of *omamori*—amulets from Japan, purchased in a Buddhist temple in Honolulu, Hawaii. They are hung in the home or worn or carried. One is for a safe and easy delivery, the other is used to protect children from maladies. Figure 7-3 is a shrine erected for the Day of the Dead celebration. This Mexican holiday is celebrated on November 2, and families gather together to remember family members and friends who have died.

- ꙮ What family stories have been passed to you from your parents and grandparents? What are your family's traditional HEALTH beliefs and practices? If you could choose two or three examples of health/HEALTH practices from your family's heritage, what would they be?

- ꙮ You may come from a family where traditional HEALTH and ILLNESS beliefs and practices constitute a significant part of your daily life. On the other hand, you may have little or no working knowledge of personally practiced "folk medicine," or traditional medicine, within your own family. In what ways does your traditional heritage influence your personal health beliefs and practices? In what ways does your own background influence your professional practice? Does it complement or disagree with contemporary teachings?

In addition to exploring the already described questions regarding the definitions of *health* and *illness*, it is beneficial to your understanding to describe how you maintain, protect, and/or restore your *health/HEALTH*. Common forms of self-medication and treatment are the use of over-the-counter medications such as acetaminophen for headaches, decongestants for colds, and occasional vitamin supplements. Initially, you may admit to using tea, honey, and lemon and hot or cold compresses for headaches and minor aches and pains. For the most part, however, people tend to look to the healthcare system for the prevention and treatment of illness.

There is an extremely rich tradition in the United States related to self-care. This includes the early use of patent medicines. Throughout most of their history, patent medicines enjoyed a free existence and were very popular with the people of the times. Some of the most popular medicines of the early 20th century contained alcohol; others contained opium and cocaine. This increased their popularity, and the practice continued until passage of the Food, Drug, and Cosmetic Act of 1938. Today, as our lives become more complex and the healthcare system becomes more complicated, costly, and difficult to access, we see a return to self-care and an increasing use of traditional and homeopathic healthcare systems (see Chapters 5 and 6).

■ Familial HEALTH Traditions

We are now ready for a transitional link, and it is time to resume climbing the steps to CULTURALCOMPETENCY. The initial links—a discussion of heritage, an overview of demographic issues, an exploration of terms such as *health* and *illness*, and a discussion of HEALTH and ILLNESS as they relate to religion and spirituality—have been presented, and what remains is the ascent! Before you read on, ask yourself the following questions regarding your health/HEALTH beliefs and practices:

- ∞ Again, what remedies and/or methods do you use to maintain, protect, and restore your health/HEALTH?
- ∞ Do you know the health/HEALTH and illness/ILLNESS beliefs and practices that were or are a part of your heritage?
- ∞ Were you ever thought to be seriously ill/ILL?
- ∞ What did your familial caregiver do to take care of you?
- ∞ Did he or she consult someone in your own ethnic or religious community to find out what was wrong?

It has been mentioned earlier in this text that the first step for developing CULTURALCOMPETENCY is to know yourself, your heritage, and the health/HEALTH and illness/ILLNESS beliefs and practices derived from your heritage—cultural, ethnic, religious, or all. It was pointed out in Chapters 5 and 6 that many daily HEALTH practices have their origins in various heritages, yet may not be thought of in this context.

The following interview procedure is useful for making you aware of the overall history and health/HEALTH belief and practice-related folklore and ethnocultural knowledge of your family. Because the ethnocultural history of each family is unique, you may want to discover more than health/HEALTH beliefs and practices with this interview. Ask your parents or grandparents questions about your family such as their surname, traditional first names, family stories, the history of family "characters" or notorious family members, how historical events affected your family in past generations, and so forth. Next, ask the person you are interviewing the questions in the Heritage Assessment, found in Appendix B. Then, in interviewing your grandmothers, great-aunts, and mother, obtain answers to the following questions:

1. What did they do to maintain health/HEALTH? What did their mothers do?
2. What did they do to protect health/HEALTH? What did their mothers do?

3. Do they wear, carry, or hang in their home objects that protect their HEALTH and home?

4. Do they follow a particular dietary regimen or refrain from eating taboo foods?

Physical, mental, and spiritual aspects are implicit in each of the next three questions:

1. What home remedies do they use to restore health/HEALTH? What did their mothers use?

2. What are their traditional beliefs regarding pregnancy and childbirth?

3. What are their traditional beliefs regarding dying and death?

There are two reasons for exploring your familial heritage. First, it draws your attention to your ethnocultural and religious heritage and the HEALTH practices derived from it. Many of your daily habits relate to early socialization practices that are passed on by parents or additional significant others. Many behaviors are both subconscious and habitual, and much of what you believe and practice is passed on in this manner. By digging into the past, remote and recent, you can recall some of the rituals you observed either your parents or your grandparents perform. You are then better able to realize their origin and significance. Many beliefs and practices are ethnically similar, and socialization patterns may tend to be similar among ethnic groups as well. Religion also plays a role in the perception of, interpretation of, and behavior in health/HEALTH and illness/ILLNESS.

The maternal side is ideal for your interview because, in today's society of interethnic, interracial, interreligious, and/or same-sex marriages and complex family structures, it is assumed that the ethnic beliefs and practices related to health/HEALTH and illness/ILLNESS of the family may be more in tune with the mother's family than with the father's. By and large, family nurturance and health/HEALTH maintenance, protection, and/or restoration have been the domain of women in most cultures and societies. The mother tends to be the gatekeeper—the person within a family who cares for family members when illness/ILLNESS occurs. She also tends to be the prime mover in protecting health/HEALTH and seeking health/HEALTH care. It is most frequently the mother who tells the child what and how much to eat and drink, when to go to bed, and how to dress in inclement weather. She shares her knowledge and experience with her offspring, but usually the daughter is singled out for such experiential sharing. However, this is not a "universal" circumstance, and in many family heritages, the father is the family caregiver. If that is true for your family, it is your paternal family whom you must interview. Given the complex familial and social changes related to family life, it behooves you to question all those involved in raising you. For example, in a same-sex partnership or marriage there may be one partner who fulfills the caretaker role.

The second reason for this examination of familial health/HEALTH practices is to sensitize you to the role your ethnocultural and religious heritage has played. You must reanalyze the concepts of health/HEALTH and illness/ILLNESS and view your own definitions from another perspective. If your familial background is presented in a class or other group setting, the peer group is able to see you in a different light. The group observes similarities and differences among its members. You discover peer beliefs and practices that you originally had no idea existed. You may then be able to identify the "why" behind many daily health/HEALTH habits, practices, and beliefs in your family. You will be amazed to discover the origins of the health/HEALTH practices. The "mysterious" behavior of a roommate or friend may be explained by reflecting on its origin. It is interesting to discover cross-ethnic practices within your own peer group, as some people believe that a given practice is an "original," done only by their family. However, many practices are cross-heritage. How often were you told to do something like the health/HEALTH maintenance practice examples that follow?

- *Austrian*—eat fresh vegetables
- *English*—keep the window open at night (even in winter) and get enough sleep
- *Ethiopian, German, Iranian, Irish, Norwegian*—cleanliness
- *Native American*—dress appropriately for the weather
- *Polish*—good personal hygiene
- *Swedish*—a daily spoonful of cod liver oil.

There are also countless traditional ways to protect health/HEALTH, including:

- *Austrian*—camphor around the neck (in the winter) in a small cloth bag to prevent measles and scarlet fever
- *Canadian*—camphor around the neck to ward off any evil spirit
- *English*—strict enforcement of lifestyle
- *French, German*—every spring, take sulfur and molasses for 3 days as a laxative to get rid of worms
- *Irish, Spanish*—Blessing of the Throat on Saint Blaise Day
- *Italian*—garlic cloves strung on a piece of string around the neck of infants and children to prevent colds and "evil" stares from other people, which, it is believed, could cause headaches and a pain or stiffness in the back or neck.

Table 7-1 lists examples of health/HEALTH restoration practices of people from several heritages. Further examples of health/HEALTH maintenance, protection, and restoration are available on the student resources site that accompanies this text. Table 7-2 gives examples of selected familial ethnocultural and religious beliefs and practices related to birth and death.

Table 7-1   Selected Examples of Common Health Problems, Methods of Restoring Heath, and the Related Heritage

Health Problem	Health Restoration	Heritage
Aches and pains	Hot Epsom salt bath	Canadian
	Hot mustard plaster	German
Acne, rashes	Apply baby's urine	Irish
Backache	Apply hot oatmeal in a sock; place a silver dollar on the sore area, light a match to it; while the match is burning, put a glass over the silver dollar and then slightly lift the glass, and this causes a suction, which is said to lift the pain out	Irish
	Hot mustard plaster	German
	Massage with alcohol	Russian
Colds	Hot boiled milk with honey	African
	Hot lemons	Canadian
	Fluids, aspirin, rest	Eastern Europe
	Chicken soup	French, Polish
	Camphor on chest and red scarves around chest	English
	Hot peppermint drink	Norway
Constipation	Ivory soap suppositories	Canadian
Cough	Shot of whiskey	Canadian
	Honey	Iranian
	Cough syrup made from honey, whiskey, and lemon	Irish
	Chicken soup, honey	Polish
	Warm milk and butter	Swedish
Earache	Warm cod liver oil in ear	England
	Few drops of warm milk in the ear	German
	Heat salt, put in stocking behind the ear	Irish
	Warm oil in ear	Swedish
Evil eye	They put some kind of plant root on fire and make the man who has the evil eye smile and the man talks about his illness	Ethiopian
Eye infections, sties	Potatoes are rubbed on eyes or a gold wedding ring is placed on them and the sign of the cross is made three times	Canadian
	Cold tea-leaf compress	German
	Hot tea bag to area	Irish
Fever	Lots of blankets and heat to make you sweat out a fever	Canadian, Swedish
	Mix whiskey, water, and lemon juice and drink before bed—causes person to perspire and break fever	German

Health Problem	Health Restoration	Heritage
	Spirits of niter on a dry sugar cube or mix with water	Irish
Headache	Boil a beef bone, break up toast in the broth, and drink	German
	Fill a soup bowl with cold water and put some olive oil in a large spoon; hold the spoon over the bowl in front of the person with the headache; while doing this, recite words in Italian and place index finger in the oil in the spoon; drop three drops of oil from the finger into the bowl; by the diameter of the circle the oil makes when it spreads in the water, the severity of the headache can be determined (larger = more severe); after this is done three times, the headache is gone	Italian
High blood pressure	Colonies of blood suckers were kept in clay, where they were born; the person with high blood pressure would have a blood sucker put on his fanny, where it would suck blood; it was thought that this would lower his blood pressure	Italian
Insect bites	Vaseline or boric acid applied to bite	Irish
	Poultice	Swedish
Insomnia	Glass of wine	Canadian
Recovery diet, build up blood	Ginseng tea	Chinese
Sinuses	Camphor placed in a pouch and pinned to the shirt	Canadian
Sore throat	Suck yolks out of eggshell	Native American
Stomach problems, cramps, colic	Baking soda	Irish
	Herbal tea	Italian
Warts	Rub raw potato on wart, run outside, and throw it over left shoulder	Canadian
Wounds, cuts	Fry chopped onions, make a compress, and apply to the infections	Austrian

■ Consciousness Raising

The experience of sharing one's familial HEALTH practices raises one's consciousness in several ways, helps participants see themselves and others in a different context, and facilitates the understanding of patients' practices.

Recognizing Similarities

In my experience, as discussion continues, people realize that many personal beliefs and practices do, in fact, differ from what they are being taught in nursing or medical education to accept as the "right" way of doing things.

Table 7-2   Examples of Selected Familial Ethnocultural and Religious Beliefs and
Practices Related to Birth and Death

Nation of Origin and Religion	Birth Beliefs	Death Beliefs
England—Christian	Baptism	Body dying
	Natural event	Everlasting life with Christ/heaven
		Funeral and prayer
Germany— Lutheran	Birth is sacred	Body dies when we die—souls go to heaven and enjoy everlasting life
	Do not take baby out until it is baptized	Celebrate person's life and the promise of eternal life
	Mother does not go to the baptism	God's will
Greece— Orthodox	After 40 days, mother and newborn go to church—baby is blessed and prayers are said to keep away the evil spirits	After a death, light a candle that burns all night
	Baptized at 2	
	Gifts given to the baby to protect it from the evil eye—charms of white and blue beads are worn on the wrist	In mourning, women wear black for the rest of their lives and men grow facial hair
		Visit grave daily; hold a special service on the 40th day
	Wrap the baby in blankets and pin to sheets to relax	
		The good go to paradise; the bad go to hell
Ireland—Catholic	Baby shower before birth, but never set up the crib until after birth	After death, the body is washed and prepared for the wake at home by a neighbor and then the wake and mass
	Men not present at birth	Blessing with oils and receive the Eucharist for the last time
	Tell of pregnancy after 3 months	Dying person wears a Rosary around the neck to keep evil spirits away and God closer
		Final separation of the soul from the body—soul lives on and is transported to God
		Wake—"a party with one less person"
Italy—Catholic	Life begins at conception	Closed casket or cremation

Nation of Origin and Religion	Birth Beliefs	Death Beliefs
Japan—Shinto	Umbilical cord saved—a lasting bond between mother and child	Cremation
	100-day-old child taken to the Shrine	
Portugal—Catholic	Throw a party for the birth of a boy (relates to the time when males were needed to work on the farms)	A party comforts the loved ones, but if one dies in a painful way, there is no celebration
	Women during pregnancy get less pretty with a girl because the baby is taking her mother's looks	Celebrate a painless death—means the person has been good and is now with Jesus
		Widow must forever wear black—this serves as a warning to other men that she has suffered a loss and is not attractive to prevent shame from being brought to her
Sicily—Catholic	Baptism	Close all shades and never go out during daylight
		Women mourn for years, wearing only black and seldom going outside

Participants begin to admit that they do not seek medical care when the first symptoms of illness appear. On the contrary, they usually delay seeking care and often elect to self-treat at home. They also recognize that there are many preventive and health maintenance acts learned in school with which they choose not to observe. Sometimes, they discover that they are following a self-imposed regimen for health-related problems and are not seeking any outside intervention.

Another facet of a group discussion is the participants' exposure to the similarities that exist among them in terms of health/HEALTH maintenance and protection. To their surprise and delight, they find that many of their daily acts—routines they take for granted—directly relate to methods of maintaining and protecting health/HEALTH.

As is common in most large groups, students seem to be shy at the beginning of this exploration. As more and more members of the group are willing to share their experiences, however, other students feel more comfortable and share more readily. A classroom tactic I have used to break the ice is to reveal an experience I had on the birth of my first child. My mother-in-law, an immigrant from Eastern Europe, drew a circle around the baby's crib with her fingers and spat on him three times to prevent the evil spirits from harming him. Once such an anecdote is shared, other participants have less difficulty in remembering similar events that took place in their own homes.

Students have a variety of feelings about the self-care practices of their families. One feeling discussed by many students is shame. A number of students express conflict in their attitudes: They cannot decide whether to believe the old ways when they have continued to be practiced, or to drop them and adopt the more modern ones they are learning in school. For example, a young man from Ethiopia revealed that he experienced angst when he had an upper respiratory infection and his mother offered him herbs from their homeland. (This is an example of cognitive dissonance.) Many admit that this is the first time they have disclosed these HEALTH beliefs and practices in public, and they are relieved and amazed to discover similarities with other students. Frequently, there is a logical explanation as to why a given practice is successful. The acts may have different names or be performed in a slightly different manner, but the uniting thread among them is to prevent ILLNESS and to maintain and/or restore HEALTH.

Transference to Patients and Others

The effects of such a verbal catharsis are long remembered and often quoted or referred to throughout the remainder of a course. The awareness we gain helps us understand the behavior and beliefs of patients and, for that matter, other people better. Given this understanding, we are comfortable enough to ask patients how they interpret a symptom and how they think it ought to be treated. We begin to be more sensitive to people who delay in seeking healthcare or fail to comply with preventive measures and treatment regimens. We come to recognize that we do the same thing. The increased familiarity with home health/HEALTH practices and remedies helps us project this awareness and understanding to the patients who are served.

Analyzed from a "scientific" perspective, the majority of these practices have a sound basis. In the area of health/HEALTH maintenance (see Table 7-1), one notes an almost universal adherence to activities that include rest, balanced diet, and exercise.

In the area of health/HEALTH protection, various differences arise, ranging from visiting a physician to wearing a clove of garlic around the neck. Although the purpose of wearing garlic around the neck is "to keep the evil spirit away," the act also forces people to stay away: What better way to cut down exposure to wintertime colds than to avoid close contact with people?

One person remembered that during her childhood her mother forced her to wear garlic around her neck. Like most children, she did not like to be different from the rest of her schoolmates. As time went on, she began to have frequent colds, and her mother could not understand why this was happening. The mother followed her child to school some weeks later and discovered that she removed the garlic on her way to school, hiding it under a rock and then replacing it on the way home. There was quite a battle between the mother and daughter! The youngster did not like this method of protection because her peers mocked her.

A discussion of home remedies is of further interest when each of the methods presented is analyzed for its possible "medical" analogy and for its prevalence among various religious and ethnic groups. Many of the practices and remedies, to the surprise and relief of students, tend to run throughout groups but have different names or contain different ingredients.

In this day of computers and sophisticated medicine, including transplants, cloning, and intricate surgery, the most prevalent need expressed by people who practice traditional medicine is to protect people and prevent "evil" from harming them or to remove the "evil" that may be the cause of their HEALTH problem. As students, we analyze and discuss a problem and its traditional treatments, and we begin to see how evil continues to be considered the cause of ILLNESS and how often the treatment is then designed to remove it.

Each person testifies to the efficacy of a given remedy. Many state that, when their grandmothers and mothers shared these remedies with them, they experienced great feelings of nostalgia for the good old days, when things seemed so simple. Some people may express a desire to return to these practices of yesteryear, whereas others openly confess that they continue to use such measures—sometimes in addition to what a healthcare provider tells them to use, or often without even bothering to consult a provider.

The goal of this kind of consciousness-raising session is to reawaken the participant to the types of health/HEALTH practices within her or his own family. The other purpose of the sharing is to make known the similarities and differences that exist as part of a cross-ethnocultural and religious phenomenon. We are intrigued to discover the wide range of beliefs that exists among our peers' families. We had assumed that people thought and believed as we did. For the first time, we individually and collectively realize that we all practice a certain amount of traditional medicine, that we all have ethnocultural-specific ways of treating ILLNESS, and that we, too, often delay in seeking professional healthcare. We learn that most people prefer to treat themselves at home and that they have their own ways of treating a particular set of symptoms—with or without a prescribed medical regimen. The previously held notion that "everybody does it this way" is shattered. The greatest challenge in this activity is to encourage students and others to think of HEALTH, rather than simply health. This exercise brings you to the window on the glass door pictured in the introduction.

Explore MediaLink

Go to the Student Resource Site at pearsonhighered.com/nursingresources for chapter-related review questions, case studies, and activities. Contents of the CulturalCare Guide and CulturalCare Museum can also be found on the Student Resource Site. Click on Chapter 7 to select the activities for this chapter.

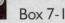

Box 7-1

Keeping Up

Folklife Centers
The following is a listing of selected folklife centers in the United States. From these centers, and others readily discovered on the World Wide Web, one may obtain films and literature related to folklife and medicine.

Alabama
The Alabama Folklife Program and The Alabama Folklife Association

Arizona
Southern Arizona Folklife Center
University of Arizona

California
Center for Study of Comparative Folklore and Mythology
University of California, Los Angeles

Kentucky
Appalshop

Missouri
Missouri Folk Arts Program

New England
Folk Arts Center of New England

Utah
The Utah Arts Council

Washington, DC
Within the federal government, resources for folklore and folklife endeavors in Washington, DC, are concentrated in four agencies:
1. The Library of Congress
2. The Smithsonian Institution
3. National Endowment for the Arts
4. National Endowment of the Humanities.

American Folklife Center
The Library of Congress
Washington, DC 20540
This center was created by Congress in 1976 to "preserve and present" American folklife. It is an educational and research program.

Archive of Folk Culture
The Library of Congress
Washington, DC 20540

The American Folklore Society

■ References

Kennet, F. (1976). *Folk medicine—Fact and fiction: Age-old cures, alternative medicine, natural remedies.* New York, NY: Crescent Books.

CHAPTER 8

Health and Illness in Modern Healthcare

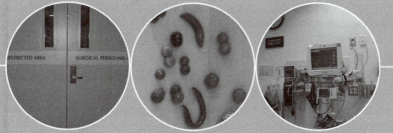

| Figure 8-1 | Figure 8-2 | Figure 8-3 |

■ Objectives

1. Discuss the professional socialization of nurses, physicians, and other members of the healthcare delivery system.
2. Describe the "culture" of the healthcare providers.
3. Summarize the costs of healthcare in the United States.
4. Identify trends in the development of today's modern healthcare system.
5. Describe problems within the healthcare system.
6. Describe the amazing maze of healthcare.
7. Identify barriers to healthcare.
8. Identify factors that determine medicine to be an institution of social control.
9. Compare and contrast modern medical care and CULTURALCARE.

The next links on the *HERITAGECHAIN* are those of the modern healthcare system. The opening images for this chapter depict the inner depths of the modern healthcare system's cultures. Figure 8-1 is an example of the doors to a surgical suite. These doors are closed to all except those sanctioned to enter and state "restricted area—surgical personnel." Few people outside of this closed system understand the intricacies of the cultures of healthcare and the meanings of its particular knowledge and rituals, beliefs, and practices. Figure 8-2 is a microbial mural in the lobby of the Centers for Disease Control and Prevention in Atlanta, Georgia. It symbolizes the numerous accomplishments that have been made in the practice of public health and the numbers of diseases that are preventable when public health knowledge, policies, and procedures are followed. Figure 8-3 is a well-equipped modern emergency department. Note the array of technological equipment in this small amount of space. The knowledge and training necessary to use these items are extensive and costly. The equipment is extremely expensive, and many institutions have many units that are equipped like this one. The personnel responsible for delivering care in technical settings are highly skilled. This image suggests one of the reasons for the extraordinary costs of healthcare to be discussed in this chapter. It has been frequently demonstrated that the high cost of healthcare is not proof of high quality (Abelson, 2007, p. A-1).

∞ What are the unique symbols of your profession within the overall culture of modern healthcare? What settings or objects would you choose to represent your experiences of modern healthcare delivery?

The links or concepts inherent in modern healthcare delivery systems include the healthcare providers' culture, the costs of healthcare, selected trends in the development of the modern healthcare system, common problems in the healthcare delivery system, the barriers to healthcare, and the differences between modern healthcare and CULTURALCARE. Each link is an overview of the given topic to familiarize you with the overall issues relevant to healthcare delivery.

"The healthcare system of this nation has been in crisis for many decades" (Knowles, 1970). Indeed, there have been extraordinary and costly advances in medical science and care since 1970—cardiac and renal transplants, technological intensive care units from newborn to illness specialty, robotic surgery, and sophisticated diagnostic procedures; but "the common everyday needs of preventive care and routine medical care are often inferior, wastefully delivered, and inequitably financed" (Knowles, 1970). What is it about our healthcare system and the people who practice within it that generated and continue to generate these comments? This chapter presents an overview of the issues inherent in the acculturation of healthcare providers and the healthcare delivery system in the United States. It begins by discussing the norms of the healthcare provider "cultures" and then examines many of the salient issues regarding the healthcare system in general.

■ The Healthcare Provider's Culture

The providers of healthcare—nurses; physicians and physician assistants; social workers; dietitians; physical, occupational, respiratory, and speech therapists; and laboratory and departmental professionals—are socialized into the culture of their profession. Professional socialization teaches the student a set of beliefs, practices, habits, likes, dislikes, norms, and rituals. Each of the professional disciplines has its own language and objects, rituals, garments, and myths, which become an inherent part of the scope of students' education, socialization, and practice. Many providers view time in their own ways, and they believe that their view of a given health and illness situation and subsequent interventions are the only possible answers to the complex questions surrounding a health-related event. The newly learned information regarding health and illness may differ in varying degrees from that of the students' heritage. As students become more and more immersed and knowledgeable in the scientific and technological domains, they may move away from their past belief systems. They certainly may move away from traditional health/HEALTH and illness/ILLNESS beliefs of the populations they serve.

Just as it is not unusual to hear providers say, "Etoh, bid, tid, im, iv," and so forth, it is not uncommon to hear patients say things such as "I have no idea what the nurses and doctors are saying!" "They speak a foreign language!" "What they are doing is so strange to me." In addition, there exists an underlying cultural norm among healthcare providers that "all must be done to save a patient, regardless of the patient's and family's wishes" and regardless of the financial consequences to the patient and family, to the healthcare system, or to society in general. A consequence of this philosophy has been the rise of iatrogenic health problems and the escalation of out-of-control healthcare costs.

Healthcare providers can be viewed by many laypeople as an alien or foreign culture or ethnic group. They have a social and cultural system; they experience "ethnicity" in the way they perceive themselves in relation to the healthcare consumer and often each other. Even if they deny the reality of the situation, many healthcare providers must understand that they are ethnocentric. Not only are they ethnocentric, but many of them are also xenophobic. To appreciate this critical issue, consider the following. A principal reason for the difficulty experienced between the healthcare provider and the consumer is that healthcare providers, in general, adhere rigidly to the modern allopathic, or Western, philosophy of healthcare. With few exceptions, they do not publicly sanction any methods of maintaining, protecting, or restoring health/HEALTH other than scientifically proven ones. Healthcare providers ordinarily fail to recognize or use any sources of medications and other therapies that have not been deemed effective by scientific means. The only types of healers that are sanctioned are those that have been educated, licensed, and certified according to the requirements of this culture.

What happens, then, when people of this belief system encounter people who have other beliefs regarding the maintenance, protection, and/or restoration of health/HEALTH? Is the provider able to meet the needs as perceived and defined by the patient? More often than not, a wall of misunderstanding arises between the two. At this point, a breakdown in communication occurs, and the consumer ends up at a disadvantage.

Providers think that they comprehend all facets of health and illness and may frequently take a xenophobic view to HEALTH and ILLNESS and traditional HEALERS. Although in training and education healthcare providers have a significant advantage over the consumer-patient, it is entirely appropriate for providers to explore other ideas regarding health/HEALTH and illness/ILLNESS and to adjust their approach to coincide with the needs of the specific patient. Healthcare providers have tried to force Western medicine on one and all, regardless of results.

The following list gives examples of the more obvious aspects of the healthcare provider's culture. In connection with later chapters, it can be referred to as a framework for comparing various other ethnic and cultural beliefs and practices.

1. *Beliefs*—standardized dualistic definitions of *health* and *illness,* and the omnipotence of technology
2. *Practices*—the maintenance of health and the protection of health or prevention of disease through such mechanisms as the avoidance of stress, the use of immunizations, and the high use of costly medications; and the annual physical examinations and diagnostic procedures, such as Pap smears, mammographies, and colonoscopies
3. *Habits*—charting, the constant use of medical jargon, the use of a systematic approach and problem-solving methodology, and observing and depending on electronic monitors and other devices
4. *Likes*—promptness, neatness and organization, patient compliance with all teaching and prescriptions
5. *Dislikes*—tardiness, disorderliness, and disorganization
6. *Customs*—professional deference and adherence to the pecking order found in autocratic and bureaucratic systems, hand washing and the ritual scrubbing procedures, the use of certain procedures attending birth and death
7. *Expectations*—Recovery no matter the cost or consequences of the therapies expended.

As noted, inherent in the socialization into the healthcare professions are countless cultural traits that are passed on both verbally and nonverbally. Remember, the doors in Figure 8-1 symbolize the closed aspects of the entire healthcare system.

▇ Healthcare Costs

There are three fundamental questions to ask regarding the costs of healthcare:

1. *What are the costs of healthcare?*
2. *How do we pay for healthcare?*
3. *Is healthcare in America better than in any other place on Earth?*

What Are the Costs of Healthcare?

This question is critical, and there are countless ways to answer it. However, it is certainly at the root of the problems we now face. The American healthcare system is both a source of national pride—if one has an expensive and adequate health insurance package or the money, it certainly is possible to get the finest medical/technological care in the world—and a source of deep embarrassment—those who are poor or uninsured may be wanting for care as people with a low family income do not have consistent health insurance. In one example alone, a 21-year-old college senior went for a checkup at a satellite clinic of a major Boston hospital. The bill for the 20-minute examination was more than $1,500 (Farragher, 2015). According to Kinney (2010), "the elephant in the room when it comes to healthcare is its cost." She explains that the inflation in healthcare costs in the United States are due to:

1. The advances in medical science and associated technology and pharmaceutical products and

2. The advent of widespread health insurance coverage (Kinney, 2010, p. 406).

The advances in technology have contributed to overall healthcare costs and expenditures.

Today, the problems of healthcare delivery have grown exponentially, and solutions are more elusive than ever. Healthcare providers in the United States administer the world's most expensive medical (illness) care system. The costs of U.S. healthcare soared from $4 billion in 1940 to $27.5 billion in 1960, to the staggering 2013 figure of $2.919 trillion (U.S. Department of Health and Human Services, 2015, p. 304). Healthcare is an enterprise that exceeds all the goods and services produced by half the states in the country. Health has become this country's biggest business, and it accounts for 17.4% (2013) of our gross domestic product. In fact, $9,255 was spent in 2013 per capita on healthcare for every man, woman, child, and fetus (U.S. Department of Health and Human Services, 2015, p. 302). In Table 8-1, you can examine the growth in national health expenditures from 1960 to 2013. Note the extreme rise in the costs of hospital care, physicians and clinical services, home healthcare, and prescription drugs over this time period.

The following are examples of the changing costs of healthcare from 1960 to 2013:

■ National health expenditures were $27.6 billion; they soared to $2,919.1 billion in 2013.

■ Hospital care expenditures were $9.0 billion; they soared to $936.9 billion in 2013.

■ Physician and clinical services expenditures were $5.6 billion; they were $586.7 billion in 2013.

■ Research funding was $0.7 billion; it rose to $46.7 billion in 2013.

Indeed, the costs of healthcare have risen and far exceed the costs of food, transportation, travel, and entertainment. However, technology has exploded, the costs of healthcare have soared, and many of the healthcare-related programs are seen as "entitlements." Yes, healthcare is vital and, as mentioned earlier, exceptional in this country for some.

Table 8-1   Selected National Health Expenditures: United States, Selected Years:
1960–2013

Expenditure Category	Year/Amount in Billions			
	1960	1980	2000	2013
National Health Expenditures	**$27.4**	**$255.8**	**$1,378.0**	**$2,919.1**
Health Consumption Expenditures	**24.8**	**235.7**	**1,290.0**	**2,754.5**
Personal healthcare	**23.4**	**217.2**	**1,165.7**	**2,468.6**
Hospital care	9.0	100.5	415.6	936.9
Professional services	**8.0**	**64.6**	**390.2**	**777.9**
Physicians and clinical services	5.6	47.7	290.9	586.7
Home healthcare	0.1	2.4	32.4	79.8
Retail outlet sales of medical products	**5.0**	**25.9**	**255.0**	**370.0**
Prescription drugs	2.7	12.0	121.2	271.1
Durable Medical Equipment	0.7	4.1	25.2	43.0
Net Cost of health insurance	1.0	9.3	64.2	173.6
Government public health activities	0.4	6.4	43.0	75.4
Investment	**2.6**	**20.1**	**88.0**	**164.8**
Research	0.7	5.4	25.5	46.7
Structures and equipment	1.9	14.7	62.5	117.9

Source: Health, United States, 2014: With Special Feature on Adults Aged 55–64, by National Center for Health Statistics, 2015, p. 304, Hyattsville, MD: Author. Retrieved from http://www.cdc.gov/nchs/data/hus/hus14.pdf

How Do We Pay for Healthcare?

The sources for paying for care in 1960 were primarily personal, made out of pocket or through private insurance. The government programs of Medicare and Medicaid were developed in 1965. Coverage shifted from the private sector to the public sector. Today, methods of third-party payments for healthcare are a complex web of insurance companies, policies, and procedures. Unlike other developed countries, the United States does not have a single-payer system. The itemized costs of services are hidden, and quite often it is impossible for a patient to get an itemized bill for hospitalization. When people get them, they are astonished at the costs but state, "My insurance covers it and it costs me nothing or minimal." However, for more and more people, the costs of healthcare have become so high that their health insurance companies either disallow desired procedures, insist patients seek other procedures, or provide only partial coverage for certain procedures. In many cases, families find themselves choosing between expensive care and financial insolvency. Even families with health insurance may find themselves facing bankruptcy if a family member experiences a catastrophic illness or injury.

On March 23, 2010, President Obama signed the Affordable Care Act. The controversial law put in place comprehensive health insurance reforms that put consumers back in charge of their healthcare. In most states, the coverage includes an end to preexisting condition exclusions for children; keeps young adults covered until age 26 under their parents' plans; ends the arbitrary withdrawal of insurance coverage; and guarantees the right to appeal the denial of payment. It ends lifetime limits on coverage and the donut holes with Medicare. It provides free preventive care, and the person has the right to choose their doctors. Emergency care can be sought as needed (U.S. Department of Health and Human Services, 2015).

Regardless of whether a person or family gets health benefits through work, buys insurance themselves, has a small business and desires to provide health coverage to their employees, has Medicaid coverage, or does not currently have insurance, the Affordable Care Act gives a better control of decisions about health coverage. It is designed to make healthcare insurance affordable by providing small businesses with a tax credit to provide coverage.

Is Healthcare in America Better Than in Any Other Place on Earth?

One method used to examine the status of a healthcare delivery system is to examine the infant mortality rate. Infant mortality is the rate of death during the first year of a child's life. The historically low rate, 5.96 per 1,000 live births in 2013, was a milestone for the United States. However, the infant mortality rates for Sweden (2.1), Japan (2.3), Finland (2.4), and the Czech Republic (2.7) are considerably lower than that of the United States (National Center for Health Statistics, 2015, p. 82). Judging by the standard of the infant mortality rate, neither the amount of money spent per capita nor the percentage expended as a percentage of our gross domestic product yields a society healthier than those of several countries such as Sweden and Finland. *The World Factbook*, published by the Central Intelligence Agency in 2015, includes estimated infant mortality rates for 2015. The entry gives the number of deaths of infants under 1 year old in a given year per 1,000 live births and ranks each country from highest to lowest number of deaths. Afghanistan, with 115.05 infant deaths per 1,000, ranks highest; Monaco, with 1.82 deaths, ranks lowest at 222; and the United States ranks 174th with 5.98 deaths (Central Intelligence Agency, 2015).

How did we get to this costly and critical situation? What factors converged to bring us to this dramatic breaking point? Because of the unprecedented growth of biomedical technology, we have witnessed the tremendous advancement in medical science and in the ability to perform an astounding variety of lifesaving procedures; now, not only can we no longer afford to finance these long-dreamed-of miracles, but the dream has become a nightmare.

The question—"Why is it that healthcare is so expensive?"—may be answered by exploring the trends in the development of the healthcare system, but factored into this analysis is also the increase in the population; the desire by healthcare providers, researchers, and vendors to cure all diseases; and the public's expectation that all illnesses can be cured. Each event has contributed to this situation, and the results are the ongoing issues we are confronting today.

■ Trends in Development of the Healthcare System

During the days of the early colonists, our healthcare system was a system of superstition and faith. It has evolved into a system predicated on a strong belief in science; the epidemiological model of disease; highly developed technology; and strong values of individuality, competition, and free enterprise. Two major forces—free enterprise and sciences—have largely shaped the problems we now face. Health problems have evolved from the epidemics of 1850 to the chronic diseases of today, notwithstanding the resurgence of tuberculosis and the AIDS epidemic. In 1850, healthcare technology was virtually nonexistent; today, it dominates the delivery of healthcare. We now take for granted such dramatic procedures as kidney, heart, and liver transplants. New technologies and bio-medical milestones are materializing daily. However, the consequences of these events are also rising daily in terms of extraordinary costs, countless practice issues and errors, and iatrogenic health problems.

The belief that healthcare is a right for all Americans is still a prominent philosophy, yet the fulfillment of that right is still in question. The trends, begun in the 1980s and early 1990s, such as the cutbacks in federal funding for health services and the attempt to turn the clock back on social programs, led to a diminished and denigrated role for the government in people's health. However, the passage of the Affordable Care Act has thrust the government into being a primary player once again. In addition, the events of September 11, 2001, have pointed out the consequences of cuts to healthcare and the enormous and compelling need to boost public health and national security efforts.

There is growing and grave concern about the realization of this basic human right of health and healthcare. Mounting social problems, such as toxic waste, homelessness, and millions of people without health insurance confound the situation. These factors all affect the delivery of healthcare. The problems of acquiring and using the healthcare system are legendary and ongoing.

The year 1960 is the benchmark being used to compare healthcare costs and significant events. A brief overview of these landmark events follows. These events have contributed to what we see today as the healthcare "nightmare." We are in a situation in which healthcare delivery has become less and less personal and more and more technological in many healthcare settings. The barriers to healthcare are increasing and, as evidenced earlier, more and more people are unable to obtain healthcare, in spite of having health insurance. The events depicted that have occurred in the healthcare system, whether within the public health or medical sector, have happened within the context of the larger societal framework. The public sector events include those related to the collective responsibility for the health of large populations in many dimensions—prevention, surveillance, disease control, and so forth—and those events, positive and negative, that affect large population cohorts. The medical events are those that include the development of diagnostic and/or therapeutic methods that are problem-specific and affect limited numbers of people. The public health events include government laws and policies that were designed initially to increase the scope of the healthcare system and later to control medical costs.

This information is further embedded in the key health system issues of the last century and the start of this decade, the key health problems, and the selected key health strategies of the time. The key issues were professionalization, infrastructure building, improved access, cost control, and market forces. The key health problems are reemerging infectious diseases, chronic diseases, and changes in modern care. The aging of the baby boomer generation is also playing a dramatic role in this situation.

Box 8-1 presents an overview in the ongoing trends in healthcare.

Box 8-1

Healthcare Trends 1900–2015

- At the turn of the 20th century, 1900–1930, efforts were underway to identify medicine as a profession and to eradicate all philosophies of care that were not under the umbrella of the Flexner definition of a profession. Agents such as quinine for malaria and the diphtheria antitoxin for immunization were discovered, and the use of radium to treat cancer began. Infectious diseases, including pneumonia and influenza, were pandemic. The main health strategy was maternal and child health, given the large numbers of new immigrants. In 1929, third-party payment for healthcare began with the creation of Blue Cross and Blue Shield.
- Between 1930 and 1960, the primary issue facing the healthcare system was infrastructure building. The passage of the Hill-Burton Act in 1946 provided funding for the building of hospitals and other healthcare resources. The system was moving forward—the development of today's extraordinarily costly tests and treatments began, and the settings for their use were built. The development of vaccines and antibiotics paved the way to a decrease in the occurrence of communicable disease, and a false sense of freedom from illness began to develop.
- The 1960s was a decade of profound change in the delivery of healthcare, public health, and available methods of treating health problems and funding new resources. For example, vaccines for polio and rubella (1961 and 1963) were developed, as were transplant procedures for the heart (1967) and liver. In 1965, President Lyndon B. Johnson's War on Poverty became the focal point of social and health policy and, among other laws, Medicare and Medicaid came into being.
- The 1970s brought even greater strides in medical technology and public health with the first test tube baby born in 1978 and the biotechnical explosion. At the end of the 1970s, efforts were developed to "control" the costs of healthcare, yet the seductiveness of the "advances" in technology, such as nuclear magnetic resonance imaging (1980), fed the desire for more development.

(continued)

Box 8-1   *Continued*

- The 1990s to the present time have presented even greater challenges to the availability and affordability of healthcare. In 1993 and 1994, President and Mrs. Clinton made an extraordinary effort to study our complex healthcare system and sought ways to reform it. That effort failed. Meanwhile, the costs of healthcare continue to soar. For example, in 2015, the Federal Drug Administration approved a virus—Imlygie—to treat advanced melanoma. The cost for this treatment is $65,000 for a course of treatment (Tedeschi, 2015).
- The Affordable Care Act was signed into law by President Barack Obama in 2010 and was enacted to increase the quality and affordability of health insurance, lower the uninsured rate by expanding public and private insurance coverage, and reduce the costs of healthcare for individuals and the government.

Grave concern is being expressed regarding the high costs of healthcare, yet the costs of durable medical supplies and medications continue to rise. On one hand, we are seeking to ever expand therapeutic miracles; on the other hand, there is shock and dismay at the ever-increasing costs of healthcare.

◼ Common Problems in Healthcare Delivery

Many problems exist within today's healthcare delivery system. Some of these problems affect all of us, and others are specific to the poor and to emerging majority populations. It has been suggested that the healthcare delivery system fosters and maintains a childlike dependence and depersonalized condition for the consumer. The following describes selected common problems experienced by many consumers of healthcare, as historically categorized by Ehrenreich and Ehrenreich (1971). The headings that follow are quoted from this book.

Finding Where the Appropriate Care Is Offered at a Reasonable Price

It may be difficult for even a knowledgeable consumer to find adequate care. If you have relocated to a new home, changed health insurance plans, or have a provider who retired, the search for a new provider may prove frustrating. Urgent care centers provide episodic acute care; however, they are not adequate for long-term primary care.

Finding One's Way Among the Many Available Types of Medical Care

A friend experienced gastric problems from time to time and initially sought help from a family physician who was unable to treat the problem adequately. She was offered several referrals but soon became frustrated by going to different providers, each with a different opinion and no real answers. She realized that she was essentially on her own in terms of securing appointments with either a gastroenterologist or a surgeon. Because she had little money to spend on a variety of physicians and limited health insurance, she decided to wait to see what would happen. She was fortunate and had few further problems.

Figuring Out What the Physician Is Doing

It is not always easy for members of the health professions to understand what is happening to them when they are ill. What must it be like for the average person, who has little or no knowledge of healthcare routines and practices?

Imagine you are a layperson who has just been relieved of all your clothes and given a paper dress to put on. You are lying on a table with strange eyes peering down at you. A sheet is thrown over you, and you are given terse directions—"breathe," "cough," "don't breathe," "turn," "lift your legs." Without warning, you may feel a cold disk on your chest or a cold hand on your back. As the physical examination process continues, you may feel a few taps on the ribs, see a bright light shining in your eye, feel a cold tube in your ear, and gag on a stick probing the inside of your mouth. What is going on? The jargon you hear is unfamiliar. You are being poked, pushed, prodded, peered at and into, and jabbed, and you do not know why. If you are female and going for your first pelvic examination, you may have no idea what to expect. Perhaps you have heard only hushed whisperings, and your level of fear and discomfort is high. Insult is added to injury when you experience the penetration of a cold, unyielding speculum: "What is the doctor doing now and why?"

Finding Out What Went Wrong

The "Patient's Bill of Rights" allows the patient the right to read his or her own medical record and to be clearly informed of all that is going to happen. But, does he or she understand the information? Suppose one enters the hospital for what is deemed to be a simple medical or surgical problem. All is well if everything goes according to expectations. However, what happens when complications develop? The more determined the patient is to discover what the problem is or why there are complications, the more he or she believes that the healthcare providers are trying to hide something. The cycle perpetuates itself, and a tremendous schism develops between provider and consumer. Quite often, "the conspiracy of silence" tends to grow as more questions are asked. A recent problem is that of "concurrent surgeries"—the surgeon is operating on two patients at the same time. Patients are generally not informed that this is happening. Nurses all too often enter into this collusion and play the role of a silent partner with the physician and the institution.

Overcoming the Built-in Racism and Male Chauvinism of Doctors and Hospitals

There is little difficulty in describing many subtle incidents of racism and male chauvinism, and classroom discussion helps identify subtle incidents of racism. For example, Black patients may be the last to receive morning or evening care, meal trays, and so forth. When this is a frequent occurrence on a floor, it is an indictment in itself. Racism also may take another tack. Is it an accident that the Black person is the last patient to receive routine care, or has he or she consciously been made to wait? Does the fact that the Black person may have to wait longest for water or a pill demonstrate racism on a conscious level, or is it subliminal?

Nurses recognize the subtle patronization of both themselves and female patients. For example, physicians frequently refer to nurses and female patients, no matter their age, as "girls," and often devalue a woman's perceptions of a situation. Once the situation is probed and spelled out, a much more realistic attitude toward the insensitivity of those who choose a racist or chauvinistic style of practicing is reached.

■ Pathways to Health Services

Figure 8-4 illustrates the amazing maze of healthcare and the variety of obstacles a patient must deal with in attempting to navigate this complex system. Indeed, the patient not only needs to navigate an internal system of a given hospital, but also needs to understand all the types of care available such as primary care, long-term care, and so forth. Just to complicate matters more deeply, many people are given information that contradicts itself—as with the diagnosis and treatment of breast cancer or the use of estrogen replacement therapy—and then asked to make choices for themselves.

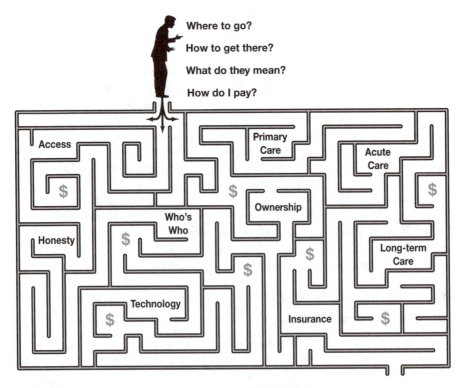

Figure 8-4 Navigating the amazing maze of healthcare.

When a health problem occurs, there is an established system whereby health-care services are obtained. The family is usually the first resource. It is in the domain of the family that the person seeks validation that what he or she is experiencing is indeed an illness. Once the belief is validated, the person seeks healthcare outside of the home. It is not unusual for a person to be receiving care from many different pro-viders, with limited or no communication among the attending caregivers. Problems and complications erupt when a provider is not aware that other providers are caring for a patient. For patients who are forced to use the clinics of a general hospital, there may be no continuity of care because resident physicians come and go each year. This is known as the level of first contact, or the entrance into the healthcare system.

The second level of care, if needed, is found at the specialist's level: in clinics, private practice, or hospitals. Obstetricians, gynecologists, surgeons, neurologists, nephrologists, and other specialists make up a large percentage of those who practice medicine. Yet, who's who and what do they do?

The third level of care is delivered within hospitals that provide inpatient care and services. Care is determined by need, whether long term (as in a psy-chiatric setting or rehabilitation institute) or short term (as in the acute care setting and community hospitals). Technology is employed in all aspects of care, and the use of extraordinary means for diagnosing and treating a problem may well be overwhelming.

An in-depth discussion of the different kinds of hospitals—voluntary or profit-making and nonprofit institutions and hospital ownership—is more appropriate to a book dealing solely with the delivery of healthcare. In our present context, the issue is, "What does the patient know about such settings, and what kind of care can he or she expect to receive?" Is the care in a propri-etary hospital different from that in a voluntary hospital? How will my insur-ance impact the care I receive? How much will it cover?

■ Barriers to Healthcare

There are countless other factors or barriers, in addition to the financial ones, that thwart a person's or family's ability to use the healthcare system to its great-est potential. The following are some examples:

- *Access.* This is when a person is unable to enter into the system because he or she lacks money, health insurance, or the ability to get to a center where healthcare is delivered. Another factor related to access is that some primary care physicians are leaving their practices, either to retire or to limit the scope of their practices to "concierge" services.
- *Age.* The person is too young or too old to enter into the system and is unaware of ways to overcome this.
- *Class.* A person may be from a class that is not part of the dominant cul-ture, limiting his or her ability to determine the need for healthcare and to understand the subtleties involved in making healthcare system choices.
- *Education.* A person may not know how to read and write English and may not read and write in his or her native tongue.

- *Gender.* Existing services may not be limited to a specific gender, affecting those who are unwilling or unable to access a system that does not deliver gender-specific care.
- *Geography.* A person may not reside near a healthcare facility, and the costs of traveling to a facility may be unaffordable.
- *Homelessness.* A person may be homeless in a place where healthcare is not provided to people who are homeless, and/or the person does not know the ways to access the system.
- *Insurance.* A person may not have health insurance, or it may be inadequate to cover the scope of the person's needs.
- *Language.* A person may not speak or understand English, and adequate interpreter services may not be available.
- *Manners.* A person's manners or expectations of the provider's manners may not be congruent.
- *Philosophy.* The philosophy of an institution may not be congruent with a person's religious or personal philosophy.
- *Prejudice.* The person seeking healthcare may sense the prejudice that the providers and institution exhibit.
- *Race.* There may be residuals of racial prejudice as part of the institution's philosophy.
- *Racism.* The institution may have specific barriers in place to not treat people from races other than the race of the owners of the facility.
- *Religion.* A patient may not desire to be treated in an institution that is not derived from his or her religious background, and there may be manifest prejudice on both sides—patient and institution. A given religion's teachings regarding HEALTH and ILLNESS may contradict modern healthcare practices.
- *SES (socioeconomic status).* The two extremes of socioeconomic status are poverty and great wealth. Poverty can limit access to care; wealth may prevent people from seeking care in institutions where they prefer to not go because of the patient population served there.
- *Technology.* A person may not be able to afford or want the plethora of diagnostic tests and therapies offered to him or her.
- *Transportation.* There may be no public transportation available from where the patient resides to the institution.

■ Medicine as an Institution of Social Control

The people of today's youth-oriented, cure-expecting, death-denying society have unusually high expectations of the healers of our time. We expect a cure; if not a cure, then a perfect recovery and/or the artificial prolongation of life as the outcome of illness. The technology of modern healthcare dominates our expectations of treatment, and our primary focus is on the curative aspects of medicine and the rising interest in prevention of chronic diseases.

As control over the behavior of a person has shifted from the family and church to a physician, "be good" has shifted to "take your medicine." The role that physicians play within society in terms of social control is ever-growing, so that conflict frequently arises between medicine and the law over definitions of accepted codes of behavior and the relative status of the two professions in governing American life. As early as 1972, Dr. Irving K. Zola used the following examples to illustrate the "medicalization" of society. His words ring true today.

Through the Expansion of What in Life Is Deemed Relevant to the Good Practice of Medicine

This factor is exemplified by the change from a specific etiological model of disease to a multicausal one. The "partners" in this new model include greater acceptance of comprehensive medicine, the use of the computer, and the practice of preventive medicine. In preventive medicine, however, the medical person must get to the layperson before the disease occurs; patients must be sought out. Thus, forms of social control emerge in an attempt to prevent disease: eating a low-cholesterol diet, avoiding stress, stopping smoking, avoiding hot dogs and processed meats such as bacon due to their alleged carcinogenic effects, and getting proper and adequate exercise. It is interesting to note that quite often the "new" forms of prevention and therapies are often abandoned for even newer methods over time.

Through the Retention of Absolute Control over Certain Technical Procedures

This is, in essence, the right to perform surgery and the right to prescribe drugs. In the lifespan of human beings, modern medicine can often determine life or death from the time prior to conception to old age through genetic counseling; abortion; assisted reproductive technologies, surgery; and other technological devices, such as computers, respirators, and life-support systems. Medicine has at its command drugs that can cure or kill—from antibiotics to the chemotherapeutic agents used to combat cancer. Modern medicine can control what medications are available for legal consumption. This, too, changes over time, an example being the legalization of marijuana for either recreational and/or medicinal use in several states.

Through the Expansion of What in Medicine Is Deemed Relevant to the Good Practice of Life

This expansion is illustrated by the use of medical jargon to describe a state of being—such as the *health* of the nation or the *health* of the economy. Any political or economic proposal or objective that enhances the "health" of those concerned wins approval.

There are numerous areas in which medicine, religion, and law overlap. For example, public health practice, law, and medicine overlap in the creation of laws that establish quarantine and the need for immunization, and in areas of sanitation and rodent and insect control. Abortion and gay marriage represent areas replete with conflict that involve politics, law, religion, and medicine. Those in favor see these issues as "rights," and opponents argue on moral and religious grounds. However, both abortion and gay marriage are legal. Another highly charged area of conflict involves the practice of euthanasia. As of this writing, the "Death with Dignity Law" has been passed in five states—Oregon, Washington, Montana, New Mexico, and California—and it is being considered in several others (Barone, 2014).

Finally, although many daily practical activities are undertaken in the name of health—taking vitamins, practicing hygiene, using birth control, engaging in dietary or exercise programs—the "diseases of the rich" (cancer, heart disease, and stroke) tend to capture more public attention and funding than the diseases of the poor (malnutrition, high maternal and infant death rates, sickle-cell anemia, and lead poisoning).

In this chapter, we have explored, in a very limited way, the culture and characteristics inherent in the socialization into the healthcare professions; many of the issues surrounding the American healthcare delivery system by examining the history and trends that led to its present character; the experiences a person may have in attempting to obtain care; and examples of the insurmountable barriers to healthcare, and how medicine is an institution of social control. In closing, it is critical to see several of the differences between medical care and CULTURALCARE. Whereas:

- Medical care is "The art and science of the diagnosis and treatment of disease and the maintenance of health"; CULTURALCARE is professional HEALTHCARE that is culturally sensitive, culturally appropriate, and culturally competent.

- Medical care defines health as the "experience of well-being and integrity of mind and body"; CULTURALCARE defines HEALTH as "the balance of the person, both within one's being—physical, mental, and spiritual—and in the outside world—natural, communal, and metaphysical."

- The goals of medical care are the prevention of disease and injury and promotion and maintenance of health, relief of pain and suffering caused by illness, care and cure of those with an illness, avoidance of premature death, and the pursuit of a peaceful death. In contrast, CULTURALCARE is the provision of care that is based on knowledge of and constructive attitudes toward the HEALTH traditions observed among diverse cultural groups and the assistance to the patient/family in pursuit of HEALTH and HEALING.

- The philosophy of allopathic care is body and mind and scientific zeal; that of CULTURALCARE is holistic care predicated on the HEALTH and HEALING traditions of a given patient/family/community.

■ Medical care creates and embraces scientific and technological developments that are sophisticated and costly; CULTURALCARE understands and respects ethnocultural HEALTH-related traditions (Hanson & Callahan, 1999).

The struggles continue as we attempt to find a balance between the high technology of the 21st century and primary preventive care and a strong public healthcare system. There must also be a balance between the forces of modern medical care and CULTURALCARE.

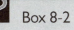

Explore MediaLink

Go to the Student Resource Site at pearsonhighered.com/nursingresources for chapter-related review questions, case studies, and activities. Contents of the CULTURALCARE Guide and CULTURALCARE Museum can also be found on the Student Resource Site. Click on Chapter 8 to select the activities for this chapter.

Box 8-2

Keeping Up

It goes without saying that much of the data presented in this chapter will be out of date when you read this text. However, at this final stage of writing, it is the most recent information available. The following resources will be most helpful in keeping you abreast of the frequent changes in healthcare events, costs, and policies:

1. The National Center for Health Statistics publishes *Health, United States,* an annual report on trends in health statistics.
2. Information regarding the Affordable Care Act can be found by searching for the Affordable Care Act.
3. Information regarding selected health statistics and other relevant information in a global context can be found in *The World Factbook,* published annually by the Central Intelligence Agency.

References

Abelson, R. (2007, June 14). In healthcare, cost isn't proof of high quality. *New York Times*, p. A-1.

Barone, E. (2014, November 3). See which states allow assisted suicide. *Time.* Retrieved from http://time.com/3551560/brittany-maynard-right-to-die-laws/

Central Intelligence Agency. (2015). *The World Factbook.* Washington, DC: Author. Retrieved from https://www.cia.gov/library/publications/the-world-factbook/index.html

Ehrenreich, B., & Ehrenreich, J. (1971). *The American health empire: Power, profits, and politics.* New York, NY: Random House, Vintage Books.

Farragher, T. (2015, October 24). Big hospitals' prices remain a big concern, check up reveals. *Boston Globe*, p. 3.

Hanson, M. J., & Callahan, D. (Eds.). (1999). *The goals of medicine: The forgotten issue in health care reform.* Washington, DC: Georgetown University Press.

Kinney, E. D. (2010). For profit enterprise in healthcare: Can it contribute to health reform? *American Journal of Law and Medicine, 36,* 405–435.

Knowles, J. (1970, January). It's time to operate. *Fortune*, p. 79.

National Center for Health Statistics. (2015). *Health, United States, 2014: With special feature on adults aged 55–64.* Hyattsville, MD: Author. Retrieved from http://www.cdc.gov/nchs/data/hus/hus14.pdf

Tedeschi, B. (2015, October 28). FDA approves virus to treat advanced melanoma. *Boston Globe*, p. 1.

U.S. Department of Health and Human Services. (2015). *Affordable Care Act: About the law.* Retrieved from http://www.hhs.gov/healthcare/about-the-law/index.html

Zola, I. K. (1972, November). Medicine as an institution of social control. *Sociological Review, 20*(4), 487–504.

Unit III

HEALTH and ILLNESS
Panoramas

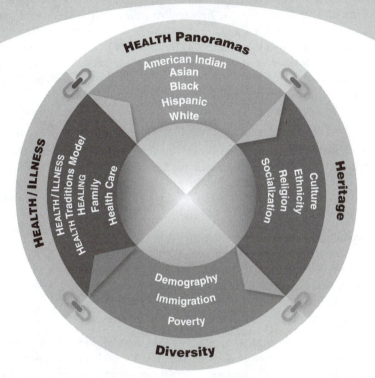

Thus far, this book has described several links in the *HERITAGECHAIN* and discussed four of the six steps to CULTURALCOMPETENCY. The first eight chapters presented the underlying theoretical rationale that is the foundation for CULTURALCOMPETENCY and brought you to the transparent door depicted in the introduction, to "observe" the various links, philosophies, concepts, and situations involved in the development of CULTURALCOMPETENCY:

- Chapter 1 presented the theoretical foundation link and rationale for the development of CULTURALCOMPETENCY.
- Chapter 2 set the theoretical foundation of the first step, *know your personal heritage*, as it reviewed the sociological components of heritage.
- Chapter 3 developed the background necessary to understand the role that the changing demographics of the larger communities have had in

society in general and specifically in the delivery of healthcare—this is the second step.

- Chapters 4, 5, and 6 explored the links of health/HEALTH, illness/ILLNESS, and curing/HEALING—the third step.
- Chapter 7 provided the opportunity to look intensely inside this door from your personal experience and presented information regarding the exciting and challenging intricacies of exploring *your* heritage and your family's health/HEALTH and illness/ILLNESS beliefs and practices. As stated, this completes the first and most important step in becoming CULTURALLYCOMPETENT.
- Chapter 8 examined the link of the "culture" of healthcare providers and that of the healthcare delivery system and introduced arguments relevant to the trends in the development of the healthcare system, common problems in the delivery of healthcare, pathways to health services, and medicine as an institution of social control and compared modern and traditional philosophies of healthcare delivery.

The chapters in this unit embrace the fifth step—traditional HEALTHCARE—and will provide a framework for learning about the communities you may be practicing in. Each chapter presents examples of the *traditional* HEALTH, ILLNESS, and HEALING beliefs and practices of selected populations, and the links introduce:

- The background of the population
- The *traditional* definitions of *HEALTH/ILLNESS/HEALING*
- *Traditional* methods of HEALTH maintenance and protection
- *Traditional* methods of HEALTH restoration
- Current health problems, and
- Health disparities in morbidity and mortality rates.

These areas can be applied in researching information regarding the populations you are caring for and working with. The World Wide Web is extremely helpful in gathering the demographic and modern health-related data applicable to a given population. Chapter 14 illustrates the journey on the Road to CULTURALCOMPETENCY and how this knowledge is vital to a person's growth and development in this discipline.

My experiences have taught me that people are thirsty for knowledge regarding *tradition*, be it their own or the traditions of others. They are eager to learn about traditions and the HEALTH traditions and other cultural events from their own ethnocultural heritage, the heritages of peers, and the heritages of other people. Thus, an effort has been exerted to maintain the integrity of older references. These are the sources of the primary data that have been gathered regarding HEALTH beliefs and practices over the 40+ years I have devoted to this text. In the race to modernity, science, technology, and "scholarly" endeavors, the HEALTH traditions of families and others may well be lost to this and future generations.

The links within the first five chapters in Unit III will present an overview of relevant historical and contemporary theoretical content that will help you:

1. Develop a level of awareness of the background and health/HEALTH problems of both the emerging majority and White ethnic populations.
2. Understand and describe selected *traditional* HEALTH beliefs and practices.
3. Understand the *traditional* pathways to HEALTHCARE.

The following exercises are inherent in Chapter 14 and are appropriate to all chapters in Unit III:

1. Familiarize yourself with some literature of the given community—that is, read literature, poetry, or a biography of a member of each of the communities.
2. Familiarize yourself with the history and sociopolitical background of each of the communities.

The questions that follow should be thoughtfully considered:

∞ What are the traditional definitions of *HEALTH* and *ILLNESS* in each of the communities? Are they alike or different?
∞ What are the traditional methods of maintaining HEALTH?
∞ What are the traditional ways of protecting HEALTH?
∞ What are the traditional ways of restoring HEALTH?
∞ Who are the traditional HEALERS? What functions do they perform?

This is an extraordinary way to build connections between communities and to see how much different ethnocultural and religious communities have in common. Because HEALTH is the metaphor for this text, it brings to the forefront a way to analyze and understand some of the variability in HEALTH and HEALTHCARE.

CHAPTER 9

HEALTH and ILLNESS in the American Indian and Alaska Native Population

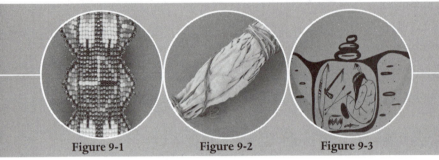

Figure 9-1   Figure 9-2   Figure 9-3

To "make medicine" is to engage upon a special period of fasting, thanksgiving, prayer, and self denial, even self-torture.

—Wooden Leg (late 19th century) Cheyenne

■ Objectives

1. Discuss the historical and demographic backgrounds of the American Indian and Alaska Native population.
2. Describe the traditional definitions of HEALTH and ILLNESS of the American Indian and Alaska Native population.
3. Explain the traditional methods of HEALING of the American Indian and Alaska Native population.
4. Discuss the practice of a traditional HEALER.
5. Describe current healthcare problems of the American Indian and Alaska Native populations.
6. Summarize the services rendered by the Indian Health Service.

This link in the *HERITAGECHAIN* examines the historical and demographic backgrounds, HEALTH and ILLNESS traditions, and healthcare issues of the American Indian and Alaska Native population in the United States. The opening images for this chapter depict objects related to traditional American Indian HEALTH beliefs and practices. Figure 9-1 is an example of intricate beadwork. The circle is divided into four quadrants and arrows are woven into this piece. Beading is a recognized method for protecting, maintaining, and restoring HEALTH. Figure 9-2 is of sage, a sacred plant commonly used in ceremonies to purify a setting (such as room, entire home, or store) or a person. The sage is ignited at the bottom, the flames are blown out, and the smoke is used in smudging. It gathers spirits to drive away negative energies and restore HEALTH. Figure 9-3, "Burial Moon," by the late Micmac artist, Philip Young, illustrates a traditional way of burying people. The body is placed in a sitting position in a shallow grave, dressed to meet the challenges of the next life. Necessary tools—a bow and arrows, a hatchet, a knife, and a bowl—are placed in the grave. The grave is then marked with three stones.

■ Background

The descendants of the original inhabitants of the North American continent and Alaska were estimated to number 5.4 million people, or 1.2% of the total population of the United States in the estimated census of 2014 (U.S. Department of Commerce, U.S. Census Bureau, 2015). When compared to "U.S. all races," the American Indian/Alaska Native (AI/AN) population lags behind in several areas, including lower educational levels and higher unemployment rates. The AI/AN population is a young population. The median age of the population is 31.4 years. The population has larger families, less health insurance, and a poverty level nearly twice that of the rest of the population. The American Indian population served by the Indian Health Service is living longer than it did 30 or even 20 years ago. In fact, statistics on age at death show that during 1972–1974, life expectancy at birth for the American Indian population was about 63.6 years and has now increased to 73.7 years, but it is still 4.4 years less than the U.S. all-races life expectancy of 78.1 years (2013 rates) (NCHS, 2015; IHS, 2015d).

The first time that American Indians were counted as a separate group was in the 1860 census, and the 1890 census was the first to count American Indians throughout the country. The counting of American Indians before 1890 was limited to those living in the general population of the various states; the American Indians residing in American Indian territory and on American Indian reservations were not included. Alaska Natives, in Alaska, have been counted since 1880, but until 1940 they were generally reported in the "American Indian" racial category. The people were enumerated separately (as Eskimo and Aleut) in 1940 in Alaska. It was not until the 1970 census that separate response categories were used to collect data on the Eskimo and Aleut population, and then only in Alaska.

The American Indian nations that are the largest populations include the Cherokee, Navajo, Latin American Indian, Choctaw, Sioux, and Chippewa. The largest Alaska Native group is Eskimo (U.S. Department of the Interior, Bureau of Indian Affairs, n.d.).

To realize the plight of today's American Indians, it is necessary to journey back in time to the years when Whites settled in this land. Before the arrival of Europeans, this country had no name but was inhabited by groups of people who called themselves nations. The people were strong both in their knowledge of the land and in their might as warriors. The Vikings reached the shores of this country about AD 1010. They were unable to settle on the land and left after a decade of frustration. Much later, another group of settlers, since termed the "Lost Colonies," were repulsed. More people came to these shores, however, and the land was taken over by Europeans.

As the settlers expanded westward, they signed "treaties of peace" or "treaties of land cession" with the American Indians. These treaties were similar to those struck between nations, although in this case the agreement was imposed by the "big" nation onto the "small" nation. One reason for treaties was to legitimize the takeover of the land that the Europeans had "discovered." Once the land was "discovered," it was divided among the Europeans, who set out to create a "legal" claim to it. The American Indians signed the resultant treaties, ceding small amounts of their land to the settlers and keeping the rest for themselves. As time passed, the number of Whites rapidly grew, and the number of Indians diminished because of wars and disease. As these events occurred, the treaties began to lose their meaning; the Europeans disregarded them. They decided that these "natives" had no real claim to the land and shifted them around like cargo from one reservation to another. Although the American Indians tried to seek just settlements through the American court system, they failed to win back the land that had been taken from them through misrepresentation. For example, in 1831, the Cherokees were fighting in the courts to keep their nation in Georgia. They lost their legal battle, however, and, like other American Indian nations after the time of the early European settlers, were forced to move westward. During this forced westward movement, many died, and all suffered. Many nations are seeking to reclaim their land through the courts (Brown, 1970; Deloria, 1969, 1974; Fortney, 1977). Several claims, such as those of the Penobscot and Passamaquoddy tribes in Maine, have been successful. The number of federally recognized tribes has increased from just over 100 as recently ago as the 1980s to the present (2015) number of 566 (U.S. Department of the Interior, Bureau of Indian Affairs, n.d.).

As the American Indians migrated westward, they carried with them the fragments of their culture. Their lives were disrupted, their land was lost, and many of their leaders and teachers perished, yet much of their history and culture somehow remained. Today, more and more American Indians are seeking to know their history. The story of the colonization and settlement of the United States is being retold with a different emphasis—now the voice of the American Indians is speaking. Institutions, such as the National Museum of the American Indian, are working to educate people about the contributions American Indians have made and continue to make to this country (National Museum of the American Indian, 2016).

American Indian people have sought ways to rebuild Indian communities and to maintain an Indian future in America. The American Indian Movement (AIM) was born in Minnesota in 1968. It is apparent that the movement has transformed policy making into programs and organizations that have served Indian people in many communities. The policies were consistently made in consultation with spiritual leaders and elders. One example of the organization's work is the National Coalition on Racism in Sports and Media, which was formed in 1971 with the purpose of fighting the potent media influence to use imagery with misconceptions of American Indians in the form of sports team identities. This leads to racial, cultural, and spiritual stereotyping (National Coalition on Racism in Sports and Media, n.d.). In fact, the movement was founded to turn the attention of Indian people toward a renewal of spirituality; at the heart of AIM is deep spirituality and a belief in the connectedness of all Indian people (Wittstock & Salinas, 2006).

American Indians live predominantly in 26 states (including Alaska), with most residing in the western part of the country as a result of the forced westward migration. Although many American Indians remain on reservations and in rural areas, many live in cities, especially on the West Coast. Oklahoma, Arizona, California, New Mexico, and Alaska have the largest numbers of American Indians (IHS, 2015f). More and more people are proclaiming their American Indian roots.

■ Traditional Definitions of HEALTH and ILLNESS

Although each American Indian nation or tribe had its own history and belief system regarding HEALTH and ILLNESS and the traditional treatment of ILLNESS, some general beliefs and practices underlie the more specific tribal ideas. The terms *HEALTH* and *ILLNESS* are used to indicate that, among traditional people, the connotations are holistic, as defined and discussed in Chapters 5 and 6. The data—collected through an ongoing review of the literature and from interviews granted by members of the groups—come from the Navajo Nation, Hopis, Cherokees, Shoshones, and New England Indians with whom I have worked closely.

The traditional American Indian belief about HEALTH is that it reflects living in "total harmony with nature and having the ability to survive under exceedingly difficult circumstances" (Zuckoff, 1995). Humankind has an intimate relationship with nature (Boyd, 1974). The Earth is considered to be a living organism—the body of a higher individual, with a will and a desire to be well. The Earth is periodically HEALTHY and less HEALTHY, just as human beings are. According to the American Indian belief system, a person should treat his or her body with respect, just as the Earth should be treated with respect. When the Earth is harmed, humankind is itself harmed; and conversely, when humans harm themselves, they harm the Earth. The Earth gives food, shelter, and medicine to humankind; for this reason, all things of the Earth belong to human beings and nature. "The land belongs to life, life belongs to the land, and the land belongs to itself." In order to maintain HEALTH, Indians must maintain their relationship with nature. "Mother Earth" is the friend of the American Indian, and the land belongs to the American Indian (Boyd, 1974).

According to American Indian belief, as explained by a medicine man, Rolling Thunder, the human body is divided into two halves, which are seen as plus and minus (yet another version of the concept that every whole is made of two opposite halves). There are also—in every whole—two energy poles: positive and negative. The energy of the body can be controlled by spiritual means. It is further believed that every being has a purpose and an identity. Every being has the power to control him- or herself and, from this force and the belief in its potency, the spiritual power of a person is kindled (Boyd, 1974).

In all American Indian cultures, disease is associated with the religious aspect of society as supernatural powers are associated with the causing and curing of disease. Disease is conceived of in a wide variety of ways. It is believed to occur due to a lack of prevention, which is given by wearing or using charms; the presence of some material object that has intruded into the body via sorcery; or the absence of the free soul from the body (Lyon, 1996, pp. 60–61). One example of an amulet is *Duklij*, turquoise or green malachite that is believed to contain supernatural qualities that ward off the evil spirits and bring rain (Lyon, 1996, p. 68).

Many American Indians with traditional orientations believe there is a reason for every sickness or pain. They believe that ILLNESS is the price to be paid either for something that happened in the past or for something that will happen in the future. In spite of this conviction, a sick person must still be cared for. Everything is seen as being the result of something else, and this cause-and-effect relationship creates an eternal chain. American Indians do not generally subscribe to the germ theory of modern medicine. ILLNESS is something that must be. Even the person who is experiencing the ILLNESS may not realize the reason for its occurrence, but it may, in fact, be the best possible price to pay for the past or future event(s) (Boyd, 1974).

The Hopi Indians associate ILLNESS with evil spirits. The evil spirit responsible for an ILLNESS is identified by the medicine man, and the remedy for the malady resides in the treatment of the evil spirit (Leek, 1975, p. 16).

Traditionally, the Navajos see ILLNESS, disharmony, and sadness as the result of one or more combinations of the following actions: "(1) displeasing the holy people; (2) annoying the elements; (3) disturbing animal and plant life; (4) neglecting the celestial bodies; (5) misuse of a sacred Indian ceremony; or (6) tampering with witches and witchcraft" (Bilagody, 1969, p. 57). If disharmony exists, disease can occur. The Navajos distinguish between two types of diseases: (1) contagious diseases, such as measles, smallpox, diphtheria, syphilis, and gonorrhea; and (2) more generalized ILLNESSES, such as "body fever" and "body ache." The notion that ILLNESS is caused by a microbe or another physiological agent is alien to the Navajos. The cause of disease, of injury to people or to their property, or of continued misfortune of any kind must be traced back to an action that should not have been performed. Examples of such infractions are breaking a taboo and contacting a ghost or witch. To the Navajos, the treatment of an ILLNESS, therefore, must be concerned with the external causative factor(s), not with the ILLNESS or injury itself (Kluckhohn & Leighton, 1962, pp. 192–193).

■ Traditional Methods of HEALING

Traditional HEALERS

The traditional HEALER of Native America is the medicine man or woman, and American Indians, by and large, have maintained their faith in him or her over the ages. The medicine men and women are wise in the ways of the land and of nature. They know well the interrelationships of human beings, the Earth, and the universe. They know the ways of the plants and animals, the sun, the moon, and the stars. Medicine men and women take time to determine first the cause of an ILLNESS and then the proper treatment. To determine the cause and treatment of an ILLNESS, they perform special ceremonies, which may take up to several days.

A medicine man or woman is also known among many people as a *Kusiut*, a "learned one." The acquisition of full shamanic powers takes many years, often as many as 30 years of training before one has the ability to cure illness. The shaman's power is accumulated through solitary vision quests and fasts repeated over the years. The purification rituals include scrubbing oneself in freezing cold water and ingesting emetics (Lyon, 1996, p. 141).

The medicine man or woman of the Hopis uses meditation in determining the cause of an ILLNESS and sometimes even uses a crystal ball as the focal point for meditation. At other times, the medicine man or woman chews on the root of jimsonweed, a powerful herb that produces a trance. The Hopis claim that this herb gives the medicine man or woman a vision of the evil that has caused a sickness. Once the meditation is concluded, the medicine man or woman is able to prescribe the proper herbal treatment. For example, fever is cured by a plant that smells like lightning; the Hopi phrase for fever is "lightning sickness" (Leek, 1975, p. 16).

The Navajo people consider disease to be the result of breaking a taboo or the attack of a witch. The exact cause is diagnosed by divination, as is the ritual of treatment. There are three types of divination: motion in the hand (the most common form and often practiced by women), stargazing, and listening. The function of the diagnostician is first to determine the cause of the ILLNESS and then to recommend the treatment—that is, the type of chant that will be effective and the medicine man or woman who can best do it. A medicine man or woman may be called on to treat obvious symptoms, whereas the diagnostician is called on to ascertain the cause of the ILLNESS. (A person is considered wise if the diagnostician is called first.) Often, the same medicine man or woman can practice both divination (diagnosis) and the singing (treatment). When any form of divination is used in making the diagnosis, the diagnostician meets with the family, discusses the patient's condition, and determines the fee.

The practice of motion in the hand includes the following rituals. Pollen or sand is sprinkled around the sick person, during which time the diagnostician sits with closed eyes and face turned from the patient. The HEALER's hand begins to move during a song. While the hand is moving, the diagnostician thinks of various diseases and various causes. When the arm begins to move in a certain way, the diagnostician knows that the right disease and its cause have been discovered and is then able to prescribe the proper treatment (Wyman, 1966, pp. 8–14). The ceremony of motion in the hand also may incorporate the use of sand paintings. (These paintings are a well-known form of art.) Four basic colors are used—white, blue, yellow, and black—and each color has a symbolic meaning. Chanting is performed as the painting is produced, and the shape of the painting determines the cause and treatment of the ILLNESS. The chants may continue for an extended time (Kluckhohn & Leighton, 1962, p. 230), depending on the family's ability to pay and the capabilities of the singer. The process of motion in the hand can be neither inherited nor learned. It comes to a person suddenly, as a gift. It is said that people able to diagnose their own ILLNESSES are able to practice motion in the hand (Wyman, 1966, p. 14).

Unlike motion in the hand, stargazing can and must be learned. Sand paintings are often but not always made during stargazing. If they are not made, it is either because the sick person cannot afford to have one done, or because there is not enough time to make one. The stargazer prays the star prayer to the star spirit, asking it to show the cause of the ILLNESS. During stargazing, singing begins, and the star throws a ray of light that determines the cause of the patient's ILLNESS. If the ray of light is white or yellow, the patient will recover; if it is red, the illness is serious. If a white light falls on the patient's home, the person will recover; if the home is dark, the patient will die (Wyman, 1966, p. 15).

Listening, the third type of divination, is somewhat similar to stargazing, except that something is heard rather than seen. In this instance, the cause of the ILLNESS is determined by the sound that is heard. If someone is heard to be crying, the patient will die (Wyman, 1966, p. 16).

The traditional Navajos continue to use medicine men and women when an ILLNESS occurs. They use this service because, in many instances, the treatment they receive from the traditional HEALERS is better than the treatment they receive from the healthcare establishment. Treatments used by singers include massage and heat treatment, the sweatbath, and use of the yucca root—approaches similar to those common in physiotherapy (Kluckhohn & Leighton, 1962, p. 230).

The main effects of the singer are psychological. During the chant, the patient feels cared for in a deeply personal way as the center of the singer's attention, since the patient's problem is the reason for the singer's presence. When the singer tells the patient recovery will occur and the reason for the ILLNESS, the patient has faith in what is heard. The singer is regarded as a distinguished authority and as a person of eminence with the gift of learning from the holy people, and is considered to be more than a mere mortal. The ceremony—surrounded by such high levels of prestige, mysticism, and power—takes the sick person into its circle, ultimately becoming one with the holy people by participating in the singing that is held on the patient's behalf. The patient once again comes into harmony with the universe and subsequently becomes free of all ILLS and evil (Kluckhohn & Leighton, 1962, p. 232).

The religion of the Navajos is one of good hope when they are sick or suffer other misfortunes. Their system of beliefs and practices helps them through the crises of life and death. The stories that are told during ceremonies give the people a glimpse of a world that has gone by, which promotes a feeling of security because they see that they are links in the unbroken chain of countless generations (Kluckhohn & Leighton, 1962, p. 233).

Many Navajos believe in witchcraft, and, when it is considered to be the cause of an ILLNESS, special ceremonies are employed to rid the individual of the evil caused by witches. Numerous methods are used to manipulate the supernatural. Although many of these activities may meet with strong social disapproval, Navajos recognize the usefulness of blaming witches for ILLNESS and misfortune. Tales abound concerning witchcraft and how the witches work. Not all Navajos believe in witchcraft, but for those who do, it provides a mechanism for laying blame for the overwhelming hardships and anxieties of life.

Such events as going into a trance can be ascribed to the work of witches. The way to cure a "witched" person is through the use of complicated prayer ceremonies that are attended by friends and relatives, who lend help and express sympathy. The victim of a witch is in no way responsible for being sick and is, therefore, free of any punitive action by the community if the ILLNESS causes the victim to behave in strange ways. However, if an incurably "witched" person is affected so that alterations in the person's established role severely disrupt the community, the victim may be abandoned (Kluckhohn & Leighton, 1962, p. 244). Box 9-1 presents selected beliefs of a traditional Cherokee medicine man.

Traditional Remedies

American Indians practice an act of purification in order to maintain their harmony with nature and to cleanse the body and spirit. This is done by total immersion in water in addition to the use of sweatlodges, herbal medicines, and special rituals. Purification is seen as the first step in the control of consciousness, a ritual that awakens the body and the senses and prepares a person for meditation. The participants view it as a new beginning (Boyd, 1974, pp. 97–100).

The basis of therapy lies in nature, hence the use of herbal remedies. Specific rituals are to be followed when herbs are gathered. Each plant is picked to be dried for later use. No plant is picked unless it is the proper one, and only enough plants are picked to meet the needs of the gatherers. Timing is crucial, and the procedures are followed meticulously. So deep is their belief in the harmony of human beings and nature that the herb gatherers exercise great care not to disturb any of the other plants and animals in the environment (Boyd, 1974, pp. 101–136).

One plant of interest, the common dandelion, contains a milky juice in its stem and is said to increase the flow of milk from the breasts of nursing mothers. Another plant, the thistle, is said to contain a substance that

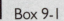

Box 9-1

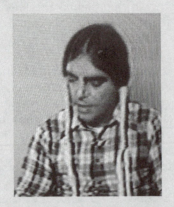

Figure 9-4 Hawk Littlejohn.

Hawk Littlejohn, 1941–2000

I had the privilege of working with Hawk Littlejohn, a traditional medicine man, in 1979 at the Boston (Massachusetts) Indian Council. He was a native of western North Carolina and a member of the Eastern Band of the Cherokee nation. He was known among the Cherokee and community at large to be a highly respected and skilled medicine man and knowledgeable in the history of the Cherokee nation. I interviewed him in June 1979. Here are several of his thoughts in his own words:

- A medicine man sees himself in my tribe as a person who is many, many things. Not just as a HEALER or not just as a priest. We like to see ourselves like the fingers on a hand. They are separated and work independently of the hand if requested to, but they're still part of the whole. And each one of these fingers can do different things. It's like when I go to visit a home and there is a child there who is suffering from malnutrition but in our medicine we're more interested in the cause not the symptom. So, I've left my role as a HEALER and a priest to a role that might turn out to be social or political to find out why the child is hungry, why this child is feeling this way. And that might be dealing with the tribal government or some kind of social situation. We elect to see ourselves as representatives of our people's needs.

- The medicine man or HEALER in my tribe is considered to be chosen by the Great Spirit. For a couple of years the medicine men check all children for unusual marks, it is not any particular mark on the body but something they consider very unusual as a sign. The unusual marks that were on me were Simian Creases, the line that goes across my hand. I'm told it is unusual to have one of these but to have two, one on each hand, is very unusual. I was perhaps two or three years old when I was chosen.

- As a child I was taught that there are three parts of us and the most obvious part is the physical aspect, then the second part is the intellectual part, and the third part is the spiritual aspect of a person. The physical is the tangible, the one we can see and touch and be with all the time. We go through acceptance of our physical being. This is what I have to walk the path of life with and I accept it for what it is. The intellectual aspect is the part that interprets things for you—dreams, visions, feelings, and what the spirit is saying to you. The spiritual aspect of a person is the slowest and the last in most cases to mature. The spiritual aspect is kept in harmony and in balance by the awareness that it is part of everything else. We believe that all life forms have a spirit and the relationship of man to all other beings

(continued)

Box 9-1   *Continued*

that are alive is a spiritual one. When all three aspects are working together it is called balance and harmony, or the center of the earth.

- Let's say a student, for example, puts a lot of emphasis on the intellect and neglects the physical and the spiritual aspect of him, we believe that there are natural forces which always try to seek a balance. For instance, if you get a cut, you heal because it is natural to try to seek balance. We believe that there are many subtle things the Great Spirit made and very obvious things that the Great Spirit made like creatures like elephants, whales, and the obvious. And then much more subtle creatures like what you call germs and viruses and when we believe that when the Great Spirit created life, he created laws to govern life, that the wolf wouldn't eat the deer in one day, that there would be laws to govern these kinds of things. One of the laws was what we call a "*skilly*." It is a being or a creature and it has no good or bad. When a person neglects the spiritual and physical part for the intellect, and does not seek balance, the *skilly* comes in and one of the effects of the *skilly* is sickness and disease.
- One of the ways to treat people is indirectly. When I go to see people we talk about their corn and their lives and they talk about my corn and my life and then we get down to the reason why I am there. They don't tell me their physical symptoms One of the things we've realized is that sickness isolates people from other people and the sickness has separated the person from the community and from his family. So we automatically try to make him or bring him back out of that isolation and one of the ways we do that is to include the family and friends in the HEALING process.
- In my tribe we have knowledge of about 500 different plants and use about 350 of them on a pretty regular basis. We see the plants as other life forms, but the commonality between all life forms is this spiritual aspect. We believe that each thing that is alive has a spirit and its spirit has a personality, so I use the spirit of the plant to cure another spirit—when the spirit of the sickness is not compatible with the spirit of the plant, the disease dissipates. We call the plants, plant people. My people's medicine started off as a trial and error, like most medicine did, using the plants. If you had a sickness that reminded them of a rabbit, for example, a plant that reminded them of a fox would be used to treat it.
- I think the solution to Indian problems is for Indian people to start identifying themselves. I see as a traditional person that one of the steps on this long journey is to gain pride and dignity in oneself. Naturally, I believe it is in traditionalism. Traditionalism is a philosophy, a way of life and living, a holistic sort of thing that we're a part of.

Source: Hawk Littlejohn, personal interview, 1979.

relieves the prickling sensation in the throats of people who live in the desert. The medicine used to hasten the birth of a baby is called *weasel medicine* because the weasel is clever at digging through and out of difficult territory (Leek, 1975, p. 17).

The use of American Indian cures and herbal remedies continues to be popular. For example, among the Oneida Indians, the following remedies are used (Knox & Adams, 1988):

Illness	Remedy
Colds	Witch hazel, sweet flag
Sore throat	Comfrey
Diarrhea	Elderberry flowers
Headache	Tansy and sage
Ear infection	Skunk oil
Mouth sores	Dried raspberry leaves

Drums are another source of treatment. Drumming, rattles, and singing accompany HEALING ceremonies. The noise consists of sounds that interfere with the negative work of the spirits of the disease. The rhythm of the drumming plays a role in altering human consciousness (Lyon, 1996, p. 67). "Drumming is essential in helping the shaman make the transition from an ordinary state of consciousness to the shamanistic state of consciousness" (p. 68). Quiet HEALING ceremonies are unheard of.

■ Current Healthcare Problems

Today, American Indians are faced with a number of health-related problems and health disparities. Many of the old ways of diagnosing and treating illness have not survived the migrations and changing ways of life of the people. Because these skills often have been lost and because modern healthcare facilities are not always available, American Indian people are frequently caught in limbo when it comes to obtaining adequate healthcare. Many of the illnesses that are familiar among White patients may manifest themselves differently in American Indian patients. *Native American people experience higher disease rates and lower life expectancy than any other racial or ethnic group in the country.* The rates of diabetes, mental illness, cardiovascular disease, pneumonia, influenza, and unintentional injuries of Indians are exponentially higher, and the infant mortality rate is greater for Indians than that of White infants. The suicide rate among young males between the ages of 15 and 24 was 29.1 per 100,000 people, and the homicide rate for males between 25 and 44 years was 15.4 per 100,000 population in 2013 (NCHS, 2015, pp. 135, 139). The impact of this is felt throughout the community. In addition, at least one third of American Indians exist in a state of abject poverty. With this destitution come poor living conditions and attendant problems, as well as diseases of the poor—including malnutrition, tuberculosis, and high maternal and infant death rates. Poverty and isolated living serve as further barriers that keep American Indians from using limited healthcare facilities even when they are available (IHS, 2015d).

The legacy of the extraordinary traumas that the American Indian people experienced over the past 340+ years, such as the early King Philip's War (1675–1676), the Trail of Tears (beginning in the early 1830s), and the massacre at Wounded Knee (1890), are historically part of the problem, as is the ongoing decimation of the land and culture (History.com Staff, 2009).

Unfortunately, traumatic experiences continue to pervade the lives of American Indian people. Despite high rates of interpersonal violence and child abuse on tribal lands, a 2014 report by the U.S. Attorney General's Office found that federal funding to support prevention and response efforts has languished (U.S. Attorney General's Office, 2014). Historical and current traumatization of the AI/AN peoples has a profound effect on their daily lives and on their approach to the modern healthcare system.

Morbidity and Mortality

The American Indian and Alaska Native people have long experienced lower health status when compared with other Americans. Lower life expectancy and the disproportionate disease burden exist perhaps because of inadequate education, disproportionate poverty, discrimination in the delivery of health services, and cultural differences. These are broad quality-of-life issues rooted in economic adversity and poor social conditions.

In 2013, American Indian and Alaska Native people had a crude birth rate of 10.3, and the largest cohort of mothers delivering babies per 1,000 women were between the ages of 20 and 24 years. The rate of infant mortality was 8.4 per every 1,000 live births, as compared to 6.0 per 1,000 for the U.S. population in 2012 (NCHS, 2015 p. 76). Table 9-1 compares selected health status indicators for all races and American Indians and Alaska Natives.

Mental Illness

The family in this population is often a nuclear family, with strong biological and large extended family networks. Children are taught to respect traditions, and community organizations are growing in strength and numbers. Many American Indians tend to use traditional medicines and HEALERS and are knowledgeable about these resources. People may frequently be treated by a traditional medicine man or woman. Several diagnostic techniques include the use of divination, conjuring, and stargazing. A sweat lodge, an enclosed, completely dark space, may be used therapeutically. Extremely hot stones, or another source of heat, are placed inside to heat the room. Inside the sweat

Table 9-1   Comparison of Selected Health Status Indicators—All Races and
American Indians and Alaska Natives: 2013

Health Indicator	All Races	American Indians and Alaska Natives
Crude birth rate per 1,000 population by race of mother, 2013	12.4	10.3
Percentage of live births to teenage childbearing women—18–19 years, 2013	5.0	**8.7**
Percentage of low birth weight per live births >2,500 grams, 2013	8.02	7.48
Infant mortality per 1,000 live births, 2012	6.0	**8.4**
Respondent-reported prevalence percent of adults: Cancer—all sites, 2012–2013, 18 years and over	5.9	4.3
Respondent-reported prevalence percent of adults: Heart Disease—2012–2013, 18 years and over	10.6	10.1
Respondent-reported prevalence percent of adults: Stroke—2012–2013, 18 years and over	2.5	3.3
Male death rates from suicide, all ages, age adjusted per 100,000 resident population, 2013	20.3	18.1
Male death rates from homicide, all ages, age adjusted per 100,000 resident population, 1999–2003	8.2	8.2

Source: Health, United States, 2014: With Special Feature on Adults Aged 55–64, by National Center for Health Statistics, 2015, Hyattsville, MD: Author, pp. 58, 61, 64, 76, 134, 135, 138, 139, 161.

lodge, participants sing sacred songs and recite prayers during the purification process (Lyon, 1996, p. 270).

"Ghost sickness" is a culture-bound syndrome that affects some American Indians. This mental health problem involves a preoccupation with death and an intense fear of ghosts and the deceased, and it is associated with witchcraft. It is thought to be caused by the touch of a ghost. The ghosts of the recently departed may cause illness or even death among the living. Symptoms include bad dreams, weakness, feelings of danger, loss of appetite, and confusion.

Methamphetamine (meth) abuse and suicide are two top concerns in Indian country. Methamphetamine is a low-cost, highly addictive stimulant. Its introduction to Indian country has destabilized and disrupted entire health and social systems. Meth is a synthetic/artificial stimulant with a number of effects on the brain and the rest of the body. People who use this chemical may display high levels of aggression and may injure or kill themselves and others. Meth also causes significant physical complications including neurological/organic brain changes. Hand in hand with meth abuse is the high suicide rate (Nieves, 2007). A wide range of general risk factors, such as "getting into trouble," have been shown to contribute to suicide in adolescents. AI/AN young people face, on average, a greater number of these risk factors, and/or the risk factors are more severe in nature. The age-adjusted suicide rate for AI/AN young men between the ages of 15 and 24 was 29.1, as compared to a rate of 17.3 for males in this age cohort in the overall population. The suicide rate for AI/AN men between the ages of 25 and 44 in 2013 was 29.1, as compared to 24.1 for all men (NCHS, 2015, pp. 138–139). The factors that protect Native youth and young adults against suicidal behavior are their sense of belonging to their culture, strong tribal spiritual orientation, and cultural continuity. The Bureau of Indian Education provides direct action services in youth suicide prevention to the community. They provide the technical assistance and monitoring regional School Safety Specialists to ensure schools comply with intervention strategies and reporting protocols to ensure student safety. A Suicide Prevention Training Initiative was initiated in 2012 (Hawk, 2011).

Alcoholism is a major mental health problem among American Indians. A comparison of the 10 leading causes of death among American Indians/Alaska Natives and the general population reveals that unintentional injuries (#3), chronic liver disease and cirrhosis (#4), and suicide (#6) rank higher as causes of death than for the population at large. Each of these causes of death is related to mental health problems, including alcoholism.

Table 9-2 compares the 10 leading causes of death between all persons and American Indians and Alaska Natives. The 2nd leading cause of death is unintentional injuries; 4th is chronic liver disease and cirrhosis; and homicide is 7th and suicide is 10th—these carry an association to alcoholism. American Indians and Alaska Natives experience injury mortality rates that are 2.4 times greater than other Americans (IHS, 2015e).

Table 9-2   **Comparison: The 10 Leading Causes of Death for American Indians and Alaska Natives and for All Persons, 2013**

American Indians and Alaska Natives	All Persons
1. Diseases of heart	1. Diseases of heart
2. Malignant neoplasms	2. Malignant neoplasms
3. Unintentional injuries	3. Chronic lower respiratory diseases
4. Diabetes mellitus	4. Unintentional injuries
5. Chronic liver disease and cirrhosis	5. Cerebrovascular diseases
6. Chronic lower respiratory disease	6. Alzheimer's disease
7. Cerebrovascular diseases	7. Diabetes mellitus
8. Suicide	8. Influenza and pneumonia
9. Influenza and pneumonia	9. Nephritis, nephrotic syndrome, and nephrosis
10. Nephritis, nephrotic syndrome, and nephrosis	10. Suicide

Source: Health, United States, 2014: With Special Feature on Adults Aged 55–64, by National Center for Health Statistics, 2015, Hyattsville, MD: Author, pp. 97, 98.

Fetal Alcohol Syndrome

"My son will forever travel through a moonless night with only the roar of the wind for company" (Dorris, 1989, p. 264). This momentous quote reflects on the tragedy of fetal alcohol syndrome, an affliction that affects countless American Indian children. Alcohol and substance use, as well as mental health issues and suicide, continue to be among the most severe health and social problems American Indians and Alaska Natives face (http://www.samhsa.gov/tribal-affairs).

Alcohol use can disrupt fetal development at any stage during a pregnancy—including at the earliest stages and before a woman knows she is pregnant—increasing the risk for the infant developing fetal alcohol syndrome (PubMed Health, n.d.).

The markings of fetal alcohol syndrome include:

- Abnormal growth in height, weight, and/or head circumference, including microcephaly
- Central nervous system problems such as behavioral and/or mental health problems, including learning disabilities and abnormal sleeping and eating patterns; and
- Appearance with a specific pattern of recognizable deformities, such as the three key facial features, a smooth philtrum, a thin vermillion border, and small palpebral fissures (Bertrand, Floyd, & Weber, 2005, p. 3).

People with FASD often have difficulty in coordination, emotional control, school work, socialization, and holding a job. They often make bad decisions, repeat the same mistakes, trust the wrong people, and do not understand the consequences of their choices and actions (PubMed Health, n.d.).

Domestic Violence

As mentioned earlier, other problems related to alcohol abuse in the American Indian people are domestic (intimate partner) violence and child maltreatment in the forms of physical, emotional, sexual abuse, and neglect (IHS, 2015b, 2015c). Abuse is not traditional in American Indian life but has evolved. True American Indian love is based on a tradition of mutual respect and the belief that men, women, and children are part of an ordered universe where the people should live peacefully. In the traditional American Indian home, children are raised to respect their parents. Intimate partner abuse toward women was not practiced. In modern times this is not the case, and women are far more vulnerable. Domestic violence has a profound effect on the community and on the family. A pattern of abuse is easily established. It begins with tension: The female attempts to keep peace but the male cannot contain himself, a fight erupts, and then the crisis arrives. The couple may make up, only to fight again. Attempts to help must be initiated, or the cycle escalates and the problem is extremely complex.

Urban Problems

Approximately 70% of American Indians and Alaska Natives live in urban areas. Although this population is not particularly dense, urban Indians share the same health problems as the general Indian population. The rates of diphtheria, tuberculosis, otitis media with subsequent hearing defects, alcohol abuse, inadequate immunization, iron-deficiency anemia, childhood developmental lags, mental health problems (including depression, anxiety, and coping difficulties), and caries and other dental problems are high. The health problems are exacerbated in terms of mental and physical hardships because of the lack of family and traditional cultural environments. Urban Indian youth are at greater risk for serious mental health and substance abuse problems, suicide, increased gang activity, teen pregnancy, abuse, and neglect (IHS, 2015f). As in all dysfunctional families, problems arise that are related to marital difficulties and financial strain, which usually are brought about by unemployment and the lack of education or knowledge of special skills. The tension often is compounded further by alcoholism.

Healthcare Provider Services

Some historical differences in healthcare relate to geographic locations. American Indians living in the eastern part of this country and in most urban areas are not covered by the services of the Indian Health Service, services that are available to American Indians living on reservations in the West. In 1923, tribal government—under the control of the Bureau of Indian Affairs—was begun by the Navajos, who established treaties with the U.S. government; but in the areas of health and education, the United States did not honor these treaties. Health services on the reservations were inadequate. Consequently, the people were sent to outside institutions for the treatment of illnesses, such as tuberculosis and mental health problems. As recently as 1930, the vast Navajo lands had only seven hospitals with 25 beds each. Not until 1955 were American Indians finally offered concentrated services with modern physicians. Only since 1965 have more comprehensive services been available to the Navajos.

■ The Indian Health Service (IHS)

The IHS, an agency within the U.S. Department of Health and Human Services, is responsible for providing federal health services to American Indians and Alaska Natives. The provision of health services to members of federally recognized tribes grew out of the special government-to-government relationship between the federal government and Indian tribes established in 1787. It is based on Article I, Section 8, of the Constitution and has been given form and substance by numerous treaties, laws, Supreme Court decisions, and executive orders. The IHS is the principal federal healthcare provider and health advocate for American Indian people. Its goal is to raise their health status to the highest possible level. The IHS provides a comprehensive health service delivery system for American Indians and Alaska Natives who are members of 566 federally recognized tribes across the

United States. The mission of the agency is to raise the physical, mental, social, and spiritual health of American Indians and Alaska Natives to the highest level. The Indian Health Service is divided into 12 physical areas of the United States; Alaska, Albuquerque, Bemidji, Billings, California, Great Plains, Nashville, Navajo, Oklahoma, Phoenix, Portland, and Tucson. Each of these areas has a unique group of tribes that they work with on a day-to-day basis. The headquarters are in Rockville, Maryland (IHS, 2015a).

The Indian Health Care Improvement Act (IHCIA), the cornerstone legal authority for the provision of healthcare to American Indians and Alaska Natives, was signed into law by President Obama on March 23, 2010, as part of the Patient Protection and Affordable Care Act. The authorization of appropriations for the IHCI expired in 2000, and IHCIA now has no expiration date.

There are several ways by which a person can show that they are eligible for IHS care. For example, a person must show Indian and/or Alaska Native descent as evidenced by factors such as being regarded by the community in which that person lives as an Indian or Alaska Native or actively participating in tribal affairs.

The Affordable Care Act will help address the health disparities by investing in prevention and wellness and increasing access to affordable health coverage. The act provides American Indians and Alaska Natives with more choices, depending on their eligibility and the coverage available in their state.

Many providers of healthcare and social services are not aware that many of the American Indians on the East Coast have dual citizenship as a result of the Jay Treaty of 1794. This treaty allows for *international citizenship* between the United States and Canada. This raises questions about whether American Indians can freely cross the border between the United States and Canada and whether the people who live in the United States are eligible for welfare or Medicaid.

■ Cultural and Communication Problems

A factor that inhibits the American Indian use of White-dominated health services is a deep, cultural problem: American Indians suffer disease when they come into contact with White healthcare providers. American Indians feel uneasy because for too many years, they have been the victims of haphazard care and disrespectful treatment. All too often, conflict arises between what the American Indians perceive their illness to be and what the physicians diagnose. American Indians, like most people, do not enjoy long waits in clinics; separation from their families; the unfamiliar, regimented environment of the hospital; or the unfamiliar behavior of the nurses and physicians, who often display demeaning and demanding attitudes. Their response to this treatment varies. Sometimes, they remain silent; other times, they leave and do not return. Many American Indians request that, if the ailment is not an emergency, they be allowed to see the medicine man or woman first and then receive treatment from a physician. Often, when a sick person is afraid of receiving the care of a physician, the medicine man or woman encourages the person to go to the hospital.

Healthcare providers must be aware of several factors when they communicate with American Indians. One is recognition of the importance of nonverbal communication. Often, American Indians observe providers and say very little. A patient may expect a provider to deduce the problem through instinct rather than by the extensive use of questions during history taking. In part, this derives from the belief that direct quoting is intrusive on individual privacy. When examining an American Indian with an obvious cough, a provider might be well advised to use a declarative statement—"You have a cough that keeps you awake at night"—and then allow time for the patient to respond to the statement.

It is American Indian practice to converse in a very low tone of voice. It is expected that the listener will pay attention and listen carefully in order to hear what is being said. It is considered impolite to say, "Huh?" or "I beg your pardon" or to give any indication that the communication was not heard. Therefore, an effort should be made to speak with patients in a quiet setting, where they will be heard more easily.

Note taking is taboo. Indian history has been passed through generations by means of verbal storytelling. American Indians are sensitive about note taking while they are speaking. When one is taking a history or interviewing, it may be preferable to use memory skills rather than to record notes. This more conversational approach may encourage greater openness between the patient and the provider.

Another factor to be considered is differing perceptions of time between the American Indian patient and the provider. Life on the reservation is not governed by the clock but by the dictates of need. When an American Indian moves from the reservation to an urban area, this cultural conflict concerning time often exhibits itself as lateness for appointments. One solution is the use of walk-in clinics.

This chapter has presented an overview of the health/HEALTH and illness/ILLNESS situation as found in the American Indian/Alaska Native communities and described many links on the *HERITAGECHAIN* related to this topic.

RESEARCH ON CULTURE

A large amount of research has been conducted among members of the American Indian and Alaska Native population. The following study is one example:

Strickland, C. J., & Cooper, M. (2011). Getting into trouble: Perspectives on stress and suicide prevention among Pacific Northwest Indian youth. *Journal of Transcultural Nursing, 22*(3), 240–247.

This descriptive, ethnographic study in a Pacific Northwest tribe seeks to gain an understanding of the life experiences of the youth in the studied community. Focus groups and observations were conducted with 30 Indian youth between the ages of 14 and 19 years. The youths were asked to discuss their stressors, sense of family and community, and hopes for the future.

(continued)

RESEARCH ON CULTURE   *Continued*

The youths reported major stress and noted that friends and family were both a support and a source of stress. The stressors included "getting into trouble." This was doing something in home, community, or society that would result in sanctions or discipline. The coping skills were found to be "speaking up for oneself," often resulting in more trouble. It was further discovered that the youth desired to "stay on track." They want to strengthen their cultural values, experience economic development, and future opportunity. The findings provide insight about the suicide risk among Indian youth.

Explore  MediaLink

Go to the Student Resource Site at pearsonhighered.com/nursingresources for chapter-related review questions, case studies, and activities. Contents of the CULTURALCARE Guide and CULTURALCARE Museum can also be found on the Student Resource Site. Click on Chapter 9 to select the activities for this chapter.

Box 9-2

Keeping Up

It goes without saying that much of the data presented in this chapter will be out of date when this text is read. However, at this final stage of writing, it is the most recent information available. The following resources will be most helpful in keeping you abreast of the frequent changes in HEALTH and ILLNESS in the American Indian and Alaska Native communities:

1. The National Center for Health Statistics publication *Health, United States*, an annual report on trends in health statistics
2. Health-related data and other statistics available from the Centers for Disease Control
3. The National Congress of American Indians
4. U.S. Department of Health and Human Services, Indian Health Service Fact Sheets
5. U.S. Department of the Interior, Bureau of Indian Affairs
6. U.S. Department of the Interior, Bureau of Indian Education.

■ References

Bertrand, J., Floyd, R. L., & Weber, M. K. (2005). Guidelines for identifying and referring persons with fetal alcohol syndrome. *MMWR, 54*(RR-11).

Bilagody, H. (1969). An American Indian looks at health care. In R. Feldman & D. Buch (Eds.), *The ninth annual training institute for psychiatrist-teachers of practicing physicians.* Boulder, CO: WICHE, No. 3A30.

Boyd, D. (1974). *Rolling thunder*. New York, NY: Random House.

Brown, D. (1970). *Bury my heart at Wounded Knee*. New York, NY: Holt.

Deloria, V., Jr. (1969). *Custer died for your sins*. New York, NY: Avon Books.

Deloria, V., Jr. (1974). *Behind the trail of broken treaties*. New York, NY: Delacorte.

Dorris, M. (1989). *The broken cord*. New York, NY: Harper & Row.

Fortney, A. J. (1977, January 23). Has White man's lease expired? *Boston Sunday Globe*, pp. 8–30.

Hawk, L. E. (2011). *Oversight field hearing: Helping our people engage to protect our youth*. U.S. Department of the Interior, Committee on Indian Affairs. Washington, DC: U.S. Senate. Retrieved from http://www.bia.gov/cs /groups/xocl/documents/text/idc015409.pdf

History.com Staff. (2009). *Native American cultures*. A&E Television Networks. Retrieved from http://www.history.com/topics/native-american-history /native-american-cultures

Kluckhohn, C., & Leighton, D. (1962). *The Navaho* (Rev. ed.). Garden City, NY: Doubleday.

Knox, M. E., & Adams, L. (1988). *Traditional health practices of the Oneida Indian*. Oshkosh, WI: University of Wisconsin, College of Nursing.

Leek, S. (1975). *Herbs: Medicine and mysticism*. Chicago, IL: Henry Regnery.

Littlejohn, H. (1979). Personal interview. Boston, MA.

Lyon, W. S. (1996). *Encyclopedia of Native American healing*. New York, NY: Norton.

National Center for Health Statistics (NCHS). (2015). *Health, United States, 2014: With special feature on adults aged 55–64*. Hyattsville, MD: Author. Retrieved from http://www.cdc.gov/nchs/data/hus/hus14.pdf

National Coalition on Racism in Sports and Media. (n.d.). http://www.aimovement .org/ncrsm/

National Museum of the American Indian. (2016). Home Page. Washington, DC: Smithsonian Institution. Retrieved from http://www.nmai.si.edu/

Nieves, E. (2007, June 9). Indian reservation reeling in weave of youth suicides and attempts. *New York Times*, p. A-9.

PubMed Health. (n.d.). *Fetal alcohol syndrome*. Retrieved from http://www.ncbi .nlm.nih.gov/pubmedhealth/PMHT0024268/

Strickland, C. J., & Cooper, M. (2011). Getting into trouble: Perspectives on stress and suicide prevention among Pacific Northwest Indian youth. *Journal of Transcultural Nursing. 22*(3), 240–247.

U.S. Attorney General's Office. (2014). *Ending violence so children can thrive: Executive summary*. Attorney General's Advisory Committee on American Indian/Alaskan Native Children Exposed to Violence. Retrieved from https://www .washingtonpost.com/r/2010-2019/WashingtonPost/2014/11/17 /National-Security/Graphics/Report_re5.pdf

U.S. Department of Commerce, U.S. Census Bureau. (2015). *Census 2014 estimates*. Retrieved from http://www.census.gov/

U.S. Department of Health and Human Services, Indian Health Service (IHS). (2015a). *Fact sheet: Basis for health services*. Retrieved from https://www.ihs .gov/newsroom/factsheets/basisforhealthservices/

U.S. Department of Health and Human Services, Indian Health Service (IHS). (2015b). *Fact sheet: Behavioral health*. Retrieved from https://www.ihs.gov /newsroom/factsheets/behavioralhealth/

U.S. Department of Health and Human Services, Indian Health Service (IHS). (2015c). *Fact sheet: Child maltreatment.* Retrieved from https://www.ihs.gov /forpatients/index.cfm/healthtopics/ChildMaltreatment/

U.S. Department of Health and Human Services, Indian Health Service (IHS). (2015d). *Fact sheet: Disparities.* Retrieved from https://www.ihs.gov /newsroom/factsheets/disparities/

U.S. Department of Health and Human Services, Indian Health Service (IHS). (2015e). *Fact sheet: Injuries.* Retrieved from https://www.ihs.gov /newsroom/factsheets/injuries/

U.S. Department of Health and Human Services, Indian Health Service (IHS). (2015f). *Fact sheet: Urban Indian Health Program.* Retrieved from https:// www.ihs.gov/newsroom/factsheets/uihp/

U.S. Department of the Interior, Bureau of Indian Affairs. (n.d.). *Who we are.* Retrieved from http://www.indianaffairs.gov/WhoWeAre/index.htm

Wittstock, L., & Salinas, E. J. (2006). *A brief history of the American Indian Movement.* Retrieved from http://www.aimovement.org/ggc/history.html

Wyman, L. C. (1966). Navaho diagnosticians. In W. R. Scott & E. H. Volkhart (Eds.), *Medical care.* New York, NY: John Wiley & Sons.

Zuckoff, M. (1995, April 18). More and more claiming American Indian heritage. *Boston Globe,* p. A8.

■ Additional Readings

Bear, S., & Bear, W. (1996). *The medicine wheel.* New York, NY: Fireside.

Catlin, G. (1993). *North American Indian portfolio.* Washington, DC: Library of Congress.

Erdrich, L. (2012). *The round house.* New York, NY: HarperCollins.

Neihardt, J. G. (1991). *When the tree flowered.* Lincoln: University of Nebraska Press (Original work published 1951).

Neihardt, J. G. (1998). *Black Elk speaks.* Lincoln: University of Nebraska Press (Original work published 1961).

Neihardt, N. (1993). *The sacred hoop.* Tekamah, NE: Neihardt.

Noble, M. (1997). *Sweet Grass: Lives of contemporary Native women of the Northeast.* Mashpee, MA: C. J. Mills.

Peltier, L. (1999). *Prison writings: My life is my sun dance.* New York, NY: St Martin's Press.

Silko, L. M. (1977). *Ceremony.* New York, NY: Penguin.

Senier, S. (2001). *Voices of American Indian assimilation and resistance.* Norman: University of Oklahoma Press.

Wiebe, R., & Johnson, Y. (1998). *Stolen life—The journey of a Cree woman.* Athens: Ohio University Press.

Wolfson, E. (1993). *From the Earth to the sky.* Boston, MA: Houghton Mifflin.

HEALTH and ILLNESS in the Asian Population

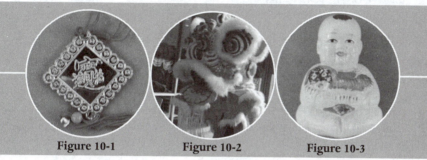

Figure 10-1   **Figure 10-2**   **Figure 10-3**

But when she arrived in the new country, the immigration officials pulled her swan away from her leaving the woman fluttering her arms and with only one swan feather for a memory.

— *Amy Tan*

■ Objectives

1. Discuss the historical and demographic background of the Asian American population.
2. Describe the traditional definitions of HEALTH and ILLNESS of the Asian American population.
3. Explain the traditional methods of HEALING of the Asian American population.
4. Describe the practice of a traditional HEALER.
5. Summarize current healthcare problems of the Asian American population.

The next link in the *HERITAGECHAIN* examines the historical and demographic backgrounds, HEALTH and ILLNESS traditions, and healthcare issues of the Asian American population in the United States. The traditional HEALTH beliefs and practices derived from China are explored, and a brief overview of Ayurvedic medicine is included. The opening images for this chapter depict objects symbolic of items used to maintain, protect, and/or restore HEALTH. Figure 10-1 is a small metal amulet with red strings that may be hung in the home or workplace to maintain balance in the space and bring good luck and good HEALTH to the people living or working there. Figure 10-2 is the Chinese Dragon who appears on January 1, the Chinese New Year, and other festive occasions. He brings physical as well as spiritual HEALTH and strength, luck, and prosperity; and he symbolizes heroism, self-confidence, excellence, perseverance, and happiness. Figure 10-3 is a smiling Buddha and a powerful spiritual symbol—many homes have shrines with the Buddha as the central figure. Family members leave offerings of fruits and rice and burn incense at the shrine.

■ Background

More than 5.3% of the population of the United States, some 18.9 million people, are people of Asian heritage (McDonnell-Smith, 2013; U.S. Department of Commerce, U.S. Census Bureau, 2014). *Asian* refers to people having origins in any of the nations of the Far East, Southeast Asia, or the Indian subcontinent (for example, Cambodia, China, India, Japan, Korea, Malaysia, Pakistan, the Philippine Islands, Thailand, and Vietnam). The Asian people are not limited to nationalities but are characterized by their diversity. More than 30 different languages are spoken, including Chinese, Japanese, Korean, Thai, Hindi, and Urdu (U.S. Department of Commerce, U.S. Census Bureau, 2014), and there are a similar number of cultures and many different religions, including but not limited to Buddhism, Confucianism, Hinduism, Islam, and Taoism. Over half of all people who reported an Asian heritage lived in three states—Hawaii, California, and Washington. The cities with the largest Asian populations are New York, Los Angeles, San Jose, San Francisco, and Honolulu. Honolulu County, Hawaii, has the highest percentage, 60.9%, of Asians in the nation (McDonnell-Smith, 2013).

This chapter focuses on the traditional HEALTH and ILLNESS beliefs and practices of the Chinese Americans, because the HEALTH and ILLNESS beliefs and practices of many of the other Asians and Pacific Islanders are derived in part from the Chinese HEALTH traditions. An overview of the Ayurvedic system of healthcare is included as it is a predecessor of Chinese medicine.

Chinese immigration to the United States began over 150 years ago. In 1850, there were only 1,000 Chinese residents in this country; in 1880, there were well over 100,000. This rapid increase occurred in part because of the discovery of gold in California and in part because of the need for cheap labor to build the transcontinental railroads. The immigrants were laborers who met the needs of the dominant society. Like many early immigrant groups, they came here intending to stay only as temporary workers. Most of the immigrants were men, and they clung closely to their customs and beliefs and stayed together in their own communities. The hopes that many had for a better life when they came to the United States did not materialize. Subsequently, many of the workers and their kin returned to China before 1930. Part of the disharmony and disenchantment occurred because the immigrants were not White and did not have the same culture, language, and habits as Whites. For these reasons, they were not welcomed, and many jobs were not open to them. For example, Chinese immigrant workers were excluded from many mining, construction, and other hard-labor jobs, even though the transcontinental railroad was constructed mainly by Chinese laborers. Between 1880 and 1930, the Chinese population declined by nearly 20%. One factor that helped perpetuate this decline in population was a series of exclusion acts halting further immigration. The people who remained behind were relegated to menial jobs, such as cooking and dishwashing. The Chinese workers first took these jobs in the West and later moved eastward throughout the United States. They tended to move to cities where they were allowed to let their entrepreneurial talents surface—their main pursuits included running small laundries, food shops, and restaurants.

The people settled in tightly knit groups in urban neighborhoods that took the name "Chinatown." Here they were able to maintain the ancient traditions of their homeland. They were hard workers and, in spite of the dull, menial jobs usually available to them, they were able to survive.

Both U.S. immigration laws and political problems in China have had an effect on the nature of today's Chinese population. When the exclusion acts were passed, many men were left alone in this country without the possibility that their families would join them. For this reason, a great majority of the men spent many years alone. In addition, the political oppression experienced by the Chinese in the United States was compounded—at a time when immigration laws were relaxed here after World War II, people were unable to return to or leave China because of that country's restrictive new regulations. By 1965, however, a large number of refugees who had relatives here were able to come to this country. They settled in the Chinatowns of America, causing the population of these areas to swell.

■ Traditional Definitions of HEALTH and ILLNESS

Chinese medicine teaches that HEALTH is a state of spiritual and physical harmony with nature. In ancient China, the task of the physician was to prevent ILLNESS. A first-class physician not only cured an ILLNESS, but could also prevent disease from occurring. A second-class physician had to wait for patients to become ill before they could be treated. The physician was paid by the patient while the patient was healthy. When illness occurred, payments stopped. Indeed, not only was the physician not paid for services when the patient became ill, but the physician also had to provide and pay for the needed medicine (Mann, 1972, p. 222).

To understand the Chinese philosophy of HEALTH and ILLNESS, it is necessary to look back at the age-old philosophies from which more current ideas have evolved. The foundation rests in the religion and philosophy of Taoism. Taoism originated with a man named Lao-Tzu, who is believed to have been born about 604 BC. The word *Tao* has several meanings: way, path, or discourse. On the spiritual level, it is the way of ultimate reality. It is the way of all nature, the primeval law that regulates all heavenly and earthly matters. To live according to the Tao, one must adapt oneself to the order of nature. Chinese medical works revere the ancient sages who knew the way and "led their lives in Tao" (Smith, 1958, pp. 175–192).

The Chinese view the universe as a vast, indivisible entity, and each being has a definite function within it. No one thing can exist without the existence of the others. Each is linked in a chain that consists of concepts related to each other in harmonious balance. Violating this harmony is like hurling chaos, wars, and catastrophes on humankind—the end result of which is ILL-NESS. Individuals must adjust themselves wholly within the environment. Five elements—wood, fire, earth, metal, and water—constitute the guiding principles of humankind's surroundings. These elements can both create and destroy each other. For example, "wood creates fire," "two pieces of wood rubbed together produce a spark," "wood destroys earth," "the tree sucks strength from the earth." The guiding principles arise from this "correspondences" theory of the cosmos (Wallnöfer & von Rottauscher, 1972, pp. 12–16, 19–21).

For a person to remain HEALTHY, his or her actions must conform to the mobile cycle of the correspondences. The exact directions for achieving this were written in such works as the *Lu Chih Ch'un Ch'iu* (*Spring and Autumn Annals*) written by Lu Pu Wei, who died circa 230 BC.

The teachings of Asian religions, including Confucianism and Buddhism, are complementary and have played a major role in the shaping of the cultural values in Asia (Smith, 1958):

- **Buddhism** teaches harmony/nonconfrontation (silence as a virtue), respect for life, moderation in behavior, self-discipline, patience, and humility. Individualism is devalued.

- **Confucianism** teaches the achievement of harmony through observing the five basic hierarchical roles and relationships of society, such as the ruler and ruled, the father and son, and between friends, and the importance of family.

- **Taoism** teaches harmony between humans and nature, charity, happiness, and a long life.

The holistic concept, as explained by Dr. P. K. Chan (1988), is an important idea of traditional Chinese medicine in preventing and treating diseases. It has two main components:

1. A human body is regarded as an integral organism, with special emphasis on the harmonic and integral interrelationship between the viscera and the superficial structures in these close physiological connections, as well as their mutual pathological connection. In Chinese medicine, the local pathological changes always are considered in conjunction with other tissues and organs of the entire body, instead of considered alone.

2. Special attention is paid to the integration of the human body with the external environment. The onset, evolution, and change of disease are considered in conjunction with the geographic, social, and other environmental factors.

Four thousand years before the English physician William Harvey described the circulatory system in 1628, *Huang-ti Nei Ching* (*Yellow Emperor's*

Book of Internal Medicine) was written. This is the first known volume that describes the circulation of blood. It described the oxygen-carrying powers of blood and defined the two basic world principles: *yin* and *yang*, powers that regulate the universe. *Yang* represents the male, positive energy that produces light, warmth, and fullness. *Yin* represents the female, negative energy—the force of darkness, cold, and emptiness. *Yin* and *yang* exert power not only over the universe, but also over human beings.

Yin and *yang* were further explained by Dr. Chan as having been originally a philosophical theory in ancient China. Later, the theory was incorporated into Chinese medicine. The theory holds that "everything in the Universe contains two aspects—*yin* and *yang*, which are in opposition and also in unison. Hence, matters are impelled to develop and change." In traditional Chinese medicine, the phenomena are further explained as follows:

- Matters that are dynamic, external, upward, ascending, and brilliant - belong to *yang*.
- Those that are static, internal, downward, descending, dull, regressive, and hypoactive are *yin*.
- *Yin* flourishing and *yang* vivified steadily is the state of health. *Yin* and *yang* regulate themselves in the basic principle to promote the normal activities of life.
- Illness is the disharmony of *yin* and *yang*, a disharmony that leads to pathological changes, with excesses of one and deficiencies of the other, disturbances of vital energy and blood, malfunctioning of the viscera, and so forth (Chan, 1988).

The various parts of the human body correspond to the dualistic principles of *yin* and *yang*. The inside of the body is *yin*; the surface of the body is *yang*. The front part of the body is *yin*; the back is *yang*. The five *ts'ang* viscera—liver, heart, spleen, lungs, and kidney—are *yang*; the six *fu* structures—gallbladder, stomach, large intestine, small intestine, bladder, and "warmer"—are *yin*. (The "warmer" is now believed to be the lymph system.) The diseases of winter and spring are *yin*; those of summer and fall are *yang*. The pulses are controlled by *yin* and *yang*. If *yin* is too strong, the person is nervous and apprehensive and catches colds easily. If the individual does not balance *yin* and *yang* properly, his or her life will be short. Half of the *yin* forces are depleted by age 40; at 40, the body is sluggish, and at 60, the *yin* is totally depleted, at which time the body deteriorates. *Yin* stores the vital strength of life. *Yang* protects the body from outside forces, and it, too, must be carefully maintained. If *yang* is not cared for, the viscera are thrown into disorder, and circulation ceases. *Yin* and *yang* cannot be injured by evil influences. When *yin* and *yang* are sound, the person lives in peaceful interaction with mind and body in proper order (Wallnöfer & von Rottauscher, 1972).

Chinese medicine has a long history. The Emperor Shen Nung, who died in 2697 BC, was known as the patron god of agriculture. He was given this title because of the 70 experiments he performed on himself by swallowing a different plant every day and studying the effects. During this period of self-experimentation, Nung discovered many poisonous herbs and rendered them harmless by the use of antidotes, which he also discovered. His patron element was fire, for which he was known as the Red Emperor. The Emperor Shen Nung was followed by Huang-ti, whose patron element was earth. Huang-ti was known as the Yellow Emperor and ruled from 2697 BC to 2595 BC. The greater part of his life was devoted to the study of medicine. Many people ascribe to him the recording of the *Nei Ching*, the book that embraces the entire realm of Chinese medical knowledge. The treatments described in the *Nei Ching*—which became characteristic of Chinese medical practices—are almost totally aimed at reestablishing balances that are lost within the body when ILLNESS occurs. Disrupted harmonies are regarded as the sole cause of disease. Surgery was rarely resorted to; when it was, it was used primarily to remove malignant tumors. The *Nei Ching* is a dialogue between Huang-ti and his minister, Ch'i Po. It begins with the concept of the Tao and the cosmological patterns of the universe and goes on to describe the powers of the *yin* and *yang*. This learned treatise discusses in great detail the therapy of the pulses and how a diagnosis can be made on the basis of alterations in the pulse beat. It also describes various kinds of fevers and the use of acupuncture (Wallnöfer & von Rottauscher, 1972, pp. 26–28).

The Chinese view their bodies as a gift given to them by their parents and forebears. A person's body is not his or her personal property. It must be cared for and well maintained. Confucius taught that "only those shall be truly revered who at the end of their lives will return their physical bodies whole and sound."

The body is composed of five solid organs (*ts'ang*), which collect and store secretions, and five hollow organs (*fu*), which excrete. The heart and liver are regarded as the noble organs. The head is the storage chamber for knowledge, the back is the home of the chest, the loins store the kidneys, the knees store the muscles, and the bones store the marrow.

The Chinese view the functions of the various organs as comparable to the functions of persons in positions of power and responsibility in the government. For example, the heart is the ruler over all other civil servants, the lungs are the administrators, the liver is the general who initiates all the strategic actions, and the gallbladder is the decision maker.

The organs have a complex relationship, which maintains the balance and harmony of the body. Each organ is associated with a color. For example, the heart—which works in accordance with the pulse, controls the kidneys, and harmonizes with bitter flavors—is red. In addition, the organs have what is referred to as an "aura," the meaning of which, in the medical context, is HEALTH. The aura is determined by the color of the organ. In the balanced, healthy body, the colors look fresh and shiny.

Disease is caused by an upset in the balance of *yin* and *yang*. The weather, too, has an effect on the body's balance and the body's relationship to *yin* and *yang*. For example, heat can be injurious to the heart, and cold is injurious to the lungs. Overexertion is harmful to the body. Prolonged sitting is harmful to the flesh and spine, and prolonged lying in bed can be harmful to the lungs.

The Chinese physician uses inspection and palpation to diagnose disease. During inspection, the Chinese physician looks at the tongue (glossoscopy), listens and smells (osphretics), and asks questions (anamnesis). During palpation, the physician feels the pulse (sphygmopalpation).

The Chinese believe that there are many different pulse types, which are all grouped together and must be felt with the three middle fingers. The pulse is considered the storehouse of the blood, and a person with a strong, regular pulse is considered to be in good health. By the nature of the pulse, the physician is able to determine various illnesses. For example, if the pulse is weak and skips beats, the person may have a cardiac problem. If the pulse is too strong, the person's body is distended (Wallnöfer & von Rottauscher, 1972).

There are six different pulses, three in each hand. Each pulse is specifically related to various organs, and each pulse has its own characteristics. According to ancient Chinese sources, there are 15 ways of characterizing the pulses. Each of these descriptions accurately determines the diagnosis. There are 7 *piao* pulses (superficial) and 8 *li* pulses (sunken). An example of an illness that manifests with a *piao* pulse is headache; anxiety manifests with a *li* pulse. The pulses also take on a specific nature with various conditions. For example, specific pulses are associated with epilepsy, pregnancy, and the time just before death.

The Chinese physician is aided in making a diagnosis by the appearance of the patient's tongue. More than 100 conditions can be determined by glossoscopic examination. The color of the tongue and the part of the tongue that does not appear normal are the essential clues to the diagnosis (Law, personal interview, October 18, 2006).

The Chinese have known breast cancer since early times. "The disease begins with a knot in the breast, the size of a bean, and gradually swells to the size of an egg. After seven or eight months it perforates. When it has perforated, it is very difficult to cure" (Wallnöfer & von Rottauscher, 1972).

■ Traditional Methods of HEALTH Maintenance and Protection

There are countless ways by which HEALTH is maintained. One example is the practices involved in daily nutrition. Foods, such as thousand-year eggs, are ingested on a daily basis. There are strict rules governing food combinations and foods that must be eaten preceding and after life events, such as childbirth and surgery. Daily exercise is also important, and many people participate in formal exercise programs, such as tai chi.

The Chinese often prepare amulets to prevent evil spirits and protect HEALTH. These amulets consist of a charm with an idol or a Chinese character painted in red or black ink and written on a strip of yellow paper. These amulets are hung over a door or pasted on a curtain or wall, worn in the hair, or placed in a red bag and pinned on clothing. The paper may be burned and the ashes mixed in hot tea and swallowed to ward off evil. Jade is believed to be the most precious of all stones because it is seen as the giver of children, HEALTH immortality, wisdom, power, victory, growth, and food. Jade charms are worn to bring HEALTH and, should they turn dull or break, the wearer will surely meet misfortune. The charm prevents harm and accidents. Children are kept safe with jade charms, and adults are made pure, just, humane, and intelligent by wearing them (Law, personal, interview, 2006).

■ Traditional Methods of HEALTH Restoration

Just as there are countless methods used to maintain and protect HEALTH, there are countless ways to restore HEALTH. The following discussion describes traditional methods of restoring HEALTH. An overview of Ayurvedic medicine is provided in Box 10-1.

Acupuncture

Acupuncture is an ancient Chinese practice of puncturing the body to cure disease or relieve pain. The body is punctured with special metal needles at points that are precisely predetermined for the treatment of specific symptoms. According to one source, the earliest use of this method was recorded between 106 BC and AD 200. According to other sources, however, it was used even earlier. This treatment modality stems from diagnostic procedures described earlier. The most important aspect of the practice of acupuncture is the acquired skill and ability to know precisely where to puncture the skin. Nine needles are used in acupuncture, each with a specific purpose. The following is a list of selected examples of needles and their purposes (Wallnöfer & von Rottauscher, 1972):

- Superficial pricking: arrowhead needle
- Massaging: round needle
- Knocking or pressing: blunt needle
- Most extensively used: filiform needle.

The specific points of the body into which the needles are inserted are known as *meridians*. The needles are thin, and the puncture barely penetrates the skin and rarely draws blood. Acupuncture is based on the concept that certain meridians extend internally throughout the body in a fixed network. There are 365 points on the skin where these lines emerge. Because all the networks merge and have their outlets on the skin, the way to treat internal problems is to puncture the meridians, which are also categorically identified in terms of *yin* and *yang*, as are the diseases. The treatment goal is to restore the balance of *yin* and *yang* (Wallnöfer & von Rottauscher, 1972). The practice of this art is far too complex to explain in great detail in these pages.

Readers may find it interesting to visit acupuncture clinics in their area. After the therapist carefully explains the art and science of acupuncture, one may be able to grasp the fundamental concepts of this ancient treatment. The practice of acupuncture is based in antiquity, yet it took a long time for it to be accepted as a legitimate method of healing by practitioners of the Western medical system. Numerous acupuncture clinics are attracting a growing number of non-Asian clients, and acupuncture is being used as a method of anesthesia and pain relief in some hospitals. Acupuncture is generally considered safe when performed by an experienced practitioner using sterile needles (NCCIH, 2015).

Moxibustion, Cupping, Bleeding, and Tui Na

Moxibustion has been practiced for as long as acupuncture. Its purpose, too, is to restore the proper balance of *yin* and *yang*. Moxibustion is based on the therapeutic value of heat, whereas acupuncture is a cold treatment. Acupuncture is used mainly in diseases in which there is an excess of *yang*, and moxibustion is used in diseases in which there is an excess of *yin*. Moxibustion is performed by heating mugwart and passing it above the skin, but never touching it, over certain specific meridians. It is used with caution, as there are meridians where it cannot be applied.

Other important traditional HEALTH restoring practices are cupping, bleeding, and a form of traditional massage, *Tui Na*:

■ Cupping involves creating a vacuum in a small glass by burning the oxygen out of it, then promptly placing the glass on the person's skin surface. Cupping draws blood and lymph to the body's surface that is under the cup. This increases the local circulation. The purpose for doing this is to remove cold and damp "evils" from the body and/or to assist blood circulation. The procedure is frequently used to treat lung congestion (Figure 10-4).

■ Bleeding, often done with the use of leeches, is performed to "remove heat from the body." Only small amounts of blood are removed.

■ Massage, *Tui Na*, "pushing and pulling," is a complex system of massage or manual acupuncture point stimulation that is used on orthopedic and neurological conditions (Ergil, 1996, pp. 208–209).

Herbal Remedies

Medicinal herbs were and are used widely in the practice of Chinese HEALING. Herbology is an interesting subject. The gathering season of an herb is important for its effect. It is believed that some herbs are more effective if gathered at night and that others are more effective if gathered at dawn. For example, it is known that a plant may not be effective if the dew has been allowed to dry on its leaves, or if the roots have been in the ground too long. The herbalist believes that the ginseng root must be harvested only at midnight in a full moon if it is to have therapeutic value. Ginseng's therapeutic value is due to its nonspecific action. Ginseng is derived from the root of a plant that resembles a person.

The release of the therapeutic properties of ginseng and its preparation are of vital importance. Ginseng must not be prepared in anything made of metal because it is believed that some of the necessary constituents are leeched out by the action of the metal. It must be stored in crockery. It is boiled in water until a sediment remains and stored in a ceramic pot. Ginseng has many uses, including

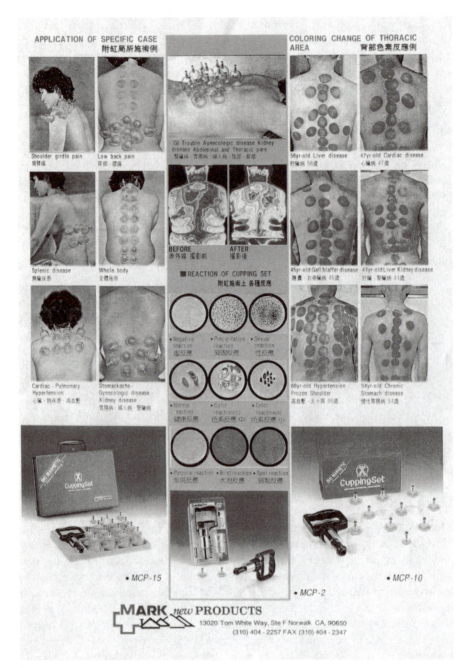

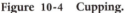

Figure 10-4 Cupping.

boosting the immune system, decreasing LDL cholesterol, lowering blood sugar, and improving agility (University of Maryland Medical Center, 2014). There are many Chinese medicinal herbs, but none is as famous as ginseng.

I bring my students to a traditional Chinese pharmacy in Boston's Chinatown where they sell herbal remedies, both over the counter and by prescription. One side wall of the pharmacy is lined with countless nonprescription remedies while the other wall is lined with drawers, each containing the different herbs that are weighed and mixed following a prescription. The Chinese doctor, whose practice is located in the pharmacy, examines the patient and writes the prescription depending on the diagnosis of the patient's problem. The cost of filling a prescription varies from a nominal $5.00 to several hundred dollars. This depends on the herbs that are used. Figures 10-5A and 10-5B illustrate the interior of this Chinese pharmacy, the drawers containing herbs, the method by which the herbs are weighed in the preparation of a prescription, and assorted over-the-counter remedies. The herbs necessary to fill the prescription are laid out on the paper, and the directions for preparing them are carefully given to the patient. In general, the preparation of the herbs involves wrapping them in cheesecloth and simmering them in water for a prescribed amount of time. The liquid is then strained, cooled, and drunk in specific amounts, at specific times each day. The amount of water and the amount of time that the herbs are boiled determines the concentration of the medicine.

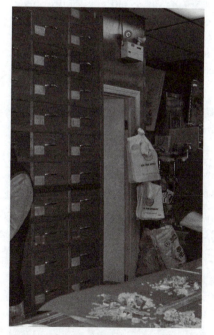

Figure 10-5A   Interior of a Chinese pharmacy; herbal prescription on counter.

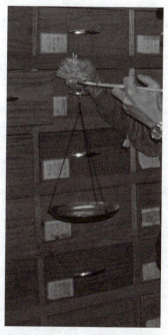

Figure 10-5B   Weighing herbs for a prescription.

In addition to herbs and plants, the Chinese use other substances with medicinal and healing properties. Popular Chinese remedies include:

- ◼ *Deer antlers*—used to strengthen bones, increase a man's potency, and dispel nightmares
- ◼ *Lime calcium*—used to clear excessive mucus
- ◼ *Quicksilver*—used externally to treat venereal diseases
- ◼ *Rhinoceros horns*—highly effective when applied to pus boils; an antitoxin for snakebites
- ◼ *Turtle shells*—used to stimulate weak kidneys and to remove gallstones

Traditional HEALERS

The Chinese physician was the primary HEALER in Chinese medicine. Physicians who had to treat women encountered numerous difficulties because men were not allowed to touch women directly who were not family members. Thus, a diagnosis might be made through a ribbon that was attached to the woman's wrist. As an alternative to demonstrating areas of pain or discomfort on a woman's body, an alabaster figure was substituted. The area of pain was pointed out on the figurine (Dolan, 1973, p. 30).

Not much is known about women doctors except that they did exist. Women were known to possess a large store of medical talent. There were also midwives and female shamans. The female shamans possessed gifts of prophecy. They danced themselves into ecstatic trances and had a profound effect on the people around them. As the knowledge that these women possessed was neither known nor understood by the general population, they were feared rather than respected. They were said to know all there was to know about life, death, and birth.

Box 10-1

Ayurvedic Medicine

Deepak Chopra describes Ayurvedic medicine as "the science of life" (Hay, 1994). He introduced it to the United States in 1984 and has emerged as one of the world's leading proponents of the innovative combination of Eastern and Western HEALING. Ayurvedic medicine (also called Ayurveda) is one of the world's oldest medical systems. It originated in India and evolved there over 3,000 years ago. It developed from Hinduism, one of the world's oldest and largest religions, and ancient Persian thoughts about HEALTH and HEALING. *Ayurveda* is built on theories of HEALTH and ILLNESS and on ways to prevent, manage, or treat HEALTH problems. It is holistic, as it integrates and balances the body, mind, and spirit. The balance is believed to lead to contentment and HEALTH and to help prevent ILLNESS, and it treats specific health problems, whether they are physical or mental. One goal of

(continued)

Box 10-1   *Continued*

Ayurvedic practice is to cleanse the body of substances that can cause disease to reestablish harmony and balance. The term "Ayurveda" combines the Sanskrit words *ayur* (life) and *veda* (science or knowledge). Many Ayurvedic practices predate written records and were handed down by word of mouth. Three ancient books known as the Great Trilogy were written in Sanskrit more than 2,000 years ago and are considered the main texts on Ayurvedic medicine—*Caraka Samhita*, *Sushruta Samhita*, and *Astanga Hridaya* (NCCIH, 2015).

In the Ayurvedic philosophy, people, HEALTH, and the universe are related, and HEALTH problems can result when the relationships are out of balance. Herbs, metals, massage, and other products and techniques are used with the intent of cleansing the body and restoring balance. Many of the Ayurvedic practices were handed down by word of mouth and were used before there were written records.

Ayurveda is the main system of healthcare in India, and variations of it have been practiced for centuries in Pakistan, Nepal, Bangladesh, Sri Lanka, and Tibet. About 70% of India's population lives in rural areas, and about two thirds of rural people still use Ayurveda and medicinal plants to meet their primary healthcare needs. In addition, most major Indian cities have an Ayurvedic college and hospital.

Examples of Traditional HEALTH Beliefs and Practices
Basic HEALTH beliefs and practices include the following.

The constitution, or HEALTH, is called the *prakriti*. The *prakriti* is thought to be a unique combination of physical and psychological characteristics and the way the body functions. It is influenced by such factors as digestion and how the body deals with waste products. The *prakriti* is believed to be unchanged over a person's lifetime.

In diagnosing a patient, the practitioner will:

- Ask about diet, behavior, lifestyle practices, and the reasons for the most recent illness and symptoms the patient had
- Carefully observe such physical characteristics as teeth, skin, eyes, and weight
- Take a person's pulse, because each *dosha* is thought to make a particular kind of pulse.

In addition to questioning, Ayurvedic practitioners use observation, touch, therapies, and advising. During an examination, the practitioner checks the patient's urine, stool, tongue, bodily sounds, eyes, skin, and overall appearance. The practitioner will also consider the person's digestion, diet, personal habits, and resilience (ability to recover quickly from illness or setbacks). As part of the effort to find out what is wrong, the practitioner may prescribe some type of treatment. The treatment is generally intended to restore the balance of a particular *dosha*. *Doshas* control activities of the body. For example, the *pitta dosha* represents the elements fire and water and is said to control hormones and the digestive system.

The practitioner develops a treatment plan and may work with the family and friends who know the patient well and can help. This helps the patient feel emotionally supported and comforted, which is considered important. Patients

(continued)

Box 10-1 *Continued*

are expected to be active participants in their treatment, because many Ayurvedic treatments require changes in diet, lifestyle, and habits. In general, treatments use several approaches, often more than one at a time.

In Ayurveda, the distinction between food and medicine is not as clear as in Western medicine, as food and diet are important components of Ayurvedic practice. There is a heavy reliance on treatments based on herbs and plants, oils (such as sesame oil), common spices (such as turmeric), and other naturally oc-curring substances. Some of the products—which may contain herbs, minerals, or metals—may be harmful, particularly if used improperly or without the direction of a trained practitioner. For example, some herbs can cause side effects or inter-act with conventional medicines. Also, ingesting some metals, such as lead, can be poisonous. Studies have examined Ayurvedic medicine, including herbal products, for specific conditions. However, there are not enough well-controlled clinical tri-als and systematic research reviews—the gold standard for Western medical re-search—to prove that the approaches are beneficial (NCCIH, 2015).

Traditional HEALERS

One example of a traditional Indian HEALER was *Sai Baba*, known as the God that descended to earth. *Sri Sai Baba*, who left his mortal body in 1918, is believed to be the living spiritual force that is drawing people from all walks of life, from all parts of the world, into his fold. It is believed that he came to serve humankind and to free them from the clutches of fear. He lived his message through the "Essence of His Being." His life and relationship with the common people was his teach-ing. He radiated a mysterious smile and a deep, inward look, of a peace that was all-understanding.

Sources: Shri SaiBaba of Shirdi: The Perfect Master of the Age, by Sai Movement, 2002, Shirdi, India: Shri SaiBaba Trust, retrieved from http://www.shrisaibabasansthan.org/, November 6, 2015; and *Ayurvedic Medicine: In Depth,* by U.S. Department of Health and Human Services, National Cen-ter for Complementary and Integrative Health, 2015, retrieved from https://nccih.nih.gov/health /ayurveda/introduction.htm, November 20, 2015.

■ Current Health Problems

In many instances, people who were born in the United States into families es-tablished here for generations are largely indistinguishable from the general population in their healthcare beliefs. Other groups, however, especially new im-migrants, differ from the general population on many social and health-related is-sues. Table 10-1 compares selected health indicators in the Asian/Pacific Islander population with people of all races. In most of the selected categories, the rates for the Asian/Pacific Islander population are lower than those for the general population. For example, Asians/Pacific Islanders have a lower rate of births to teenage childbearing women, a lower infant mortality rate, a lower incidence of cancer, and lower rates of homicide and suicide. Table 10-2 compares the causes of death in the Asian population with that of all persons in 2013.

Table 10-1   Comparison of Selected Health Status Indicators: 2013 All Races and Asian Americans

Health Indicator	All Races	Asian Americans
Crude birth rate per 1,000 population by race of mother, 2013	12.4	14.3
Percentage of live births to teenage childbearing women—18–19 years, 2013	5.0	1.4
Percentage of low birth weight per live births >2,500 grams, 2013	8.02	8.34
Infant mortality per 1,000 live births, 2012	6.0	4.1
Respondent-reported prevalence percent of adults: Cancer—all sites, 2012–2013, 18 years and over	5.9	3.4
Respondent-reported prevalence percent of adults: Heart Disease—2012–2013, 18 years and over	10.6	6.4
Respondent-reported prevalence percent of adults: Stroke—2012–2013, 18 years and over	2.5	1.8
Male death rates from suicide, all ages, age adjusted per 100,000 resident population, 2013	20.3	9.1
Male death rates from homicide, all ages, age adjusted per 100,000 resident population, 1999–2003	8.2	2.3

Source: *Health, United States, 2014: With Special Feature on Adults Aged 55–64*, by National Center for Health Statistics, 2015, Hyattsville, MD: Author, pp. 58, 59, 61, 64, 76, 134, 135, 138, 139, 161.

Poor health, however, continues to be found among some Asians partly because of poor working and crowded living conditions. Many people work long hours in restaurants and laundries and receive the lowest possible wages for their hard work. Many cannot afford even minimal, let alone preventive,

Table 10-2   Comparison: The 10 Leading Causes of Death for Asian or Pacific Islander and for All Persons, 2013

Asian or Pacific Islander	All Persons
1. Malignant neoplasms	1. Diseases of heart
2. Diseases of heart	2. Malignant neoplasms
3. Cerebrovascular diseases	3. Chronic lower respiratory diseases
4. Unintentional injuries	4. Unintentional injuries
5. Diabetes mellitus	5. Cerebrovascular diseases
6. Influenza and pneumonia	6. Alzheimer's disease
7. Chronic lower respiratory diseases	7. Diabetes mellitus
8. Alzheimer's disease	8. Influenza and pneumonia
9. Nephritis, nephrotic syndrome, and nephrosis	9. Nephritis, nephrotic syndrome, and nephrosis
10. Suicide	10. Suicide

Source: *Health, United States, 2014: With Special Feature on Adults Aged 55–64*, by National Center for Health Statistics, 2015, Hyattsville, MD: Author, pp. 97–98.

healthcare. Americans of Asian heritage frequently experience unique barriers, including linguistic and cultural differences, when they try to access the unfamiliar healthcare system.

Language difficulties and adherence to native Chinese culture compound problems already associated with poverty, crowding, and poor health. Many people still prefer the traditional forms of Chinese medicine and seek help from Chinatown "Chinese physicians" who treat them with traditional herbs and other methods. Often, Asian people do not seek help from the Western system at all unless symptoms are completely unmanageable. Others use Chinese methods in conjunction with Western methods of healthcare, although the Chinese find many aspects of Western medicine distasteful. For example, they cannot understand why so many diagnostic tests, some of which are painful, are necessary. They do, however, accept the practice of immunization and the use of x-rays.

Chinese people may not understand why the often frequent taking of blood samples, considered routine in Western medicine, is necessary. Blood is seen as the source of life for the entire body, and it is believed that blood is not regenerated. The Asian reluctance to have blood drawn for diagnostic tests may have its roots in the revered teachings of Confucius. The Chinese people also believe that a good physician should be able to make a diagnosis simply by examining a person. Consequently, they do not react well to the often painful procedures used in Western diagnostic workups. Some people—because of their distaste for the drawing of blood—leave the Western system rather than tolerate the pain. The Chinese have deep respect for their bodies and believe that it is best to die with their bodies intact. For this reason, many people refuse surgery or consent to it only under the direst circumstances. This reluctance to undergo intrusive surgical procedures has deep implications for those concerned with providing healthcare to Asian Americans.

The hospital is an alien place to many of the Asian people. Not only are the customs and practices strange, but also the patients often are isolated from the rest of their people, which enhances the language barrier and feelings of helplessness. Something as basic as food creates another problem. Hospital food is strange to Asian patients and is served in an unfamiliar manner. The typical Asian patient rarely complains about what bothers him or her. Often the only indication that there may be a problem is an untouched food tray and the silent withdrawal of the patient. Unfortunately, the silence may be regarded by the nurses as reflecting good, complacent behavior, and the healthcare team exerts little energy to go beyond the assumption. The Asian patient who says little and complies with all treatment is seen as stoic, and there is little awareness that deep problems may underlie this "exemplary" behavior. Ignorance on the part of healthcare workers may cause the patient a great deal of suffering.

Much action has been taken in recent years to make Western healthcare more available and appealing to Asian populations. In Boston, for example, there is a health clinic staffed primarily by people who speak Chinese dialects and other Asian languages. Most of the common health-related pamphlets have been translated into Chinese languages and into Vietnamese, Cambodian, and Laotian, and they are distributed to the patients. Booklets on such topics as breast self-examination and smoking cessation are available. The care is personal, and the patients are made to feel comfortable. Unnecessary and painful tests are avoided as much as possible. In addition, the clinic, which is open for long hours, provides social services and employment placements and is quite popular with the community. Although it began as a part-time, storefront operation, the clinic is now housed in its own building.

The following is a synopsis of cultural beliefs regarding mental health and illness, possible causes of mental illness, and methods of preventing mental illness among people of Asian origin. Lack of knowledge or skills in mental health therapy is seen in the Asian communities, as mental illness is much ignored in medical classics. Two points must be noted: the importance placed on the family in caring for the mentally ill, and the tendency to identify mental illness in somatic terms. There is a tremendous amount of stigma attached to mental illness. Asian patients tend to come to the attention of mental health workers late in the course of their illness, and they come with a feeling of hopelessness (Lin, 1982, pp. 69–73).

One example of cross-cultural therapy is the Japanese practice of Morita therapy. This 70-year-old treatment originated from a treatment for shinkeishitsu, a form of compulsive neurosis with aspects of neurasthenia. The patient is separated from the family for 1 to 2 weeks and taught that one's feelings are the same as the Japanese sky and instantly changeable. One cannot be responsible for how one feels, only for what one does. At the end of therapy, the patient focuses on what is being done and less on his or her inner feelings, symptoms, concerns, or obsessive thoughts (Yamamoto, 1982, p. 50). In addition, there are countless culture-bound mental HEALTH syndromes that may be identified in the Asian communities:

- *Hwa-byung*—fear of death, tiredness resulting from the imbalance between reality and anger
- *Koro*—the occurrence of sudden, intense anxiety when a man believes his penis is folding into his body and causes death
- *Taijin kyofusho*—guilt about possibly offending others (Paniagua, 2000).

This chapter has presented an introductory overview of selected cultural phenomena, HEALTH traditions, and health issues of people from Asian heritages. Needless to say, a bigger picture of the phenomenon could fill many books. However, given the significant number of new Asian immigrants, especially from China and India, this beginning discussion is very necessary.

RESEARCH ON CULTURE

A large amount of research has been conducted among members of the Asian American populations. The study described in the following article is one example:

Lee, J., & Bell, K. (2011). The impact of cancer on family relationships among Chinese patients. *Journal of Transcultural Nursing, 22*(3), 225–234.

(continued)

RESEARCH ON CULTURE *Continued*

This qualitative research study examined the impact of cancer on family relationships among members of a Chinese cancer support group. There were 96 participants at group meetings over an 8-month span of time—40% of whom were family members. The methods used included participant observation, and in-depth interviews with seven group members were held. The interview schedule is published in the article.

The findings were that family members were an integral part of the support group. Patients expressed concern about family members, and family members identified "equal suffering" when they cared for patients. There was a strong emphasis on the need to conceal emotion. Patients were also anxious about burdening their family members.

The authors concluded that the findings highlight the need for practitioners to focus on the entire family when they develop interventions to help cancer patients cope. They recommend that research should focus on gender differences in Chinese families' experiences of cancer as well as possible differences that may be found based on length of immigration.

Explore  MediaLink

Go to the Student Resource Site at pearsonhighered.com/nursingresources for chapter-related review questions, case studies, and activities. Contents of the CULTURALCARE Guide and CULTURALCARE Museum can also be found on the Student Resource Site. Click on Chapter 10 to select the activities for this chapter.

Box 10-2

Keeping Up

It goes without saying that much of the data presented in this chapter may be out of date when you read this text. However, at this final stage of writing, it is the most recent information available. The following resource will be most helpful in keeping you abreast of the frequent changes in healthcare events, costs, and policies:

The National Center for Health Statistics publication Health, United States—an annual report on trends in health statistics U.S. Census.

References

Chan, P. K. (1988, August 3). Herb specialist, interview by author, New York City. Dr. Chan prepared a supplemental written statement in Chinese and English for inclusion in this text.

Dolan, J. (1973). *Nursing in society: A historical perspective.* Philadelphia, PA: W. B. Saunders. National Center for Health Statistics.

Ergil, K. V. (1996). China's traditional medicine. In M. S. Micozzi (Ed.), *Fundamentals of complementary and alternative medicine.* New York, NY: Churchill Livingstone.

Hay, V. (1994). An interview with Deepak Chopra. *A Magazine of People and Possibilities* (online). Retrieved from http://www.intouchmag.com/chopra.html

Lee, J., & Bell, K. (2011). The impact of cancer on family relationships among Chinese patients. *Journal of Transcultural Nursing, 22*(3), 225–234.

Lin, K. M. (1982). Cultural aspects in mental health for Asian Americans. In A. Gaw (Ed.), *Cross-cultural psychiatry.* Boston, MA: John Wright.

Mann, F. (1972). *Acupuncture.* New York, NY: Vintage Books.

McDonnell-Smith, M. (2013). Asians are fastest-growing U.S. ethnic group, Blacks are slowest, reports U.S. Census Bureau. *DiversityInc.* Retrieved from http://www.diversityinc.com/diversity-and-inclusion/asians-are-fastest-growing-u-s-ethnic-group-in-2012-blacks-are-slowest-reports-u-s-census-bureau/

National Center for Health Statistics. (2015). *Health, United States, 2014: With special feature on adults aged 55–64.* Hyattsville, MD: Author. Retrieved from http://www.cdc.gov/nchs/data/hus/hus14.pdf

Paniagua, F. A. (2000). Culture-bound syndromes, cultural variations, and psychopathology. In I. Cuéllar & F. A. Paniagua (Eds.), *Handbook of multicultural mental health: Assessment and treatment of diverse populations* (pp. 140–141). New York, NY: Academic Press. Retrieved from https://www.msu.edu/course/sw/850/stocks/pack/u02/cltsyndr.pdf

Sai Movement. (2002). *Shri SaiBaba of Shirdi*: The perfect master of the age. Shirdi, India: *Shri SaiBaba* Trust. Retrieved from http://www.shrisaibabasans than.org/

Smith, H. (1958). *The religions of man.* New York, NY: Harper & Row.

University of Maryland Medical Center. (2014). *American ginseng.* Retrieved from http://umm.edu/health/medical/altmed/herb/american-ginseng

U.S. Department of Commerce, U.S. Census Bureau. (2014). *Quickfacts 2014.* Retrieved from http://quickfacts.census.gov/qfd/states/00000.html

U.S. Department of Health and Human Services, National Center for Complimentary and Integrative Health (NCCIH). (2015). *Ayurvedic medicine: In depth.* Retrieved from https://nccih.nih.gov/health/ayurveda/introduction.htm

Wallnöfer, H., & von Rottauscher, A. (1972). *Chinese folk medicine* (M. Palmedo, Trans.). New York, NY: American Library.

CHAPTER 11 HEALTH and ILLNESS in the Black Population

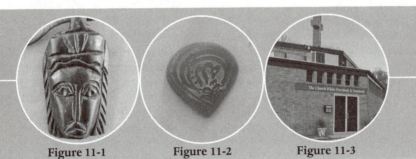

Figure 11-1   **Figure 11-2**   **Figure 11-3**

God speed the day when human blood shall cease to flow!
In every clime be understood, the claims of human brotherhood,
And each return for evil, good, not blow for blow;
That day will come all feuds to end, and change into a faithful friend each foe.

——————————————— —*Frederick Douglass, 4th of July Speech (1852)*

■ Objectives

1. Discuss the historical and demographic backgrounds of the Black or African American population.

2. Describe the traditional definitions of HEALTH and ILLNESS of the Black or African American population.

3. Explain the traditional methods of HEALING of the Black or African American population.

4. Describe the practice of a traditional HEALER.

5. Analyze current healthcare problems of the Black or African American population.

The next link in the *HERITAGECHAIN* provides an overview the historical and demographic backgrounds, HEALTH and ILLNESS traditions, and healthcare issues of the Black or African American population in the United States. Figure 11-1 is an African amulet that may be worn for HEALTH protection. Figure 11-2 is an Islamic amulet that may be worn in a satchel as a necklace or carried in a pocket or purse for HEALTH protection. Figure 11-3 is the St. George Beth El Church in Flint, Michigan. The sign over the door proclaims, "The Church Where Everybody Is Somebody."

"Black or African American" as defined in the 2010 census refers to a person having origins in any of the Black racial groups of Africa. The Black racial category includes people who marked the "Black, African American, or Negro" checkbox on the census form. It also includes respondents who marked Sub-Saharan African entries, for example, Kenya and Nigeria; and Afro-Caribbean entries such as Haiti and Jamaica. The 2013 census estimates showed that the U.S. population on April 1, 2014, was 318.9 million people, of which 44.5 million people, or 13.2%, identified as Black or African American alone. Blacks grew at a slower rate than most other major races and ethnic groups in the country. New York had the largest Black population with 3.7 million people; and Cook County, Illinois, had the largest of any county, with 1.3 million people (McDonnell-Smith, 2013).

▪ Background

"Black" is used in this chapter's text to refer to the Black or African American population, but "Black or African American" is used in content derived from government data, tables, and figures. This follows the pattern used by the Census Bureau. Most members of the present Black American community have their roots in Africa, and the majority of them descend from people who were brought here as slaves from the west coast of Africa. The largest importation of slaves occurred during the 17th century, which means that Black people have been living in the United States for many generations (Allen & Majidi-Ahi, 1989, p. 148). Presently, a number of Blacks are immigrating to the United States from African countries (such as Sudan and Ghana) and from the Dominican Republic, Haiti, and Jamaica.

Blacks are represented in every socioeconomic group; however, 3.2 million Black or African American people lived below the poverty level in 2013 (NCHS, 2015, p. 57). Furthermore, over half of Black Americans live in urban areas surrounded by the symptoms of poverty—crowded and inadequate housing, poor schools, and high crime rates. Kotlowitz (1991) described the Henry Horner Homes in Chicago as "16 high-rise buildings which stretch over eight blocks and at last census count housed 6,000 people, 4,000 of whom are children." This situation persists, and the degree of social and economic change between 1990 and 2013 has been minimal. Davis (2013) presents an in-depth exploration of the consequences of this persistent poverty and of living in these dire conditions. He writes of domestic violence, drug addiction, and street violence. He also describes methods used to turn this situation around (Davis, 2013). Genero (1995) writes of the resiliency of black families and describes how people go on with the ordinary business of everyday living—caring for the elderly, raising and educating children, celebrating festive occasions, and so forth. She points out that "daily functioning requires a high level of motivation, commitment, tenacity, and creativity" (p. 32).

According to some sources, the first Black people to enter this country arrived a year earlier than the Pilgrims, in 1619. Although the first Blacks who came to the North American continent did not come as slaves, between 1619 and 1860, more than 4 million people were transported here as slaves. One need read only a sampling of the many accounts of slavery to appreciate the tremendous hardships that the captured and enslaved people experienced during that time. Not only was the daily life of the slave very difficult, but the experience of being captured, shackled, and transported in steerage was devastating. Many of those captured in Africa died before they arrived here. The strongest and healthiest people were snatched from their homes by slave dealers and transported en masse in the holds of ships to the North American continent. In general, Black captives were not taken care of or recognized as human beings and were treated accordingly. Once here, they were sold and placed on plantations and in homes all over the country—it was only later that the practice was confined to the South. Families were separated; children were wrenched from their parents and sold to other buyers. Some slave owners bred their slaves much as farmers breed cattle today, purchasing men to serve as studs, and judging women based on whether they would produce the desired stock with a particular man (Haley, 1976). However, in the midst of all this inhuman and inhumane treatment, the Black family grew and survived. Gutman (1976), in his careful documentation of plantation and family records, traces the history of the Black family from 1750 to 1925 and points out the existence of families and family or kinship ties before and after the Civil War, dispelling many of the myths about the Black family and its structure. Despite overwhelming hardships and enforced separations, the people managed in most circumstances to maintain both family and community awareness.

The people who came to America from West Africa brought a rich variety of traditional beliefs and practices and came from religious traditions that respected the spiritual power of ancestors. They worshiped a diverse pantheon of gods who oversaw all aspects of daily life, such as the changes of the seasons, the fertility of nature, physical and spiritual personal HEALTH, and communal success. Initiation rites and naming rituals, folktales and HEALING practices, dance, song, and drumming were a part of the religious heritage. Many aspects of today's Christian religious practices are believed to have originated in these practices. For example, Catholicism and Voodoo are seen as syncretic religions. In addition, it has been estimated that between 10% and 30% of the slaves brought to America between 1711 and 1808 were Muslim.

The people brought their prayer practices, fasting and dietary practices, and their knowledge of the Qur'an (Eck, 1994).

Ostensibly, the Civil War ended slavery, but in many ways it did not emancipate Blacks. Daily life after the war was fraught with tremendous difficulty, and Black people—according to custom—were stripped of their civil rights. In the South, Black people were overtly segregated, most living in conditions of extreme hardship and poverty (Blackmon, 2008). Those who migrated to the North over the years were subject to all the problems of fragmented urban life: poverty, racism, and covert segregation (Bullough & Bullough, 1972, p. 43; Kain, 1969, pp. 1–30).

The historic problems of the Black community need to be appreciated by the healthcare provider who attempts to juxtapose modern practices and traditional health and illness beliefs. In addition, healthcare providers must be aware of the ongoing and historical events in the struggle for civil rights that affect people's lives. Box 11-1 highlights several events in the early history of this struggle. In 2007, the Supreme Court ruled in *Parents v. Seattle Schools* and *Meredith v. Jefferson Schools* that public schools cannot consider race when making student school assignments. This may be viewed as an effort to strike down *Brown v. Board of Education*, the landmark ruling of 1954. Also, in 2007, James Ford Seale, a Mississippi Klansman, was sentenced to three life terms in prison for the Moore/Dee murder of 1964. Countless race-based events have occurred since 2007, such as the killings of several black men, including: the 2012 shooting of Trayvon Martin in Florida; the fatal police shootings in 2014 of Michael Brown in Ferguson, Missouri, that led to national unrest; and the death of Eric Garner in New York City. In November 2015, the president of the University of Missouri was forced to resign when the student body and athletes united in protest over several unanswered racial insults on the campus.

It is hard to believe that nearly 60 years have passed since the teenage students known today as the "Little Rock Nine" integrated Central High School in Little Rock, Arkansas (Figure 11-4). I vividly remember the scenes on television in 1957 of nine brave teenagers, my age at the time, trying to enter the school; the cadre of hostile, angry White people spitting at them and hollering epitaphs; and the heavily armed soldiers protecting the teens. These images seared my consciousness and left an indelible imprint on my life. The activities that I accomplished each day—getting up in the morning, walking to school, attending classes, being with my friends, and so forth—were completely disrupted for the students. I remember thinking that this was not Europe; this was not Armenia, or Russia, or Germany; this was happening in "my backyard," in the United States. People who could be my neighbors violated everything that I had been taught about human dignity and respect. Two years later, my "little sister" in nursing school was one of the Little Rock Nine—I learned firsthand the damage this event wrought on her life and, I believe, on the lives of all of us. Central High School had acquired a most personal meaning.

Box 11-1

Highlights of the Civil Rights Movement

1954	*Brown v. Board of Education*—segregation in public schools found to be illegal by this landmark Supreme Court ruling
1955	Rosa Parks refuses to give up her seat on a bus in Montgomery, Alabama, and the bus boycott in Alabama begins
	Emmett Till murdered in Mississippi
1957	Central High School, Little Rock, Arkansas, integrated by the "Little Rock Nine"
1959	Sit-ins at lunch counters
1961	Segregation of interstate bus terminals ruled unconstitutional
	Freedom Riders attacked
	James Meredith is the first Black student to enroll at the University of Mississippi
1962	Civil rights movement formally organized
1963	Dr. Martin Luther King Jr. writes the seminal "Letter from Birmingham Jail," in which he argues that people have the moral duty to disobey unjust laws
	March on Washington led by Dr. Martin Luther King Jr.
1964	Killing of Charles Moore and Henry Dee
	Civil Rights Act passed
1965	Malcolm X assassinated
	Voting Rights Act is passed
1965–1968	Over 100 race riots in American cities
1968	Dr. Martin Luther King Jr. is assassinated
1991	Beating of Rodney King
1992	Major race riots in Los Angeles
1995	Million Man March
2007	*Parents v. Seattle Schools* and *Meredith v. Jefferson Schools*
	Jena, Louisiana—Black high school students held for beating a White student and tried as adults
2008	James Ford Seale convicted and sentenced to three life prison terms for his role in the Moore/Dee murders in 1964
	Senator Edward Kennedy (D-MA) introduces the Civil Rights Act of 2008, which includes provisions that ensure federal funds are not used to subsidize discrimination, holding employers accountable for age discrimination, and improving accountability for other violations of civil rights and workers' rights
2009	In the Supreme Court case *Ricci v. DeStefano*, a lawsuit brought against the city of New Haven, Connecticut, where firefighter tests to determine promotions were discarded, the Supreme Court ruled (5–4) in favor of the firefighters, saying New Haven's "action in discarding the tests was a violation of Title VII of the Civil Rights Act of 1964"
2013	The Voting Rights Act of 1965 came under fire, and the Supreme Court invalidated sections of it (Barnes, 2013).

Source: E. Brunner and E. Haney, *Civil Rights Timeline: Milestones in the Modern Civil Rights Movement.* © 2000–2012. Reprinted by permission of Pearson Education, Inc., Upper Saddle River, New Jersey.

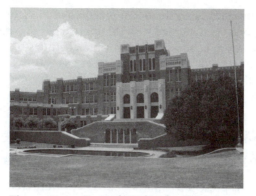

**Figure 11-4   Central High School, Little
Rock, Arkansas.**

■ Traditional Definitions of HEALTH and ILLNESS

According to Jacques (1976), the traditional definition of HEALTH stems from the African belief about life and the nature of being. To the African, life was a process rather than a state. The nature of a person was viewed in terms of energy force rather than matter. All things, whether living or dead, were believed to influence one another. Therefore, one had the power to influence one's destiny and that of others through the use of behavior, whether proper or otherwise, as well as through knowledge of the person and the world. When one possessed HEALTH, one was in harmony with nature; ILLNESS was a state of disharmony. Traditional Black belief regarding HEALTH did not separate the mind, body, and spirit.

Disharmony—that is, ILLNESS—was attributed to a number of sources, primarily demons and evil spirits. These spirits were generally believed to act of their own accord, and the goal of treatment was to remove them from the body of the ILL person. Several methods were employed to attain this result, in addition to voodoo, which is discussed in the next section. The traditional healers, usually women, possessed extensive knowledge of the use of herbs and roots in the treatment of ILLNESS. Apparently, an early form of smallpox immunization was used by slaves. Women practiced inoculation by scraping a piece of cowpox crust into a place on a child's arm. These children appeared to have a far lower incidence of smallpox than those who did not receive the immunization.

The old and the young were cared for by all members of the community. The elderly were held in high esteem because African people believed that the living of a long life indicated that a person had the opportunity to acquire much wisdom and knowledge. Death was described as the passing from one realm of life to another (Jacques, 1976, p. 117) or as a passage from the evils of this world to another state. The funeral was often celebrated as a joyous occasion, with a party after the burial. Children were passed over the body of the deceased, so that the dead person could carry any potential illness of the child away with him or her.

Many of the preventive and treatment practices of Black people have their roots in Africa but have been merged with the approaches of Native Americans, to whom the Blacks were exposed, and with the attitudes of Whites, among whom they lived and served. Then, as today, ILLNESS was treated in a combination of ways. Methods found to be most useful were handed down through the generations.

■ Traditional Methods of HEALTH Maintenance and Protection

The following sections present examples of practices employed presently or in earlier generations to maintain and protect HEALTH and to treat various types of maladies to restore HEALTH. This discussion cannot encompass all the types of care given to and by the members of the Black community but instead presents a sample of the richness of the traditional HEALTH practices that have survived over the years.

Essentially, HEALTH is maintained with proper diet—that is, eating three nutritious meals a day, including a hot breakfast. Rest and a clean environment also are important. Laxatives were and are used to keep the system "running" or "open."

Asafetida is a rotten gum resin that looks like a dried-out sponge and has an unforgettable vile odor that is worn around the neck to prevent contagious diseases. Cod liver oil is taken to prevent colds. A sulfur-and-molasses preparation is used in the spring because it is believed that at the start of a new season, people are more susceptible to illness. This preparation may be rubbed up and down the back or taken internally to cleanse the intestines. A physician is not consulted routinely and is not generally regarded as the person to whom one goes for the prevention of disease.

Copper or silver bracelets may be worn around the wrist from the time a woman is a baby or young child. These bracelets are believed to protect the wearer as she grows. If for any reason these bracelets are removed, harm befalls the owner. In addition to granting protection, these bracelets indicate when the wearer is about to become ill: the skin around the bracelet turns black, alerting the woman to take precautions against the impending illness. These precautions consist of getting extra rest, praying more frequently, and eating a more nutritious diet.

■ Traditional Methods of HEALTH Restoration

The most common method of treating ILLNESS is prayer. The laying on of hands is described quite frequently. Rooting, a practice derived from voodoo, also is mentioned by many people. In rooting, a person (usually a woman who is known as a "root-worker") is consulted as to the source of a given ILLNESS, and she then prescribes the appropriate treatment. Magic rituals often are employed (Davis, 1998).

The following home remedies have been reported by some Black people as being successful in the treatment of disease:

1. Sugar and turpentine are mixed together and taken by mouth to get rid of worms. This combination can also be used to cure a backache when rubbed on the skin from the navel to the back.

2. Numerous types of poultices are employed to fight infection and inflammation. The poultices are placed on the part of the body that is painful or infected to draw out the cause of the affliction. One type of poultice is made of potatoes. The potatoes are sliced or grated and placed in a bag, which is placed on the affected area of the body. The potatoes turn black; as this occurs, the disease goes away. It is believed that, as these potatoes spoil, they produce a penicillin mold that is able to destroy the infectious organism. Another type of poultice is prepared from cornmeal and peach leaves, which are cooked together and placed either in a bag or in a piece of flannel cloth. The cornmeal ferments and combines with an enzyme in the peach leaves to produce an antiseptic that destroys the bacteria and hastens the healing process. A third poultice, made with onions, is used to heal infections, and a flaxseed poultice is used to treat earaches.

3. Herbs from the woods are used in many ways. Herb teas are prepared—for example, from goldenrod root—to treat pain and reduce fevers. Sassafras tea frequently is used to treat colds. Another herb boiled to make a tea is the root or leaf of rabbit tobacco.

4. Bluestone, a mineral found in the ground, is used as medicine for open wounds. The stone is crushed into a powder and sprinkled on the affected area. It prevents inflammation and is used to treat poison ivy.

5. To treat a "crick" in the neck, two pieces of silverware are crossed over the painful area in the form of an X.

6. Ingest nine drops of turpentine on a sugar cube 9 days after intercourse as a contraceptive.

7. Cuts and wounds can be treated with sour or spoiled milk that is placed on stale bread, wrapped in a cloth, and placed on the wound.

8. Salt and pork (salt pork) placed on a rag can be used to treat cuts and wounds.

9. A sprained ankle can be treated by placing clay in a dark leaf and wrapping it around the ankle.

10. A remedy for treating colds is hot lemon water with honey.

11. When congestion is present in the chest and the person is coughing, the chest is rubbed with hot camphorated oil and wrapped with warm flannel.

12. An expectorant for colds consists of chopped raw garlic, chopped onion, fresh parsley, and a little water, all mixed in a blender.

13. Hot toddies are used to treat colds and congestion. These drinks consist of hot tea with honey, lemon, peppermint, and a dash of brandy or whatever alcoholic beverage the person likes and is available. Vicks Vaporub also is swallowed.

14. A fever can be broken by placing raw onions on the feet and wrapping the feet in warm blankets.

15. Boils are treated by cracking a raw egg, peeling the white skin off the inside of the shell, and placing it on the boil. This brings the boil to a head.

16. Garlic can be placed on the ill person or in the room to remove the "evil spirits" that have caused the illness.

Folk Medicine

In many traditional Black communities, folk medicine previously practiced in Africa may still be employed. The methods have been tried and tested and are still relied on. HEALERS or voodoo practitioners make no class or status distinctions among their patients, treating everyone fairly and honestly. This tradition of equality of care and perceived effectiveness accounts for the faith placed in the practices of the HEALER and in other methods. In fact, the home remedies used by some members of the Black community have been employed for many generations. Another reason for their ongoing use is that hospitals are distant from people who live in rural areas. By the time they might get to the hospital, they would be dead, yet many of the people who continue to use these remedies live in urban areas close to hospitals—sometimes even world-renowned hospitals. Nonetheless, the use of folk medicine persists, and many people avoid the local hospital except in extreme emergencies.

Traditional Methods of HEALING

Voodoo, or Voudou.   *Voodoo,* or American voudou, is a belief system often alluded to but rarely described in any detail (Davis, 1998). At various times, patients may mention terms such as *fix, hex,* or *spell.* It is not clear whether voodoo is fully practiced today, but there is some evidence in the literature that there are people who still believe and practice it to some extent (Wintrob, 1972). It also has been reported that many Black people continue to fear voodoo and believe that when they become ILL they have been "fixed." Voodoo involves two forms of magic: white magic, described as harmless; and black magic, which is quite dangerous. Belief in magic is, of course, ancient (Hughes & Bontemps, 1958, pp. 184–185).

Voodoo came to this country about 1724, with the arrival of slaves from the West African coast, who had been sold initially in the West Indies. The people who brought voodoo with them were "snake worshippers." Vodu, the name of their god, with the passage of time became *voodoo* (also *hoodoo*), an all-embracing term that included the god, the sect, the members of the sect, the priests and priestesses, the rites and practices, and the teaching (Tallant, 1946, p. 19). Leaders of the voodoo sect tended to be women, and stories abound in New Orleans about the workings of the sect and the women who ruled it—such as Marie Laveau.

In 1850, the practice of voodoo reached its height in New Orleans. At that time, the beliefs and practices of voodoo were closely related to beliefs about HEALTH and ILLNESS. For example, many ILLNESSES were attributed to a "fix" that was placed on one person out of anger. Gris-gris, the symbols of voodoo, were used to prevent ILLNESS or to give ILLNESS to others. Some examples of commonly used gris-gris follow (Tallant, 1946, p. 226):

1. *Good gris-gris:* powders and oils that are highly and pleasantly scented. The following are examples of good gris-gris: love powder, colored and scented with perfume; love oil, olive oil to which gardenia perfume has been added; and luck water, ordinary water that is purchased in many shades (red is for success in love, yellow for success in money matters, blue for protection and friends).

2. *Bad gris-gris:* oils and powders that have a vile odor. The following are examples of bad gris-gris: anger powder, war powder, and moving powder, which are composed of soil, gunpowder, and black pepper, respectively.

3. *Flying devil oil:* olive oil that has red coloring and cayenne pepper added to it.

4. *Black cat oil:* machine oil.

In addition to these oils and powders, a variety of colored candles, as in Figure 11-5, are used; the color of the candle symbolizes the intention. For

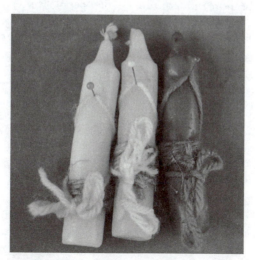

Figure 11-5   Voodoo candles.

example, white symbolizes peace; red, victory; pink, love; yellow, driving off enemies; brown, attracting money; and black, doing evil work and bringing bad luck (Tallant, 1946, p. 226).

There are a number of Catholic saints or relics to whom or to which the practitioners of voodoo attribute special powers. Portraits of Saint Michael, who makes possible the conquest of enemies; Saint Anthony de Padua, who brings luck; Saint Mary Magdalene, who is popular with women who are in love; the Virgin Mary, whose presence in the home prevents illness; and the Sacred Heart of Jesus, which cures organic illness, may be prominently displayed in the homes of people who believe in voodoo (Tallant, 1946, p. 228). These gris-gris are available today and can be purchased in stores in many American cities.

Other Practices

Many Blacks believe in the power of some people to HEAL and help others, and there are many reports of numerous HEALERS among the communities. This reliance on HEALERS reflects the deep religious faith of the people. (Maya Angelou vividly describes this phenomenon in her book *I Know Why the Caged Bird Sings*.) For example, many Blacks followed the Pentecostal movement long before its present more general popularity. Similarly, people often went to tent meetings and had an all-consuming belief in the HEALING powers of religion.

Another practice takes on significance when one appreciates its historical background: the eating of Argo starch. "Geophagy," or eating clay and dirt, occurred among the slaves, who brought the practice to this country from Africa. In *Roots*, Haley (1976) mentions that pregnant women were given clay because it was believed to be beneficial to both the mother and the unborn child (p. 32). In fact, red clays are rich in iron. When clay was not available, dirt was substituted. In more modern times, when people were no longer living on farms and no longer had access to clay and dirt, Argo starch became the substitute (Dunstin, 1969). The following was reported by a former student:

> It was my fortune, or misfortune to be born into a family that practiced geophagy (earth eating) and pica (eating Argo laundry starch). Even before I became pregnant I showed an interest in eating starch. It was sweet and dry, and I could take it or leave it. After I became pregnant, I found I wanted not only starch, but bread, grits, and potatoes. I found I craved starchy substances. I stuck to starchy substances and dropped the Argo because it made me feel sluggish and heavy.

It is believed that anemia arose from this practice of substituting non–iron-rich clays or starch for red clays that contain iron.

Many Black Americans and new immigrants from African countries are Muslims. Box 11-2 presents an overview of Islam and information that health-care providers in all settings should know.

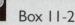

Box 11-2

Black Muslims

There about 5.5 million Muslims in the United States, and 511,000 households. Many members of the Black community are practicing Muslims. The religion of Islam is the acceptance of and obedience to the teachings of God, which He revealed to His last prophet, Muhammad. The Five Pillars of Islam are the framework of Muslim life. They are the testimony of faith, prayer, giving *zakat* (support of the needy), fasting during the month of Ramadan, and the pilgrimage to Mecca once in a lifetime for those who are able.

The people may be descendants of the earlier people who were Muslims and came to America as slaves, or they may have chosen to convert to Islam. It is difficult to generalize in any way about American Muslims because the people come from all walks of life—converts, immigrants, factory workers, doctors, professionals, and so forth. In addition, there are many African immigrants from countries such as the Sudan who are practicing Muslims, and countless people from Islamic countries are seeking healthcare services in the United States. The community is unified by a common faith.

Religious beliefs are an important part of the Muslim lifestyle, and healthcare providers should be familiar with them:

- Muslims are taught that a "person is what he or she eats." Islamic dietary restrictions consist of eating a strictly Halal diet, and a newly admitted patient who refuses to eat should be asked if the hospital's ordinary diet interferes with his or her religious beliefs. The rules of a Halal diet include not eating pork or any pork products (such as nonbeef hamburger and ham). Islamic law teaches that certain foods affect the way a person thinks and acts. Therefore, one's diet should consist of food that has a clean, positive effect. Muslims do not drink alcohol because they feel that it dulls the senses and causes illness. Halal foods are produced using equipment that is cleansed according to Islamic law.
- Muslims pray five times a day. Each prayer does not take more than a few minutes and is offered at dawn, noon, midafternoon, sunset, and night. Prayer may take place in almost any setting, such as in fields, offices, factories, universities, or hospitals. Prayer in Islam is a direct link between the worshipper and God. Before a person prays, he or she must be clean and the hands and feet are washed. Prayers are generally said in a prostrate position on a carpet on the floor.
- Muslims fast for a 30-day period during the year (fast of Ramadan). Ramadan is a special time—a month of prayer and repentance. Nothing is taken by mouth from just before sunrise until after sundown. Muslims who are ill, small children, and pregnant women are exempt from this rule. When a person is following the fast, institutions must provide the environment for the safe observance of the practice.

(continued)

Box 11-2   *(continued)*

There is also a practice of modesty, with women covering their heads with scarves, *hijabs*, and wearing long dresses, *jibabs*. The need for gender-specific care—that is, males caring for male patients and females caring for female patients—must be adhered to.

The Muslim lifestyle is strictly regulated. According to those who have practiced the religion for many generations, this stems in part from the need for self-discipline, which many Black people have not had because of living conditions associated with urban decay and family disintegration. Muslims believe in self-help and assist in uplifting each other. The Muslim lifestyle is not so rigid that the people do not have good times. Good times, however, are tempered with the realization that too much indulgence in sport and play can present problems. To Muslims, life is precious: if a person needs a transfusion to live, it will be accepted. Because of the avoidance of pork or pork products, however, it is important to understand that a Muslim with diabetes will refuse to take insulin that has a pork base. If the insulin is manufactured from the pancreas of a pig, it is considered unclean and will not be accepted. There are preparations of insulin and/or other products that can be prescribed.

Many Muslim communities differ in their practice and philosophy of Islam. Members of some communities dress in distinctive clothing—for example, the women wear long skirts and a covering on the head at all times. Other communities are less strict about dress. Some adherents do not follow the Halal diet and are allowed to drink alcoholic beverages in moderation.

Sources: A Brief Illustrated Guide to Understanding Islam, by I. A. Ibrahim, 1996, Houston, TX: Darussalam, retrieved from http://www.islam-guide.com/, November 24, 2015; *The Religion of Islam*, by Office of Dawah, 2006–2008, Rawdah: Author, retrieved from http://www.islamreligion .com/, November 24, 2015; and *Arab Households in the United States 2006–2010*, by M. Asi and D. Beaulieu, 2013, retrieved from http://www.census.gov/library/publications/2013/acs /acsbr10-20.html, November 24, 2015.

■ Current Health Problems

Health Differences Between Black and White Populations

Morbidity.   Many Black people experience wide, deep health disparities—factors such as the lack of access to health services, low income, and a tendency to self-treat illness and to wait until symptoms are so severe that a doctor must be seen (Weissman et al., 2011). Table 11-1 compares selected health status indicators for Blacks or African Americans and all races. It illustrates that the birth rate is higher, the percentage of teenage births to women aged 18–19 is higher, the percentage of low birth weight babies is higher, and the infant mortality rate is double that of all races (NCHS, 2015).

Sickle-cell Anemia.   The sickling of red blood cells is a genetically inherited trait that is hypothesized to have originally been an African adaptation to fight

Table 11-1   Comparison of Selected Health Status Indicators: 2013 All Races
and Black or African Americans

Health Indicator	All Races	Black or African American
Crude birth rate per 1,000 population by race of mother, 2013	12.4	**14.5**
Percentage of live births to teenage childbearing women—18–19 years, 2013	5.0	7.6
Percentage of low birth weight per live births >2,500 grams, 2013	8.02	12.76
Infant mortality per 1,000 live births, 2012	6.0	**10.9**
Respondent-reported prevalence percent of adults: Cancer—all sites, 2010–2013, 18 years and over	5.9	4.8
Respondent-reported prevalence percent of adults: Heart Disease—2012–2013, 18 years and over	10.6	10.7
Respondent-reported prevalence percent of adults: Stroke—2012–2013, 18 years and over	2.5	3.7
Male death rates from suicide, all ages, age adjusted per 100,000 resident population, 2013	20.3	9.3
Male death rates from homicide, all ages, age adjusted per 100,000 resident population, 1999–2003	8.2	**31.6**

Source: Health, United States, 2014: With Special Feature on Adults Aged 55–64, by National Center for Health Statistics, 2015, Hyattsville, MD: Author, pp. 58, 61, 64, 76, 134, 135, 138, 139, 161.

malaria. This condition occurs in Africans/Blacks and causes the normal, disk-like red blood cell to assume a sickle shape. Sickling results in hemolysis and thrombosis of red blood cells because these deformed cells do not flow properly through the blood vessels. Sickle-cell disease comprises the following blood characteristics:

1. The presence of two hemoglobin-S genes (Hb SS)
2. The presence of the hemoglobin-S gene with another abnormal hemoglobin gene (e.g., Hb SC, Hb SD)
3. The presence of the hemoglobin-S gene with a different abnormality in hemoglobin synthesis.

Some people (carriers) have the sickle-cell trait (Hb SS, Hb SC, or others) but do not experience symptoms of the disease.

The clinical manifestations of sickle-cell disease include hemolysis, anemia, and states of sickle-cell crises, in which severe pain occurs in the areas of the body where the thrombosed red cells are located. The cells also tend to clump in abdominal organs, such as the liver and the spleen. At present, statistics indicate that only 50% of children with sickle-cell disease live to adulthood. Some children die before the age of 20, and some suffer chronic, irreversible complications during their lifetime (NHLBI, 2015a).

Sickle-cell anemia can occur only when two people who carry sickle-cell trait have a child together. It is possible to detect the sickle-cell trait in healthy adults and to provide genetic counseling about their risk of bearing children with the disease. However, for many people, this is not an option. The cost of genetic counseling, for example, may be prohibitive (NHLBI, 2015b).

Mortality.   Blacks born in 2000 in the United States will live, on average, 5.7 fewer years than Whites. The life expectancy for a Black person born in 2007 was 73.6 years, whereas for a White person born in 2007, it was 78.4 years.

The leading three chronic diseases that are causes of death for African Americans are the same as those for all persons, but the mortality rates are greater in other diseases. For example:

- Unintentional injuries are the 4th leading cause of death in the Black or African population, 5th among all persons.
- Diabetes mellitus is the 5th leading cause of death in the Black or African population and is 7th among all persons.
- Homicide is the 6th leading cause of death in the Black or African population and is not noted as one of the 10 leading causes of death for all persons.
- Human immunodeficiency virus (HIV) disease is the 9th leading cause of death in the Black or African population and is not noted as one of the 10 leading causes of death for all persons (NCHS, 2015).

Another critical factor is that there are 1.5 million missing Black men between the ages of 25 and 54, and there are only 83 Black men for every 100 Black women not in jail. The largest gap is in Ferguson, Missouri, where there are 40 missing Black men for every 100 Black women. The men are missing either because of early death or because of incarceration. This absence has profound implications because it disrupts family formation, in that marriage rates are lower and rates of childbirth are higher out of marriage (Wolfers, Leonhardt, & Quealy, 2015). Black women are more than three times as likely as White women to be incarcerated in prison or jail. More than two thirds of Black children have at least one or both parents under some form of community or correctional supervision (Gaston, 2015). Table 11-2 lists the 10 leading causes of death for Black Americans and compares them with the causes of death for the general population in 2013.

Mental Health

The family often has a matriarchal structure, and there are many single-parent households headed by females, but there are strong and large extended family networks. There is a continuation of tradition and a strong church affiliation within the families and community. Members of the community may be treated by a traditional Voodoo priest, the "Old Lady" ("granny" or "Mrs. Markus"), or other traditional healers, and herbs are frequently used to treat mental symptoms. Several diagnostic techniques include the use of biblical phrases and/or

Table 11-2   Comparison of the 10 Leading Causes of Death for Black or African
American and for All Persons, 2014

Black or African American	All Persons
1. Diseases of heart	1. Diseases of heart
2. Malignant neoplasms	2. Malignant neoplasms
3. Cerebrovascular diseases	3. Cerebrovascular diseases
4. Unintentional injuries	4. Chronic lower respiratory diseases
5. Diabetes mellitus	5. Unintentional injuries
6. Chronic lower respiratory diseases	6. Alzheimer's disease
7. Nephritis, nephrotic syndrome, and	7. Diabetes mellitus
nephrosis influenza and pneumonia	8. Influenza and pneumonia
8. Homicide	9. Nephritis, nephrotic syndrome, and
9. Septicemia	nephrosis
10. Alzheimer's disease	10. Septicemia

Source: Health, United States, 2014: With Special Feature on Adults Aged 55–64, by National Center for Health Statistics, 2015, Hyattsville, MD: Author, p. 97.

material from old folk-medical books, observation, and/or entering the spirit of the patient. The therapeutic measures include various rituals, such as the reading of bones, the wearing of special garments, or some rituals from voodoo (Spurlock, 1988, p. 173). In addition, there are countless culture-bound mental HEALTH syndromes that may be identified in the Black community:

■ West Africa and Haiti—*Boufée delirante*—the sudden outburst of agitated and aggressive behavior, confusion, or occasional hallucinations

■ Southern United States and Caribbean groups—Falling-Out—sudden collapse without warning

■ North African countries—Zar—person is possessed by a spirit and may shout, weep, laugh, hit his or her head against the wall, or sing

■ West Africa—Brain Fog—physical and mental exhaustion, difficulty concentrating, memory loss, irritability, and sleeping and appetite problems (Fontaine, 2003, p. 119).

Blacks and the Healthcare System

To some, receiving healthcare is all too often a degrading and humiliating experience. Some Blacks fear or resent health clinics. When they have a clinic appointment, they usually lose a day's work because they have to be at the clinic at an early hour and often spend many hours waiting to be seen by a physician. They often receive inadequate care, are told what their problem is in incomprehensible medical jargon, and are not given an identity, being seen rather as a body segment ("the appendix in treatment room A"). Such an experience creates a tremendous feeling of powerlessness and alienation from the system. In some parts of the country, segregation and racism are overt. In light of this situation, it is no wonder that some Black people prefer to use time-tested home remedies rather than be exposed to the humiliating experiences of hospitalization.

Another reason for the ongoing use of home remedies is poverty. Indigent people cannot afford the high costs of American healthcare. Quite often—even with the help of Medicaid, Medicare, and provisions of the Affordable Care Act—the hidden costs of acquiring health services, such as absence from work, transportation, and/or child care, are a heavy burden. As a result, Blacks may stay away from clinics or outpatient departments or receive their care with passivity while appearing to the provider to be evasive. Some Black patients believe that they are being talked down to by healthcare providers and that the providers fail to listen to them. They choose, consequently, to "suffer in silence." Many of the problems that Blacks relate in dealing with the healthcare system can apply to anyone, but the inherent racism within the health system cannot be denied. Currently, efforts are being made to overcome these barriers, and since the 1960s, and the passage of the Affordable Care Act, healthcare services available to Blacks and other people of color have improved. A growing number of community health centers have emphasized health maintenance and promotion, and community residents serve on the boards.

Among the services provided by community health centers is an effort to discover children with high blood levels of lead in order to provide early diagnosis of and treatment for lead poisoning. Once a child is found to have lead poisoning, the law requires that the source of the lead be found and eradicated. Only apartments free of lead paint can be rented to families with young children. Apartments that are found to have lead paint must be stripped and repainted with nonlead paint. Lead poisoning is an environmental disease, and its long-term consequences are a public health crisis for African Americans (Needleman, 1999). For example, Freddie Gray, the young man who died in police custody in Baltimore, was one of thousands of children in Baltimore with toxic levels of lead in their blood. This resulted from years of living in substandard housing. Behavior problems, ADHD, and irreversible brain and central nervous damage can result from lead poisoning (Schumaker & Schelier, 2015).

Lead poisoning continues to be a serious health issue. It has become a critical problem in Flint, Michigan, due to contaminated drinking water. Flint's population is 56% Black, with an infant mortality rate of 38/100,000 (22 of every 38 being Black babies), and a poverty rate of 39.7% (Spector, 2014). In April 2014, the state changed the water supplying the city of Flint from a clean, potable, pristine water source to contaminated water from the Flint River. It quickly became apparent that residents drinking the water were becoming ill with rashes, but it was not until the fall of 2015 that officials confirmed the water was contaminated with lead. By that time, the blood lead levels in young children were rising, and more lead had leached into the water from corroded lead water pipes. The children, the poor, the elderly, and the Black community are the people most harmed by this event (Smith, 2016).

Another ongoing effort by the community health centers is to inform Blacks who are at risk of producing children with sickle-cell anemia that they are carriers of this genetic disease. This program is fraught with conflict because many people prefer not to be screened for the sickle-cell trait, fearing they may become labeled once the tendency is discovered.

Birth control is another problem that is recognized with mixed emotions. To some, especially women who want to space children or who do not want to have numerous children, birth control is a welcome development. People who believe in birth control prefer selecting the time when they will have children, how many children they will have, and when they will stop having children. To many other people, birth control is considered a form of "Black genocide" and a way of limiting the growth of the community. Health workers in the Black community must be aware of both sides of this issue and, if asked to make a decision, remain neutral. Such decisions must be made by the patients themselves.

Special Considerations for Healthcare Providers

White healthcare providers know far too little about how to care for a Black person's skin or hair, or how to understand both Black nonverbal and verbal behavior.

Physiological Assessment. Examples of possible physiological problems include the following (in observing skin problems, it is important to note that skin assessment is best done in indirect sunlight) (Bloch & Hunter, 1981):

1. *Pallor.* There is an absence of underlying red tones; the skin of a brown-skinned person appears yellow-brown, and that of a black-skinned person appears ashen gray. Mucous membranes appear ashen, and the lips and nailbeds are similar.

2. *Erythema.* Inflammation must be detected by palpation; the skin is warmer in the area, tight, and edematous, and the deeper tissues are hard. Fingertips must be used for this assessment, as with rashes, since they are sensitive to the feeling of different textures of skin.

3. *Cyanosis.* Cyanosis is difficult to observe in dark-colored skin, but it can be seen by close inspection of the lips, tongue, conjunctiva, palms of the hands, and soles of the feet. One method of testing is pressing the palms. Slow blood return is an indication of cyanosis. Another sign is ashen-gray lips and tongue.

4. *Ecchymosis.* History of trauma to a given area can be detected from a swelling of the skin surface.

5. *Jaundice.* The sclera are usually observed for yellow discoloration to reveal jaundice. This is not always a valid indication, however, since carotene deposits can also cause the sclera to appear yellow. The buccal mucosa and the palms of the hands and soles of the feet may appear yellow.

Several skin conditions are of importance in Black patients (Sykes & Kelly, 1979):

1. *Keloids.* Keloids are scars that form at the site of a wound and grow beyond the normal boundaries of the wound. They are sharply elevated and irregular and continue to enlarge.

2. *Pigmentary disorders.* Pigmentary disorders, areas of either postinflammatory hypopigmentation or hyperpigmentation, appear as dark or light spots.

3. *Pseudofolliculitis.* "Razor bumps" and "ingrown hairs" are caused by shaving too closely with an electric razor or straight razor. The sharp point of the hair, if shaved too closely, enters the skin and induces an immune response as to a foreign body. The symptoms include papules, pustules, and sometimes even keloids.

4. *Melasma.* The "mask of pregnancy," melasma, is a patchy tan to dark-brown discoloration of the face more prevalent in dark pregnant women.

Hair Care Needs.   The care of the hair of Blacks is not complicated, but special consideration must be given to help maintain its healthy condition (Bloch & Hunter, 1981):

1. The hair's dryness or oiliness must·be assessed, as well as its texture (straight or extra curly) and the patient's hairstyle preference.

2. The hair must be shampooed as needed and groomed according to the person's preference.

3. Hair must be combed well, with the appropriate tools, such as a "pic" or comb with big teeth, before drying to prevent tangles.

4. If the hair is dry and needs oiling, the preparations that the person generally uses for this purpose ought to be on hand.

5. Once dry, the hair is ready to be styled (curled, braided, or rolled) as the person desires.

Additional Considerations.   The majority of the members of the healthcare profession are steeped in a middle-class White value system. In clinical settings, providers are being helped to become familiar with and understand the value systems of other ethnic and socioeconomic groups. They are being taught to recognize the symptoms of illness in Blacks and to provide proper skin and hair care. The following are guidelines that a healthcare provider can follow in caring for members of the Black community:

1. The education of an ever-increasing number of Blacks in the health professions must continue to be encouraged.

2. The needs of the patient and family must be assessed realistically.

3. When a treatment or special diet is prescribed, every attempt must be made to ascertain whether it is consistent with the patient's physical needs, cultural background, income, and religious practices.

4. The patient's belief in and practice of folk medicine must be respected; the patient must not be criticized for these beliefs. Every effort should be made to assist the patient to combine folk treatment with standard Western treatment, as long as the two are not antagonistic. Many people who have a strong belief in folk remedies continue to use them with or without medical sanction.

5. Providers should be familiar with formal and informal sources of help in the Black community. The formal sources consist of churches, social clubs, and community groups. The informal ones include the men and women who provide assistance and care for members of their community in an informal way.

6. The beliefs and values of the healthcare provider should not be forced on the patient.

7. The treatment plan and the reasons for a given treatment must be shared with the patient in an understandable manner.

This chapter has presented an all-too-brief overview of health and illness issues in the Black or African American community by examining the historical and demographic backgrounds, HEALTH and ILLNESS traditions, and healthcare issues the community experiences.

RESEARCH ON CULTURE

A large amount of research has been conducted among members of the Black population. The study described in the following article is one example:

Wilson, D. W. (2007). From their own voices: The lived experience of African American registered nurses. *Journal of Transcultural Nursing, 18*(2), 142–149.

This phenomenological study describes the lived experiences of African American nurses who provide care to individuals, families, and communities in southeast Louisiana. The sample consisted of 13 nurses whose ages ranged from 40 to 62, with an average age of 49.53. Their nursing experience ranged from 8 to 39 years and they were educated in ad, diploma, and baccalaureate programs. Four of the informants had earned master's degrees in nursing. The essential themes found in the study were that the participants' experiences included connecting with the patients through the delivery of holistic nursing care and "proving yourself." Holistic care included respect for the patients' cultural backgrounds and the realization that in many ways they were vitally important in meeting the needs of the patients and families. They believed that they were also important in meeting the spiritual and religious needs of patients. The nurses also participated in patient teaching and advocacy. The incidental themes included fulfilling a dream, being invisible and voiceless, surviving and persevering, and mentoring and role modeling. The author recommends that, if the nursing profession is to promote nursing care that is congruent with the needs of culturally diverse patients, it must increase the representation of African American registered nurses.

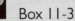

Explore MediaLink

Go to the Student Resource Site at pearsonhighered.com/nursingresources for chapter-related review questions, case studies, and activities. Contents of the CULTURALCARE Guide and CULTURALCARE Museum can also be found on the Student Resource Site. Click on Chapter 11 to select the activities for this chapter.

Box 11-3

Keeping Up

It goes without saying that much of the data presented in this chapter may be out of date when you read this text. However, at this final stage of writing, it is the most recent information available. The following resources will be most helpful in keeping you abreast of the frequent changes in healthcare events, costs, and policies:

1. The National Center for Health Statistics publishes *Health, United States*, an annual report on trends in health statistics.
2. Health-related data and other statistics are available from the Centers for Disease Control and Prevention (CDC).
3. The Substance Abuse and Mental Health Services Administration (SAMHSA) provides information regarding several topics, including behavioral health equity for blacks or African Americans, mental illness, drug misuse, and suicide prevention.

◼ References

Allen, L., & Majidi-Ahi, S. (1989). Black American children. In J. T. Gibbs (Ed.), *Children of color*. San Francisco, CA: Jossey-Bass.

Asi, M., & Beaulieu, D. (2013). *Arab households in the United States 2006–2010*. Retrieved from http://www.census.gov/library/publications/2013/acs/acsbr10-20.html

Barnes, R. (2013). Supreme Court stops key part of Voting Rights Act. *The Washington Post*. Retrieved from https://www.washingtonpost.com/politics/supreme-court-stops-use-of-key-part-of-voting-rights-act/2013/06/25/26888528-dda5-11e2-b197-f248b21f94c4_story.html

Blackmon, D. A. (2008). *Slavery by another name*. New York, NY: Doubleday.

Bloch, B., & Hunter, M. L. (1981, January–February). Teaching physiological assessment of Black persons. *Nurse Educator*, 26.

Bullough, B., & Bullough, V. L. (1972). *Poverty, ethnic identity, and health care*. New York, NY: Appleton-Century-Crofts.

Brunner, B., & Haney, E. (2009). *Civil rights timeline: Milestones in the modern civil rights movement*. Upper Saddle River, NJ: Pearson Education. Retrieved from http://www.infoplease.com/spot/civilrightstimeline1.html

Davis, R. (1998). *American voudou—Journey into a hidden world*. Denton: University of North Texas Press.

Davis, S. (2013). *Living and dying in brick city*. New York, NY: Spiegel & Grau.

Dunstin, B. (1969). Pica during pregnancy. Chap. 26 in *Current concepts in clinical nursing*. St. Louis, MO: Mosby.

Eck, D. (1994). *African religion in America: On common ground*. New York, NY: Columbia University Press.

Fontaine, K. L. (2003). *Mental health nursing* (5th ed.). Upper Saddle River, NJ: Prentice Hall.

Gaston, H. K. (2015). Mass incarceration's impact on black and Latino women and children. *Huffington Post Black Voices*. Retrieved from http://www.huffingtonpost.com/herron-keyon-gaston/mass-incarcerations-impact-black-latino_b_6702900.html

Genero, N. P. (1995). Culture, resiliency, and mutual psychological development. In H. A. McCubbin, E. A. Thompson, A. I. Thompson, & J. A. Futrell (Eds.), *Resiliency in ethnic minority families* (Vol. 2). Madison: University of Wisconsin System.

Gutman, H. G. (1976). *The Black family in slavery and freedom, 1750–1925*. New York, NY: Pantheon.

Haley, A. (1976). *Roots*. New York, NY: Doubleday.

Hughes, L., & Bontemps, A. (Eds.). (1958). *The book of negro folklore*. New York, NY: Dodd, Mead.

Ibrahim, I. A. (1996). *A brief illustrated guide to understanding Islam*. Houston, TX: Darussalam. Retrieved from http://www.islam-guide.com/

Jacques, G. (1976). Cultural health traditions: A Black perspective. In M. Branch & P. P. Paxton (Eds.), *Providing safe nursing care for ethnic people of color*. New York, NY: Appleton-Century-Crofts.

Kain, J. F. (Ed.). (1969). *Race and poverty*. Englewood Cliffs, NJ: Prentice Hall.

Kotlowitz, A. (1991). *There are no children here: The story of two boys growing up in the other America*. New York, NY: Doubleday.

McDonnell-Smith, M. (2013). Asians are fastest-growing U.S. ethnic group, Blacks are slowest, reports U.S. Census Bureau. *DiversityInc*. Retrieved from http://www.diversityinc.com/diversity-and-inclusion/asians-are-fastest-growing-u-s-ethnic-group-in-2012-blacks-are-slowest-reports-u-s-census-bureau/

National Center for Health Statistics (NCHS). (2015). *Health, United States, 2014: With special feature on adults aged 55–64*. Hyattsville, MD: Author. Retrieved from http://www.cdc.gov/nchs/data/hus/hus14.pdf

National Heart, Lung, and Blood Institute (NHLBI). (2015a). *What is sickle cell disease?* Retrieved from http://www.nhlbi.nih.gov/health/health-topics/topics/sca

National Heart, Lung, and Blood Institute (NHLBI). (2015b). *How can sickle cell disease be prevented?* Retrieved from http://www.nhlbi.nih.gov/health/health-topics/topics/sca/prevention

Needleman, H. L (1999). *History of lead poisoning in the world*. Retrieved from http://www.biologicaldiversity.org/campaigns/get_the_lead_out/pdfs/health/Needleman_1999.pdf

Office of Dawah. (2006–2008). *The religion of Islam*. Rawdah: Author. Retrieved from http://www.islamreligion.com/

Schumaker, E., & Schelier, A. (2015). Lead poisoning is still a public health crisis for African-Americans. *HuffPost Better Black Health*. Retrieved from http://

www.huffingtonpost.com/2015/07/13/black-children-at-risk-for-lead
-poisoning-_n_7672920.html

Smith, M. (2016). Flint wants safe water, and someone to answer for its crisis. *The New York Times*. Retrieved from http://www.nytimes.com/2016/01/10 /us/flint-wants-safe-water-and-someone-to-answer-for-its-crisis.html?_r=0

Spector, R. (2014). *The other side of health care*. Flint, MI: Hurley Hospital Grand Rounds.

Spurlock, J. (1988). Black Americans. In L. Comas-Diaz & E. E. H. Griffith (Eds.), *Cross-cultural mental health*. New York, NY: John Wiley & Sons.

Sykes, J., & Kelly, A. P. (1979, June). Black skin problems. *American Journal of Nursing*, 1092–1094.

Tallant, R. (1946). *Voodoo in New Orleans* (7th printing). New York, NY: Collier.

Webb, J. Y. (1971). Letter, Dr. J. R. Krevans to Y. Webb, February 15, 1967. Reported in *Superstitious influence—Voodoo in particular—Affecting health practices in a selected population in southern Louisiana*. Paper, New Orleans, LA.

Weissman, J. S., Betancourt, J. R., Green, A. R., Meyer, G. S., Tan-McGrory, A., Nudel, J. D., ..., Carillo, J. E. (2011). *Commissioned paper: Healthcare Disparities Measurement*. National Quality Forum. Retrieved from https:// www2.massgeneral.org/disparitiessolutions/z_files/Disparities%20Commis- sioned%20Paper.pdf

Wilson, D. W. (2007). From their own voices: The lived experience of African American registered nurses. *Journal of Transcultural Nursing*, *18*(2), 142–149.

Wintrob, R. (1972). Hexes, roots, snake eggs? M.D. vs. occults. *Medical Opinion*, *1*(7), 54–61.

Wolfers, J., Leonhardt, D., & Quealy, K. (2015, April 20). 1.5 million miss- ing black men. *The New York Times*. Retrieved from http://www.nytimes .com/interactive/2015/04/20/upshot/missing-black-men.html?hp&action =click&pgtype=Homepage&module=second-column-region&region=top -news&WT.nav=top-news&abt=0002&abg=0&_r=1

HEALTH and ILLNESS in the Hispanic Populations

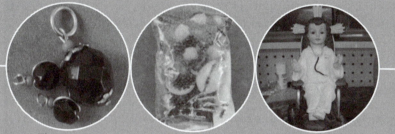

Figure 12-1   Figure 12-2   Figure 12-3

My heart is in the earth ...

—*Greenhaw (2000)*

◼ Objectives

1. Discuss the historical and demographic backgrounds of the Hispanic American population.
2. Describe the traditional definitions of HEALTH and ILLNESS of the Hispanic American population.
3. Explain the traditional methods of HEALING of the Hispanic American population.
4. Describe the practice of a traditional HEALER.
5. Summarize current healthcare problems of the Hispanic American population.

◼ Background

The next link in the *HERITAGECHAIN* provides an overview the historical and demographic backgrounds, HEALTH and ILLNESS traditions, and healthcare issues of the Hispanic American community. Figure 12-1 is a cluster of small jet stone amulets. Depending on the age and size of the person, one bead is worn as a necklace for protection from the *mal ojo*—evil eye or *envidia*, envy of others. Figure 12-2 is a small packet of seeds, amulets, a shell and a *mano mila-groso*. It is carried in a pocket or purse for protection. Figure 12-3 is a statue of the *Santo Nino*, Holy Child, dressed in a healthcare provider's white uniform and wearing a stethoscope. It is in front of the shelves of the over the counter herbal remedies in a *botanica*, pharmacy, in Los Angeles, California. A practic-ing CURANDERO, or traditional HEALER, works in the establishment.

The largest emerging majority group in the United States is composed of the Hispanic or Latino populations. According to the 2014 census esti-mates, 17.3% of the population is of Hispanic or Latino origin (U.S. Depart-ment of Commerce, U.S. Census Bureau, 2015). In fact, more than half of the growth in the total U.S. population between 2000 and 2013 was due to the increase in the Hispanic population. The largest Hispanic population is in California, and other large populations are in several counties in New Mexico and in Texas along the Mexican border. Hispanics are the nations' second largest ethnic group behind non-Hispanic whites (McDonnell-Smith, 2013). About three quarters of Hispanics reported as Mexican, Puerto Rican, or Cuban origin.

The terms *Hispanic* and *Latino* are used interchangeably in the Census estimates of 2014 and refer to a person of Cuban, Mexican, Puerto Rican, South or Central American, or other Spanish culture or origin regardless of race (U.S. Department of Commerce, U.S. Census Bureau, 2015). The people of Mexican origin comprise 63% of the Hispanic or Latino population.

This section has presented a descriptive overview of the Hispanic popu-lations as a whole; the next section describes the Mexican, or Mesoamerican, population. The term *Mesoamerican* is inclusive in that it describes peoples with Mexican and Central and South American origins (Carmack, Gasco, & Gossen, 1996, p. xvii). There is much confusion as to what their proper name is and, for the purposes of this chapter, overall government designations of *Hispanic* or *Latino* will be used for the aggregate populations and Spanish or Iberian origins and *Mexican* or *Mesoamerican* to refer to people who have a history and origins south of the U.S.-Mexico border.

■ Mexicans

The United States shares a 2,000-mile-long border with Mexico, which, in spite of walls and tightened security, remains easily crossed in both directions. The flow of people, goods, services, and ideas across it has a powerful impact on both countries.

Figure 12-4 shows the fence, or wall, as it appears in Nogales, Arizona. It is an enormous structure that will eventually hug all 2,000 miles of the U.S.-Mexico border. Here, you can see that it abuts the yards of families resid-ing on the Mexican side of the border. The U.S. federal government is planning to complete building a wall such as this across the entire 2,000 miles of the U.S.-Mexico border. This has been a controversial issue for many years.

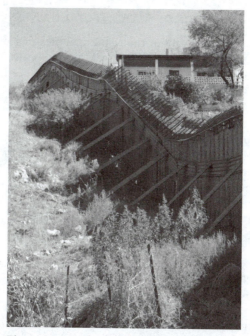

Figure 12-4   The fence along the U.S.-
Mexico border; Mexico is on
the right side.

The Mexicans have been in the United States for a long time, moving from Mexico and later intermarrying with Indians and Spanish people in the southwestern parts of what is now the United States. Santa Fe, New Mexico, was settled in 1609. Most of the descendants of these early settlers now live in Arizona, California, Colorado, New Mexico, and Texas. A large number of Mexicans also live in Illinois, Indiana, Kansas, Michigan, Missouri, Nebraska, New York, Ohio, Utah, Washington, and Wisconsin, where most arrived as migrant farmworkers. While located there as temporary farmworkers, they found permanent jobs and stayed. Contrary to the popular views that Mexicans live in rural areas, most live in urban areas. Mexicans are employed in all types of jobs. Few, however, have high-paying or high-status jobs in labor or management. The majority work in factories, mines, and construction; others are employed in agricultural work and service areas. At present, only a small—though growing—number are employed in clerical and professional areas. The number of unemployed in this group is high, and the earnings of those employed are well below the national average. The education of Mexicans, like that of most minorities in the United States, lags behind that of most of the population. Many Mexicans fail to complete high school. In the past few years, this situation has begun to change, and Mexican children are being encouraged to stay in school, go on to college, and enter the professions.

Traditional Definitions of HEALTH and ILLNESS

There are conflicting reports about the traditional meaning of HEALTH among Mexicans. Some sources maintain that HEALTH is considered to be purely the result of "good luck" and that a person loses his or her health if that luck changes (Welch, Comer, & Steinman, 1973, p. 205). Some people describe HEALTH as a reward for good behavior. Seen in this context, HEALTH is a gift from God and should not be taken for granted. People are expected to maintain their own equilibrium in the universe by performing in the proper way, eating the proper foods, and working the proper amount of time. The protection of HEALTH is an accepted practice that is accomplished with prayer, the wearing of religious medals or amulets, and the keeping of relics in the home. Herbs and spices can be used to enhance this form of prevention, as can exemplary behavior (Lucero, 1975). ILLNESS is seen as an imbalance in an individual's body or as punishment meted out for wrongdoing. The causes of ILLNESS can be grouped into five major categories:

1. *The body's imbalance.* Imbalance may exist between "hot" and "cold" or "wet" and "dry." The theory of hot and cold was taken to Mexico by Spanish priests and was fused with Aztec beliefs. The concept actually dates to the early Hippocratic theory of disease and four body humors. The cause of disease is mentioned as the disrupted relationship among these humors (Lucero, 1975; Castro, 2001).

   There are four body humors, or fluids: (1) blood, hot and wet; (2) yellow bile, hot and dry; (3) phlegm, cold and wet; and (4) black bile, cold and dry. When all four humors are balanced, the body is HEALTHY. When any imbalance occurs, an ILLNESS is manifested (Currier, 1966). These concepts, of course, provide one way of determining the remedy for a particular ILLNESS. For example, if an ILLNESS is classified as hot, it is treated with a cold substance. A cold disease, in turn, must be treated with a hot substance. Food, beverages, animals, and people possess the characteristics of hot and cold to various degrees. Hot foods cannot be combined; they are to be eaten with cold foods. There is no general agreement as to what is a hot disease or food and what is a cold disease or food. The classification varies from person to person, and what is hot to one person may be cold to another (Saunders, 1958, p. 13). Therefore, if a Mexican patient refuses to eat the meals in the hospital, it is wise to ask precisely what the person can eat and what combinations of foods he or she thinks would be helpful for the existing condition. It is important to note that *hot* and *cold* do not refer to temperature but are descriptive of a particular substance itself.

   For example, after a woman delivers a baby, a hot experience, she cannot eat pork, which is considered a hot food. She must eat something cold to restore her balance. Penicillin is a hot medication; therefore, it may be believed that it cannot be used to treat a hot disease. The major problem for the healthcare provider is to know that the rules, so to speak, of hot and cold vary from person to person. If healthcare providers understand the general nature of the hot and cold imbalance, they will be able to help the patient reveal the nature of the problem from the patient's perspective and manage it accordingly.

2. *Dislocation of parts of the body.* Two examples of "dislocation" are *empacho* and *caida de la mollera* (Nall & Spielberg, 1967). *Empacho* is believed to be caused by a ball of food clinging to the wall of the stomach (Castro, 2001, p. 89). Common symptoms of this illness are stomach pains and cramps. *Empacho* is treated by rubbing and gently pinching the spine. Prayers are recited throughout the treatment. Another, more common, cause of such illness is thought to be lying about the amount of food consumed. A 20-year-old Hispanic woman experienced the acute onset of sharp abdominal pain. She complained to her friend, and together they diagnosed the problem as *empacho* and treated it by massaging her stomach and waiting for the pain to dissipate. It did not, and they continued folk treatment for 48 hours. When the pain did not diminish, they sought help in a nearby hospital. The diagnosis was acute appendicitis. The young woman nearly died and was quite embarrassed when she was scolded by the physician for not seeking help sooner.

   Caida de la mollera (fallen fontanel) is a more serious illness. It occurs in infants and young children younger than 1 year old who are dehydrated (usually because of diarrhea or severe vomiting) and whose anterior fontanelle is depressed below the contour of the skull. Much superstition and mystery surround this problem. Some of the poorly educated and rural people, in particular, may believe that it is caused by a nurse's or physician's having touched the baby's head. This can be understood if we take into account that (1) an infant's fontanelle becomes depressed if the infant is dehydrated; and (2) when physicians or nurses measure an infant's head, they touch this area. If a mother takes her baby to a physician for an examination and sees the physician touch the child's head, and if the baby gets sick thereafter with *caida de la mollera*, it might be very easy for the woman to believe it is the fault of the physician's or nurse's touch. Unfortunately, epidemics of diarrhea are common in the rural and urban areas of the Southwest, and a number of children tend to be affected. One case of severe dehydration that leads to *caida de la mollera* may create quite a stir among the people. The folk treatment of this illness has not been found to be effective. Unfortunately, babies are rarely taken to the hospital in time, and the mortality rate for this illness is high (Lucero, 1975; Torres, 2005).

3. *Magic or supernatural causes outside the body.* Witchcraft or possession is considered to be culturally patterned role playing, a safe

vehicle for restoring oneself. Witchcraft or possession legitimizes acting out bizarre behavior or engaging in incoherent speech. Hispanic tradition, especially in the borderlands (the geographic area along the U.S.-Mexico border), blends the medieval heritage of medieval Castilian and English traditions with Mexican Indian folk beliefs (Kearney & Medrano, 2001, p. 119). *Brujas* (witches) use black, or malevolent, magic, while *curanderos* use white, or benevolent, magic. Spells may be cast to influence a lover or to get back at a rival, and cards are read to tell the future. *Herbrias* sell herbs, amulets, and talismans (Kearney & Medrano, 2001, p. 117).

A lesser disease that is caused from outside the body is *mal ojo*. *Mal ojo* means "bad eye," and it is believed to result from excessive admiration on the part of another. General malaise, sleepiness, fatigue, and severe headache are the symptoms of this condition. The folk treatment is to find the person who has caused the illness by casting the "bad eye" and having him or her care for the afflicted person (Nall & Spielberg, 1967). The belief in the evil eye, *mal de ojo*, can be traced back to the mid-1400s and Spain (Kearney & Medrano, 2001, p. 118; Torres, 2005). It has origins that go back even further in many parts of the world. This belief remains popular today.

4. **Strong emotional states.** *Susto* is described as an illness arising from fright. It afflicts many people—males and females, rich and poor, rural dwellers and urbanites. It involves soul loss: The soul is able to leave the body and wander freely. This can occur while a person is dreaming or when a person experiences a particularly traumatic event. The symptoms of the disease are: (1) restlessness while sleeping; (2) listlessness, anorexia, and disinterest in personal appearance when awake, including disinterest in both clothing and personal hygiene; and (3) loss of strength, depression, and introversion. The person is treated by *curandero* (a folk healer, discussed earlier and in the section on *curanderismo*), who coaxes the soul back into the person's body. During the healing rites, the person is massaged and made to relax (Rubel, 1964; Torres, 2005, pp. 39–42).

5. **Envidia.** *Envidia*, or envy, is also considered to be a cause of illness and bad luck. Many people believe that to succeed is to fail. That is, when one's success provokes the envy of friends and neighbors, misfortune can befall the person and his or her family. For example, a successful farmer, just when he is able to purchase extra clothing and equipment, is stricken with a fatal illness. He may well attribute the cause of this illness to the envy of his peers. A number of social scientists have, after much research, concluded that the "low" economic and success rates of Mexicans can ostensibly be attributed to belief in *envidia* (Lucero, 1975).

Religious Rituals

Magico-religious practices are quite common among the Mexican population. The more severe an illness, the more likely these practices will be used. There are four types of practices:

1. *Making promises.* A *promesa* may be made to God or to a saint; for example, a person may promise to donate money to a cause if he or she recovers from an ILLNESS (CASTRO, 2001, P. 158).

2. *Visiting shrines.* Many people make pilgrimages to shrines to offer prayers and gifts. This practice has origins in Jerusalem and later Spain, with the visits to Santiago de Compostela starting in the 11th century (Kearney & Medrano, 2001, p. 110).

3. *Offering medals and lighting candles.* This includes pinning small medals on statues of saints and lighting the candles in a church (Castro, 2001, p 158).

4. *Offering prayers.* Special prayers may be said at home, in churches, or in shrines (Nall & Spielberg, 1967).

It is not unusual for the Mexican people residing near the southern border of the continental United States, and in places further away, to return home to Mexico on religious pilgrimages. The location of one pilgrimage is Espinoza, Mexico, where *El Nino Fidencio* resided. The lighting of candles also is a frequently observed practice. Beautiful candles made of beeswax and tallow can be purchased in many stores, particularly grocery stores and pharmacies such as Sr. Garcia's *Yerberia*, located in Mexican neighborhoods (Figures 12-5, 12-6, and 12-7). Many homes have shrines with statues and pictures of saints. The candles are lit here and prayers are recited. Some homes have altars with statues and pictures on them and are the focal point of the home. Some Mexicans are devoted to the Virgin de San Juan del Valle and make pilgrimages to the shrine in San Juan, Texas. Figure 12-8 is a *retalbo*—a painting on wood or a piece of metal that illustrates a HEALING miracle. You can see the ill person lying in bed, the person praying, and the Virgin (Castro, 2001, p. 205).

In Catholic churches in communities with Hispanic populations, such as San Antonio, Texas, or Chimayo, New Mexico (Figure 12-9), it is not unusual to see statues covered with flowers and votive figures, such as those in Figures 12-10 and 12-11. These miniature articles are known in Spanish as *milagros*, meaning "miracles," *ex-votos*, or *promesas*. They are offered to a saint in thanks for answering a person's prayers for HEALING, success, a good marriage, and so forth. The *milagros* are made from wax, wood, bone, or a variety of metals and are an integral part of an ancient folk tradition found in many cultures (Egan, 1991, pp. 1–2). This practice, too, originated in Spain, and even today one can see and purchase these objects in countless churches (Kearney & Medrano, 2001, p. 115).

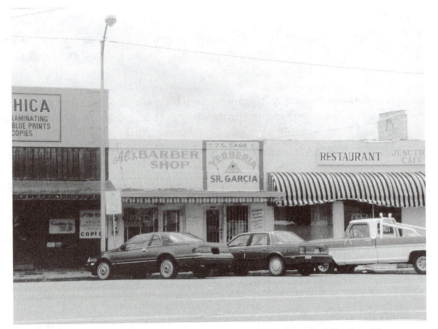

Figure 12-5 A traditional community resource *Yerberia* in Mission, Texas.

Curanderismo

There are no specific rules for knowing who in the community uses the services of folk healers. Not all Mexicans do, and not all Mexicans believe in their teachings and practices. Initially, it was thought that only the poor used a folk healer, or *curandero*, because they were unable to get treatment from the larger, institutionalized healthcare establishments. It now appears, however, that the use of HEALERS occurs widely throughout the Mexican population. Some people try to use HEALERS exclusively, whereas others use them along with modern medical care. The HEALERS do not usually advertise, but they are well known throughout the population because of informal community and kinship networks.

Curanderismo is defined as a medical system (Maduro, 1976; Torres, 2005). It is a coherent view with historical roots that combine Aztec, Spanish, spiritualistic, homeopathic, and scientific elements. It is practiced all over the southwestern United States, Mexico, and many South American countries (Torres, 2005, p. 3). There are *curanderos* practicing in Spain, and there are established communities of *curanderos* in close proximity to Madrid and Granada.

The *curandero(a)* is a holistic healer. The people who seek help from them do so for social, physical, and psychological purposes. The *curandero(a)* can be either a "specialist" or a "generalist," a full-time or part-time practitioner. Mexicans who believe in *curanderos* consider them to be religious figures.

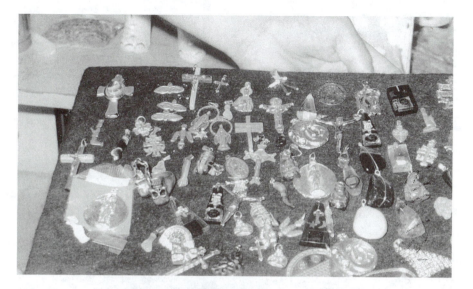

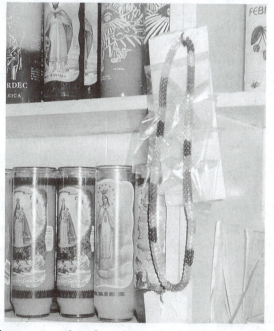

Figures 12-6 and 12-7   Samples of amulets and candles sold in Sr. Garcia's *Yerberia*.

A *curandero(a)* may receive the "gift of healing" through three means:

1. He or she may be "born" to heal. In this case, it is known from the moment of a *curandero(a)* 's birth that something unique about this person means that he or she is destined to be a healer.
2. He or she may learn by apprenticeship—that is, the person is taught the ways of healing, especially the use of herbs.

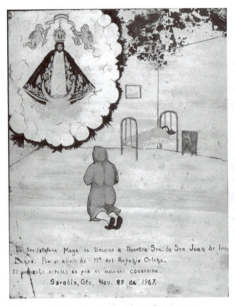

Figure 12-8 A *retalbo* that depicts a person praying to the Virgin of San Juan de la Valle for the HEALING of a loved one.

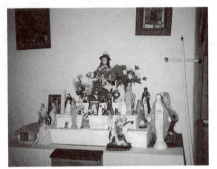

Figure 12-9 An altar in *El Santuario de Chimayo*, Chimayo, New Mexico.

3. He or she may receive a "calling" through a dream, trance, or vision by which contact is made with the supernatural by means of a "patron" (or "caller"), who may be a saint. The "call" comes either during adolescence or during the midlife crisis. This "call" is resisted at first. Later, the person becomes resigned to his or her fate and gives in to the demands of the "calling" (Torres, 2005).

Other folk healers include the *materia*, or spirit channeler, and the *partera*, or lay midwife. The *parteras* continue to practice today, but their numbers are dwindling. Box 12-1 describes the scope of the *partera*'s practice.

HEALTH Restoration

The most popular form of HEALTH restoration used by folk healers involves herbs, especially when used as teas. The *curandero* knows what specific herbs to use for a problem. This information is revealed in dreams, in which the "patron" gives suggestions.

Because the *curandero* has a religious orientation, much of the treatment includes elements of both the Catholic and Pentecostal rituals and artifacts: offerings of money, penance, confession, the lighting of candles, praying for *milagros* (little miracles), and the laying on of hands. Massage is used in illnesses such as *empacho*.

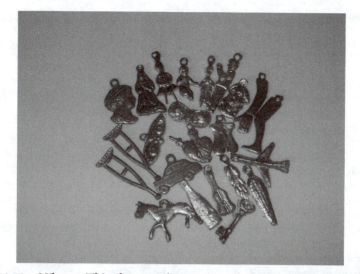

Figure 12-10 *Milagros.* This photograph is an example of the assortment of various miniature articles that may be purchased for the nominal cost in *botanicas* or in a marketplace from traditional people. In this image are crutches, a head, a woman, children and a baby, an arm, a leg, eyes, breasts, a torso, a heart, a car, a horse, a key, and a whisky bottle, among others. When a person is experiencing a problem with one of these anatomical areas or objects, he or she may pray for recovery; make a *promesa* to a saint; and, when the person's prayer is answered, take the *milagro* to a church and place it near the saint the person prayed to.

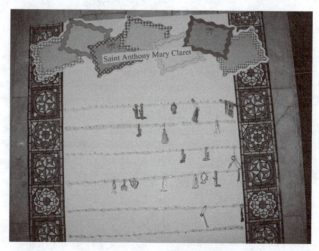

Figure 12-11 *Milagros* placed at the shrine of Saint Anthony in the Church of the Sacred Heart of Mary in San Antonio, Texas.

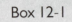

Box 12-1

Parteras

In Mexico and South Texas, there is a long history of the use of midwives, or *parteras*. The practice of midwifery predates the Spanish explorer Cortes. The goddess Tlozoteotl was the goddess of childbirth, and the midwives were known as *Tlamatqui-Tuti*. A *partera* is viewed as a HEALER by many members of the Mexican American and Mexican communities. She (most are women, although currently obstetricians from Mexico are providing this service in South Texas) is described as an individual who has the ability to HEAL and is outgoing, warm, gentle, caring, and cooperative. The *partera*'s duties include: (1) giving advice to the pregnant woman; (2) giving physical aid, such as treating any illness the woman experiences during pregnancy; (3) guiding the woman through her pregnancy in terms of nutrition or activities she can and cannot do; and (4) being in attendance during labor and delivery.

Patients are most often referred to *parteras* by their friends or relatives, and a *partera* with a good reputation is always busy. Some *parteras* receive referrals from the health department with which they register, some advertise in the local newspaper or telephone book, and some have signs on their homes or clinics (Figure 12-12). The *parteras* must now be licensed midwives, and their practice, though smaller, continues to attract many women.

The *parteras* avoid delivering women with high blood pressure, anemia, a history of diabetes, multiple babies, and transverse presentations. Some *parteras* also prefer to send women with breech presentations to the hospital. If an unfamiliar woman in labor appears at their door in the middle of the night who is very poor with no place to go to deliver, most claim they will take her in.

Most *parteras* keep records of their deliveries. Included in these records are such data as the name of the mother, date, time of admission, stage of labor, time in labor, contractions, time of delivery, presenting part, time of delivery and condition of the placenta, and physical condition of the mother and baby.

The amount of prenatal care the *parteras* deliver ranges from a lot to a little. In general, the mothers seek assistance during their 3rd or 4th month of pregnancy. When the *partera*'s assistance is sought, the mother is sent either to the health department or to a doctor for routine blood work. The *partera* is able to follow the mother's case and gives her advice and massages. One important service that the *partera* performs is the repositioning of the fetus in the womb through massage.

A *partera* may give several forms of advice to the pregnant woman. For example, she may advise the woman who is experiencing pica (the craving for and ingestion of nonfood substances, such as clay and laundry starch) to purchase solid milk of magnesia in Mexico. The milk of magnesia tastes like clay, thereby satisfying the pica, and is not considered harmful. The mother with food cravings is advised to satisfy them. The mothers are also instructed:

1. Not to lift heavy objects
2. To take laxatives to prevent constipation
3. To exercise often by walking frequently
4. Not to cross their legs, and
5. Not to bathe in hot water.

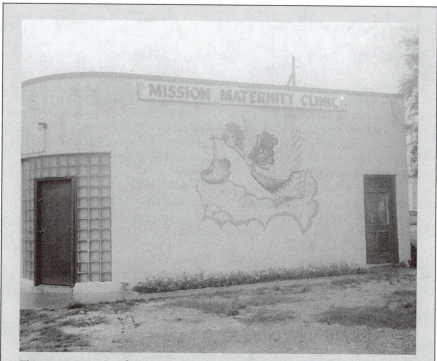

Figure 12-12   Sign for a *partera*.

The reason for the last two admonitions is the belief that crossing the legs and taking hot baths can cause the baby to assume the breech position.

If the *partera* knows the exact date of the mother's last period, she is able to estimate accurately when the woman is going to deliver by calculating 8 lunar months and 27 days from the onset of the last period.

With the onset of labor, the mother contacts the *partera*. She goes to the birthing place—the home or clinic of the *partera*—or the *partera* goes to her home. The mother is examined vaginally to determine how far along in labor she is and the position of the baby. She is instructed to shower and to empty her bowels—with an enema, if necessary—and she is encouraged to walk and move around until the delivery is imminent. Once the mother is ready to deliver, she is put to bed. Most of the mothers are delivered lying down in bed. If the mother chooses to do so, however, she is delivered in a squatting or sitting position. Several home remedies may be used during labor, including *comino* (cumin seed) tea or *canela* (cinnamon) tea to stimulate labor.

The baby is stimulated if needed, and the mucus is removed from the mouth and nose as needed with the use of a bulb syringe. The cord is clamped, tied with cord ties, and cut with scissors that have been boiled and soaked in alcohol. The stump is then treated with merbromin (Mercurochrome), alcohol, or a combination of the two. The baby is weighed, and sometime after the delivery, it is bathed. Most *parteras* bind both the mother and the baby. The baby may be fed oregano

(continued)

Box 12-1 (*continued*)

or cumin tea right after birth or later to help it spit up the mucus. Eyedrops are instilled in the baby's eyes, in compliance with state laws (silver nitrate is used most frequently).

The *partera* stays at the mother's home for several hours after the delivery and then returns to check the mother and the baby the next day. If the mother delivers at the home of the *partera*, she generally stays 12 to 14 hours.

There are several ways of disposing of the placenta. It may just be placed in a plastic bag and thrown in the trash, or it may be buried in the yard. Some placentas are buried with a religious or folk ceremony. There are several folk reasons for the burial of the placenta. The placenta must be buried so that the animals will not eat it. If it is eaten by a dog, the mother will not be able to bear any more children. If it is thrown in the trash, the mother's womb may become "cold." If the baby is a girl, the placenta is buried near the home, so the daughter will not go far away. If it is a boy, it is buried far away from the home to ensure the child's independence.

The practice of the *partera* continues in a limited way. *Parteras* in the state of Texas are licensed and registered as "direct entry midwives" (DEM). There are 267 DEMs in Texas; 11 practice in the Rio Grande Valley's most populated counties, Hidalgo and Cameron. In Hidalgo County, there was a total of 17,353 births in 2012, with 295 of the babies delivered by DEMs. The majority of these babies, 271, were born to women who came from out of state. Cameron County saw a total of 8,268 births in 2012, with 50 babies delivered by DLMs. The majority of these babies, 47, were born to women who came from out of state (Texas Department of State Health Services, 2014).

The practice of the *partera* in the Rio Grande Valley is the life of the past, the present, and the future: "a way of life *de ayer, hoy y mañana*" (Castillo, 1982).

Sources: Adapted from *Cultural Diversity in Health and Illness*, by R. Spector, 4th ed., 1996, Stamford, CT: Appleton & Lange, pp. 305–325; and J. Castillo, former director, Division of Health Related Professions, personal letter, April 6, 1982, Brownsville, TX: Texas Southmost College.

Cleanings, the removal of negative forces or spirits, or *limpias*, are done in two ways. The first is by passing an unbroken egg over the body of the ILL person. The second method entails passing herbs tied in a bunch over the body. The back of the neck, which is considered a vulnerable spot, is given particular attention.

In contrast to the depersonalized care Mexicans expect to receive in medical institutions, their relationship with and care by the *curandero(a)* are uniquely personal, as described in Table 12-1. This special relationship between Mexicans and the *curanderos* may well account for folk healers' popularity. In addition to the close, personal relationship between patient and healer, other factors may explain the continuing belief in *curanderismo*:

Table 12-1 Comparison Between *Curanderos, Parteras,* and Other Traditional Healers and Allopathic Healthcare Providers

Curanderos, Parteras, and Other Traditional HEALERS	Allopathic Healthcare Providers
1. Maintain informal, friendly, affective relationship with entire family	1. Businesslike, formal relationship; deal only with the patient
2. Make house calls day or night	2. Patient must go to physician's office or clinic, and only during the day; may have to wait for hours to be seen; home visits are rarely made
3. For diagnosis, consult with head of house, create a mood of awe, talk to all family members; are not authoritarian, have social rapport, build expectation of cure	3. Rest of family is usually ignored; deal solely with the ill person, and may deal only with the sick part of the patient; authoritarian manner creates fear
4. Are generally less expensive than physicians	4. More expensive than *curanderos*
5. Have ties to the "world of the sacred"; have rapport with the symbolic, spiritual, creative, or holy force	5. Secular; pay little attention to the religious beliefs or meaning of an illness
6. Share the worldview of the patient— that is, speak the same language, live in the same neighborhood or in some similar socioeconomic conditions, may know the same people, understand the patient's lifestyle	6. Generally do not share the worldview of the patient—that is, may not speak the same language, do not live in the same neighborhood, do not understand the patient's socioeconomic conditions or lifestyle

1. The mind and body are inseparable.

2. The central problem of life is to maintain harmony, including social, physical, and psychological aspects of the person.

3. There must be harmony between the hot and cold, wet and dry. The treatment of ILLNESS should restore the body's harmony, which has been lost.

4. The patient is the passive recipient of disease when the disease is caused by an external force. This external force disrupts the natural order of the internal person, and the treatment must be designed to restore this order. The causes of disharmony are evil and witches.

5. A person is related to the spirit world. When the body and soul are separated, soul loss can occur. This loss is sometimes caused by *susto,* a disease or illness resulting from fright, which may afflict individuals from all socioeconomic levels and lifestyles.

6. The responsibility for recovery is shared by the ILL person, the family, and the *curandero(a).*

7. The natural world is not clearly distinguished from the supernatural world. Thus, the *curandero(a)* can coerce, curse, and appease the spirits. The *curandero(a)* places more emphasis on his or her connections with the sacred and the gift of healing than on personal

properties. (Such personal properties might include social status, a large home, and expensive material goods.)

Several types of emotional illnesses are found among the traditional people from Hispanic communities. These are further divided into **mental illness** (in which the illness is not judged) and **moral illness** (in which others can judge the victim). The causes of mental illness and examples of the illness they cause are as follows:

- Heredity—epilepsy (*epilepsia*)
- Hex—evil eye (*mal ojo*)
- Worry—anxiety (*tirisia*)
- Fright—hysteria (*histeria*)
- Blow to the head—craziness (*locura*).

The causes of moral illness and examples of the illness they cause are as follows:

- Vice—use of drugs (*drogadicto*)
- Character weakness—alcoholism (*alcoholismo*)
- Emotions—jealousy (*celos*) and/or rage (*coraje*) (Spencer et al., 1993, p. 133).

Ethnopharmacologic teas may be used to treat these maladies, and amulets may be worn or religious rituals followed to prevent or treat them. The following are examples of herbs that may be purchased in grocery stores, markets, and *botanicas*, and are used as teas to treat the listed maladies:

- Camomile tea, *Manzanilla*, used to cure fright
- Spearmint tea, *Yerb Buena*, used to treat nervousness
- Orange leaves, *Te de narranjo*, used as a sedative to treat nervousness
- Sweet basil, *Albacar*, used to treat fright and to ward off evil spirits (Spencer et al., 1993, p. 133).

The HEALTH beliefs and practices discussed here are prevalent today (2015). I recently spoke with an immigrant from a small village in Mexico and inquired about *curanderismo*. She was excited to know that I was familiar with the practice and was proud to share her knowledge and experiences.

Box 12-2 describes the practices of *Santeria*—a Hispanic healthcare system similar to but different from *Curanderismo*.

People seeking healthcare may go to a physician, a folk practitioner, or both. The general progression of seeking care is as follows:

1. The person seeks advice from a daughter, mother, grandmother, or neighbor woman. These sources are consulted because the women of this culture are the primary healers and dispensers of medicine at the family level.

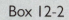

Box 12-2

Santeria

People with an Afro-Caribbean heritage share countless HEALTH beliefs and practices with the Hispanic people from Mexico, Central, and South America. However, the traditional HEALTH practices that evolved in the Caribbean—particularly Puerto Rico, Cuba, and the Dominican Republic—have several subtle differences. For example, many traditional people may believe that primarily evil spirits and forces cause physical and mental illness, and treatment may be sought from a *Santero(a)* rather than a *Curandero(a)*. *Santeria* is the form of Latin American magic that had its birth in Nigeria, the country of origin of the Yoruba people, who were brought to the New World as slaves over 400 years ago. The *Santeria*, or *santero*, uses storytelling and medicinal herbs as a way of helping people cope with day-to-day difficulties and HEALTH problems (Flores-Peña, personal interview, April 9, 1991). The people brought with them their traditional African religion, which was in time synchronized with the Catholic religion and images and the indigenous peoples of the islands. The believers continued to worship in the traditional way, especially in Puerto Rico, Cuba, and the Dominican Republic. The Yorubas identified their gods—*Orishas*—with the Christian saints and invested in these saints the same supernatural powers of gods. The following is a selected list of Orishas, the saint they represent, and the health problem they are related to:

- Chango represents Saint Barbara, and the health problem is violent death.
- Ifa represents Saint Anthony, and he brings fertility.
- Obatala represents the Crucified Christ, and bronchitis is the health problem (Gonzalez-Wippler, 1987; Riva, 1990).

Santeria is a structured system consisting of *espiritismo* (spiritualism), which is practiced by gypsies and mediums that claim to have *facultades* (sacred abilities). These special *facultades* provide them with the "license" to practice. The status or positions of the practitioners form a hierarchy: The head is the *babalow*, a male; second is the *presidente*, the head medium; and third are the *santeros*. Novices are the "believers." The *facultades* are given to the HEALER from protective Catholic saints, who have African names and are known as protectors, *protecciones*. *Santeria* can be practiced in storefronts, basements, homes, and even college dormitories. *Santeros* dress in white robes for ceremonies and wear special beaded bracelets or necklaces as a sign of their identity.

The traditional HEALER is known as a *santero* and is an important person, one who respects the patient and does not gossip about either the patient or his or her problems. Anyone can pour his or her heart out with no worry of being labeled or judged. The *santero* is able to tell a person what the problem is, prescribe the proper treatment, and tell the person what to do, how to do it, and when to do it. The following are examples of the health problems the *Santero(a)* may encounter:

- *Ataque* is screaming, falling to the ground, wildly moving arms and legs, and hysterical crying. It ends spontaneously.

(continued)

Box 12-2 *(continued)*

- *Empacho* is an ailment that occurs when food is believed to form into a ball and cling to the stomach, causing pain. The folk treatment consists of strong abdominal massage and medication.
- *Fatigue* is an ailment with asthma-like symptoms, and it is usually treated with modern medicine.
- *Mal ojo* is a sudden, unexplained illness in a usually well child or person that is prevented by wearing an amulet.
- *Pasmo*, a form of paralysis, usually is caused by an upset in the hot-cold balance.

A limited number of *santeros* place advertisements in local Spanish daily newspapers. Some of the more industrious ones distribute flyers in the streets. Others maintain a low profile, and patients visit them because of their well-established reputations.

I visited a *santero* in Los Angeles, California, with the hope of his granting me an interview. Instead, he argued that if I wanted to know about his practice I should "sit," so I did. He proceeded to examine my head and palms, throw and read cowrie shells, tell me a story, and asked me to interpret it. Once this was accomplished, he recommended certain interventions. His manner was extremely calming and, when he interpreted the story with me, I discovered his uncanny ability to read and understand my habits and behaviors (Flores-Peña, personal interview, April 9, 1991).

2. If the advice is not sufficient, the person may seek help from a *senoria* (a woman who is especially knowledgeable about the causes and treatment of illness).

3. If the *senoria* is unable to help, the person goes to a more sophisticated folk practitioner, a *curandera* or an *espiritista*. If the problem is "psychiatric," a *santero* may be consulted. These names describe similar people—those who obtain their knowledge from spirits and treat illness according to the instructions of the spirits. Herbs, lotions, creams, and massage often are used.

4. If the person is still not satisfied, he or she may go to a physician.

5. If the physicians' treatment is not satisfactory, the person may return to a folk practitioner. He or she may seek medical help sooner than step 4, or may go back and forth between the two systems.

Not all people from Hispanic heritages use the folk system. However, healthcare providers should remember that people who appear to have delayed seeking healthcare have most likely counted on curing their illness through the culturally known and well-understood folk process. Often when people disappear (or "elope") from the established health system, they may have elected to return to the folk system. Those who elope from the larger, institutionalized medical system may visit a *botanica* (Figures 12-13 and 12-14). In these

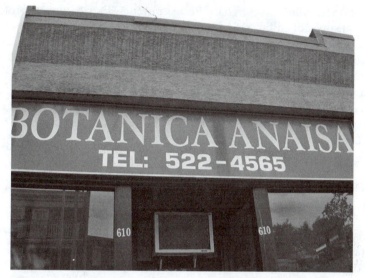

Figure 12-13   A *botanica* in Boston, Massachusetts. There are several *botanicas* in the Boston metropolitan area. The *botanicas* are visited primarily by people from Puerto Rico, the Dominican Republic, Mexico, and other Hispanics residing in the area. They sell numerous herbs and herbal preparations, amulets of all sorts, *milagros*, and statues of saints. A *santera* works in this *botanica*, and she is available to people to give advice and sell herbal remedies.

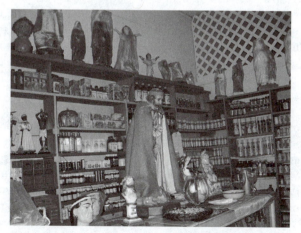

Figure 12-14   Interior of a *botanica* in Boston, Massachusetts.

small *botanicas*, one can purchase herbs, potents, Florida water, ointments, and incense prescribed by spiritualists. Some of these *botanicas* are so busy that each customer is given a number and is assisted only after the number is called (Mumford, 1973). There are countless *botanicas* located in one small area of New York City. A colleague and I visited a *botanica* in Boston that was similar to a pharmacy. The owner explained the various remedies that were for sale. We were allowed to purchase only over-the-counter items because we did not have a spiritualist's prescription for herbs. The store also sold amulets, candles, religious statues, cards, medals, and relics.

■ Current Health Problems in the Hispanic Population

The Hispanic health profile is marked by diversity, and people of the Hispanic community experience perhaps the most varied set of health issues encountered by any of the emerging majority populations. The diversity in health problems is intertwined with the effects of socioeconomic status as well as with geographic and cultural differences. The most important health issues for Hispanics are related to these demographic facts: The population is young and has a high birth rate.

Table 12-2 compares selected health status indicators between all races and Hispanics. The leading causes of death among Hispanic Americans illustrate differences between their health experiences and those of the total population, as can be seen in Table 12-3.

Hispanics experience a number of barriers when seeking healthcare. The most obvious one is language. In spite of the fact that Spanish-speaking people constitute one of the largest minority groups in this country, few healthcare deliverers speak Spanish. This is especially true in communities in which the number of Spanish-speaking people is relatively small. Hispanics who live in these areas experience tremendous frustration because of the language barrier. Even in large cities, there are far too many occasions when a sick person has to rely on a young child to act not only as a translator, but also as an interpreter. One way of sensitizing young nursing students to the pain of this situation is to ask them to present a health problem to a person who does not speak or understand a word of English. Needless to say, this is extremely difficult; it is also embarrassing. People who try this rapidly comprehend and appreciate the feelings of patients who are unable to speak or understand English. (After this experience, two of my students decided to take a foreign-language elective.) Language will continue to be a problem until: (1) there are more physicians, nurses, and social workers from the Spanish-speaking communities; and (2) more of the present deliverers of healthcare learn to speak Spanish.

A second critical barrier that Hispanic people encounter is poverty. The diseases of the poor—for example, tuberculosis, malnutrition, cancer, diabetes, and lead poisoning—all have high incidences among Spanish-speaking populations. Poverty is predominantly prevalent among migrant farmworkers. A profile of migrant workers in 2010 showed that 90% of the workers seen in the migrant labor health centers were Hispanic, and 8 out of 10 workers lived below the federal poverty level. Not only are the people at risk for the diseases mentioned, but

Table 12-2   Comparison of Selected Health Status Indicators: 2013 All Races and Hispanic or Latino Americans

Health Indicator	All Races	Hispanic Americans
Crude birth rate per 1,000 population by race of mother, 2013	12.4	**16.7**
Percentage of live births to teenage childbearing women—18–19 years, 2013	5.0	7.1
Percentage of low birth weight per live births >2,500 grams, 2013	8.02	7.09
Infant mortality per 1,000 live births, 2012	6.0	**5.1**
Respondent-reported prevalence percent of adults: Cancer—all sites, 2012–2013, 18 years and over	5.9	3.6
Respondent-reported prevalence percent of adults: Heart Disease—2012–2013, 18 years and over	10.6	8.0
Respondent-reported prevalence percent of adults: Stroke—2012–2013, 18 years and over	2.5	2.6
Male death rates from suicide, all ages, age adjusted per 100,000 resident population, 2013	20.3	**9.3**
All male death rates from homicide, all ages, age adjusted per 100,000 resident population, 2013	8.2	7.3

Source: Health, United States, 2014: With Special Feature on Adults Aged 55–64, by National Center for Health Statistics, 2015, Hyattsville, MD: Author, pp. 58, 59, 62, 64, 76, 134, 135, 138, 139, 161.

Table 12-3   Comparison of the 10 Leading Causes of Death for Hispanic or Latino and for All Persons: 2014

Hispanic or Latino	All Persons
1. Malignant neoplasms	1. Diseases of heart
2. Diseases of heart	2. Malignant neoplasms
3. Unintentional injuries	3. Chronic lower respiratory diseases
4. Cerebrovascular diseases	4. Unintentional injuries
5. Diabetes mellitus	5. Cerebrovascular diseases
6. Chronic liver diseases and cirrhosis	6. Alzheimer's disease
7. Chronic lower respiratory diseases	7. Diabetes mellitus
8. Alzheimer's disease	8. Influenza and pneumonia
9. Influenza and pneumonia	9. Nephritis, nephrotic syndrome, and nephrosis
10. Nephritis, nephrotic syndrome, and nephrosis	10. Suicide

Source: Health, United States, 2014: With Special Feature on Adults Aged 55–64, by National Center for Health Statistics, 2015, Hyattsville, MD: Author, pp. 97, 98.

also the occupational hazards of agricultural work, primarily from insecticides, are extraordinary (Boggess & Bogue, 2014; Brennan, Economos, & Salerno, 2015).

A final barrier to adequate healthcare is the time orientation of Hispanic Americans. To Hispanics, time is a relative phenomenon. Little attention is given to the exact time of day. The frame of reference is wider, and the issue is whether it is day or night. The American healthcare system, on the other hand, places great emphasis on promptness. Healthcare providers demand that clients arrive at the exact time of the appointment—despite the fact that clients are often kept waiting. Health system workers stress the client's promptness rather than their own. In fact, they tend to deny responsibility for the waiting periods by blaming them on the "system." Many facilities commonly schedule all appointments for 9:00 a.m. when it is clearly known and understood by the staff members that the doctor will not even arrive until 11:00 a.m. or later. The Hispanic person frequently responds to this practice by arriving late for appointments or failing to go at all. They prefer to attend walk-in clinics, where the waits are shorter. They also much prefer going to traditional healers.

This chapter has presented a succinct overview of the historical and demographic backgrounds, traditional definitions of HEALTH and ILLNESS, traditional methods of HEALING, the scope of practice of the traditional HEALER, and the current health problems of Hispanic Americans.

RESEARCH ON CULTURE

Much research has been conducted among members of the Hispanic American population. The following article describes one such study:

> Brennan, K., Economos, J., & Salerno, M. M. (2015). Farmworkers make their voices heard in the call for stronger protections from pesticides. *NEW SOLUTIONS: A Journal of Environmental and Occupational Health Policy*, 1–15. Retrieved from http://new.sagepub.com/content/early/2015/09/15/1048291115604428.full.pdf+html?ijkey=wTkf/PSHH/7b2&keytype=ref&siteid=spnew

This study is a collection of the stories of farmworkers who have been exposed to pesticides and the consequences of these exposures. Farm work, one of the most vital occupations in the labor force, is among the most grueling and hazardous occupations. In 1992, the U.S. Environmental Protection Agency (EPA) promulgated the Worker Protection Standard (WPS) as the primary set of regulations protecting the nation's 1 million–2 million farmworkers, many of whom are Hispanic, from occupational pesticide exposure. The farmworkers quoted in this study are an underrepresented, poorly protected, and disenfranchised population. Their voices articulate the compelling need for stronger workplace protections and enforcement measures to reduce the health risks for workers, families, and communities. New regulations were proposed in 2014, and the farmworkers responded in public hearings. Their verbatim comments in this study articulate the need for stronger workplace protections and enforcement measures to reduce health risks for workers, families, and communities.

Explore  MediaLink

Go to the Student Resource Site at pearsonhighered.com/nursingresources for chapter-related review questions, case studies, and activities. Contents of the CULTURALCARE Guide and CULTURALCARE Museum can also be found on the Student Resource Site. Click on Chapter 12 to select the activities for this chapter.

Box 12-3

Keeping Up

It goes without saying that much of the data presented in this chapter may be out of date when it is read. However, at this final stage of writing, it is the most recent information available. The following resources will be most helpful in keeping you abreast of the frequent changes in healthcare events, costs, and policies:

1. The National Center for Health Statistics publishes *Health, United States*, an annual report on trends in health statistics.
2. Health-related data and other statistics are available from the Centers for Disease Control.
3. To follow immigration information, consult the U.S. Department of Commerce Economics and Statistics Administration, Office of Homeland Security.
4. The National Center for Farmworker Health (Boggess & Bogue, 2014) and the Migrant Clinicians Network (2015) provide information about the health of migrant farmworkers.

■ References

Boggess, B. C., & Bogue, H. O. (2014). A profile of migrant health: An analysis of the uniform data system, 2010. National Center for Farmworker Health. Retrieved from http://www.ncfh.org/uploads/3/8/6/8/38685499/aprofileofmigranthealth.pdf

Brennan, K., Economos, J., & Salerno, M. M. (2015). Farmworkers make their voices heard in the call for stronger protections from pesticides. *NEW SOLUTIONS: A Journal of Environmental and Occupational Health Policy*, 1–15. Retrieved from http://new.sagepub.com/content/early/2015/09/15/1048291115604428.full.pdf+html?ijkey=wTkf/PSHH/7b2&keytype=ref&siteid=spnew

Carmack, R. M., Gasco, J., & Gossen, G. H. (1996). *The legacy of Mesoamerica*. Upper Saddle River, NJ: Prentice Hall.

Castillo, J., former director, Division of Health Related Professions. (1982, April 6). Personal letter. Brownsville: Texas Southmost College.

Castro, R. G. (2001). *Chicano folklore*. Oxford, England: Oxford University Press.

Currier, R. L. (1966, March). The hot-cold syndrome and symbolic balance in Mexican and Spanish-American folk medicine. *Ethnology, 5*, 251–263.

Egan, M. (1991). *Milagros*. Santa Fe: Museum of New Mexico Press.

Gonzalez-Wippler, M. (1987). *Santeria—African magic in Latin America*. New York, NY: Original.

Greenhaw, W. (2000). *My heart is in the earth*. Montgomery, AL: River City.

Kearney, M., & Medrano, M. (2001). *Medical culture and the Mexican American borderlands*. College Station: Texas A&M University Press.

Lucero, G. (1975, March). *Health and illness in the Mexican community*. Lecture given at Boston College School of Nursing.

Maduro, R. J. (1976, January). *Curanderismo: Latin American folk healing*. Conference, San Francisco, CA.

McDonnell-Smith, M. (2013). Asians are fastest-growing U.S. ethnic group, Blacks are slowest, reports U.S. Census Bureau. *DiversityInc*. Retrieved from http://www.diversityinc.com/diversity-and-inclusion/asians-are-fastest-growing-u-s-ethnic-group-in-2012-blacks-are-slowest-reports-u-s-census-bureau/

Migrant Clinicians Network. (2015). *Pesticides*. Retrieved from http://www.migrantclinician.org/issues/occupational-health/pesticides.html

Mumford, E. (1973, November–December). Puerto Rican perspectives on mental illness. *Mount Sinai Journal of Medicine, 40*(6), 771–773.

Nall, F. C., II, & Spielberg, J. (1967). Social and cultural factors in the responses of Mexican-Americans to medical treatment. *Journal of Health and Social Behavior, 8*, 302.

National Center for Health Statistics. (2015). *Health, United States, 2014: With special feature on adults aged 55–64*. Hyattsville, MD: Author. Retrieved from http://www.cdc.gov/nchs/data/hus/hus14.pdf

Riva, A. (1990). *Devotions to the saints*. Los Angeles, CA: International Imports.

Rubel, A. J. (1964, July). The epidemiology of a folk illness: Susto in Hispanic America. *Ethnology, 3*(3), 270–271.

Saunders, L. (1958). Healing ways in the Spanish southwest. In E. G. Jaco (Ed.), *Patients, physicians, and illness*. Glencoe, IL: Free Press.

Spector, R. (1996). *Cultural diversity in health and illness* (4th ed.). Stamford, CT: Appleton & Lange.

Spencer, R. T., Nichols, L. W., Lipkin, G. B., Henderson, H. S., & West, F. M. (1993). *Clinical pharmacology and nursing management* (4th ed.). Philadelphia, PA: Lippincott.

Texas Department of State Health Services. (2014). *Migration for birth 2012*. Retrieved from http://www.dshs.state.tx.us/chs/pubs/Migration-for-Birth/

Torres, E. (2005). *Curandero: A life in Mexican folk healing*. Albuquerque: University of New Mexico Press.

U.S. Department of Commerce, U.S. Census Bureau. (2015). *American Community Survey (ACS). 2014 ACS 1-year estimates*. Retrieved from https://www.census.gov/programs-surveys/acs/technical-documentation/table-and-geography-changes/2014/1-year.html

Welch, S., Comer, J., & Steinman, M. (1973, September). Some social and attitudinal correlates of health care among Mexican Americans. *Journal of Health and Social Behavior, 14*, 205.

CHAPTER 13

HEALTH and ILLNESS in the White Populations

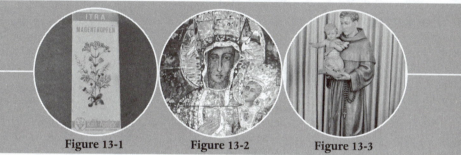

| Figure 13-1 | Figure 13-2 | Figure 13-3 |

Labour to keep alive in your Breast that Little Spark of Celestial Fire Called Conscience.

———————————————— —*George Washington, in J. Needleman (2003)*

■ Objectives

1. Discuss the historical and demographic backgrounds of selected populations within the White non-Hispanic population.
2. Compare and contrast the traditional definitions of HEALTH and ILLNESS of selected populations within the White non-Hispanic population.
3. Discuss the traditional methods of HEALING of selected populations within the White non-Hispanic population.
4. Describe current health status and problems of the White non-Hispanic population.

This link in the *HERITAGECHAIN* provides an overview of the historical and demographic backgrounds, HEALTH and ILLNESS traditions, and healthcare issues of selected communities within the White non-Hispanic European American populations. As with the other chapters in this unit, this is meant to be an overview of these topics, and space severely limits the amount of content that can be included. Figure 13-1 is a common German herbal preparation, *Magentropfen*. This over-the-counter preparation is taken to treat nausea, vomiting, and flatulence. Figure 13-2 is an image of a mosaic icon of the Virgin of Czestochowa, Poland, found in a small Catholic Church in Czestochowa, Texas. Many miracles are associated with icons of the Virgin of Czestochowa, and images of her are found in many Polish churches. Figure 13-3 is an image of Saint Anthony of Padua. He is known as the patron saint of finding lost things or people. He is honored annually the last weekend in August in an elaborate festival in Boston, Massachusetts.

■ Background

The 2015 census estimates showed that the U.S. population on April 1, 2014, was 318.9 million. Out of the total population, 77.4% identified as White and 62.1% reported they were White alone, not Hispanic or Latino. The White population increased at a slower rate than the total population (U.S. Department of Commerce, U.S. Census Bureau, 2015a).

Members of White European American communities have been immigrating to this country since the very first settlers came to the shores of New England. This population has diverse and multiple origins. The recent literature in the area of ethnicity and health/HEALTH has focused on people of color, and little has been written about the HEALTH traditions of the White non-Hispanic ethnic communities. In this chapter, an introductory overview of the differences in traditional HEALTH beliefs and practices, by ethnicity, is presented. Given that we are talking about 62.1% to 77.4% of the American population, from many diverse countries and with diverse ethnocultural and religious heritages, the enormity of the task of attempting to describe each difference is readily apparent. Instead, this chapter presents an overview of the relevant demographics of the White non-Hispanic population, highlights some of the basic beliefs of selected groups (those groups with which I have had the greatest exposure), and presents a comparison of the health status of Whites to the whole population as well as the census cohorts. The overview includes not only library research but also firsthand interviews and observations of people in their daily experiences with the healthcare delivery system, both as inpatients and as community residents receiving primary and home care.

The major groups migrating to this country between 1820 and 1990 included people from Germany, Italy, the United Kingdom, Ireland, Austria-Hungary, Canada, and Russia; they comprised a majority of the total immigrant population. However, in 1970, the numbers of immigrants from Europe began to decrease. Presently (2015), Europeans comprise only 11.9% of new immigrants (U.S. Department of Commerce, U.S. Census Bureau, 2015a).

The 1980 census was the first to include a question about ancestry. The U.S. Census Bureau uses the term ancestry to refer to a person's ethnic origin or descent, roots, heritage, or the place of birth of the person or the person's parents or ancestors before their arrival in the United States. Some ethnic identities, such as "German," can be traced to geographic areas outside the United States, while other ethnicities, such as "Pennsylvania Dutch" or "Cajun," evolved in the United States. Table 13-1 illustrates the numbers of people

Table 13-1   Population by Selected Ancestry Group: 2009–2013

Ancestry	Numbers Identifying Themselves as This Ancestry (millions)
German	47.7
Irish	34.6
English	25.8
Italian	17.4
Polish	9.6
French (except Basque)	8.7
Scottish	5.5

Source: American FactFinder: Selected Social Characteristics in the United States, from U.S. Department of Commerce, U.S. Census Bureau, 2015b, retrieved from http://factfinder.census.gov/faces/tableservices/jsf/pages/productview .xhtml?pid=ACS_13_5YR_DP02&src=pt, November 25, 2015.

claiming ancestry from European countries. The responses to the question of ancestry were a reflection of the ethnic group(s) with which persons identified, and respondents were able to indicate their ethnic group regardless of how many generations they were removed from it.

An additional facet to note is that in many states, such as New Mexico, Texas, and Hawaii, the non-Hispanic White population is now a minority. The state with the highest percentage White non-Hispanic population is Maine, whereas California has the largest White non-Hispanic population of any state (McDonnell-Smith, 2013).

The following discussion focuses on selected White ethnic groups and attempts to describe some of the history of their migration to America, the areas where they now live, the common beliefs regarding health/HEALTH and illness/ILLNESS, some kernels of information regarding family and social life, and problems that members from a given group may have in interacting with healthcare providers. The intention is not to create a vehicle for stereotyping, but to whet your appetite to search out more information about the people in your care, given the vast ethnocultural and religious differences among Whites living in the United States.

■ German Americans

The following material, relating to both the German American and Polish American communities, was obtained from research conducted in southeastern Texas in May 1982 and updated over time. It is by no means indicative of the HEALTH and ILLNESS beliefs of the entire German American and Polish American communities. It is included here to demonstrate the type of data that can be gleaned using an "emic" (a description of behavior dependent on the person's categorization of the action) approach to collecting data. It cannot be generalized, but it allows you to grasp the diversity of beliefs that surround us (Lefcowitz, 1990, p. 6).

Since 1830, more than 7 million Germans have immigrated to the United States. There are presently 47.7 million Americans who claim German ancestry, the largest ancestry population in the United States. California, Texas, and Pennsylvania have the largest numbers of people with German ancestry. The Germans represent a cross section of German society and have come from all social strata and walks of life. Some people immigrated to escape poverty, others for religious or political reasons, and still others came to take advantage of the opportunity to open up new lands in the Midwest for farming. Many were recruited to come here, as were the Germans who settled in the German enclaves in Texas. The immigrants represented all religions, but primarily included Lutherans, Catholics, and Jews. German immigrants represented the rich and the poor, the educated and the ignorant, and were of all ages. Present-day descendants are farmers, educators, and artists. The Germans brought to the United States the cultural diversity and folkways they observed in Germany. The tradition of the Christmas tree and the festivals of Corpus Christi, *Kinderfeste* (children's feast) and *Sangerfeste* (singing festival), all originated in Germany (Conzen, 1980, pp. 405–425). The German Americans introduced the first kindergartens.

The Germans began to migrate to the United States in the 17th century and have contributed 15.2% of the total immigration population. They are the least visible ethnic group in the United States, and people often are surprised to discover that there is such a large Germanic influence in this country. In some places, however, the German communities maintain strong identification with their German heritage. For example, the city of Fredericksburg, Texas, maintains an ambience of German culture and identity. Some people born there who are fourth generation and later continue to learn German as their first spoken language (Spector, 1983).

The German ethnic community is the second largest in the state of Texas and is exceeded only by the Mexican community. Germans have been immigrating to Texas since 1840 and continue to arrive. They are predominantly Catholic, Lutheran, and Methodist, and many have maintained their German identity. The major German communities in Texas are Victoria, Cuero, Gonzales, New Braunfels, and Fredericksburg.

During the European freedom revolutions of 1830 and 1848, Texas was quite popular, especially in Germany, and was seen as a "wild and fabulous land." For tradition-bound German families, however, their abandonment of the homeland was difficult. They were attracted, however, by the hopes of economic and social improvement and political idealism. An additional reason for the mass migration was the overpopulation of Germany and the immigrants' desire to escape an imminent European catastrophe. By the 1840s, several thousand northern Germans had come to Texas, and another large migration occurred in 1890. This second cluster of people came because there was severe crop failure in Russian-occupied Germany, and the Russian language had become a required subject in German schools. Other German migrations occurred from 1903 to 1905.

The Germans found pleasure in the ordinary things of everyday life. They were tied together by the German language because it bound them to the past, entertaining them with games, riddles, folk songs and literature, and folk wisdom. The greatest amusement was singing and dancing. Religion for the Lutherans, Catholics, and Methodists was a part of everyday life. The year was measured by the church calendar; observance of church ritual paced the milestones of the lifecycle. The Germans believed that each individual was a "part of the fabric of humanity," that "history was a continued process," and "everything had a purpose as mankind strove to something better" (Lich, 1982, pp. 33–72).

The Germans had a penchant for forming societies and clubs, the longest lasting of which are the singing societies. The first was organized in 1850 and exists still today. The Germans brought with them their customs and traditions; their cures, curses, and recipes; and their tools and ways of building (Lich, 1982).

Health and Illness

Among the Germans, health is described as more than not being ill, but as a state of well-being—physically and emotionally—the ability to do your duty; positive energy to do things; and the ability to do, think, and act the way you would like, to go and congregate, to enjoy life. Illness may be described as the absence of well-being: pain, malfunction of body organs, not being able to do what you want, a blessing from God to suffer, and a disorder of body imbalance.

Causes of Illness

Most German Americans believe in the germ theory of infection and in stress-related theories. Other causes of illness are identified, however, such as drafts, environmental changes, and belief in the evil eye and punishment from God.

The methods of maintaining health include the requirement of dressing properly for the season, proper nutrition, and the wearing of shawls to protect oneself from drafts—also, the taking of cod-liver oil, exercise, and hard work. Methods for preventing illness include wearing an asafetida bag around the neck in the winter to prevent colds, scapulars, religious practices, sleeping with the windows open, keeping closet doors closed, and cleanliness.

The use of home remedies to treat illnesses and physical injuries continues to be practiced. The following are examples of commonly used home remedies:

- **Black draught** or **castor oil** may be taken for constipation.
- **Chicken soup** may be taken for diarrhea or vomiting and also for a sore throat.
- **Teas** may be used, such as:
  - **Peppermint** for stomachaches
  - **Salbec** for a toothache, and
  - **Chamomile compresses** for ringworm.
- **Honey and milk** or **lemon juice and whiskey** may be used to treat a cough or cold.

- **Goose fat** may be rubbed on the chest for congestion.
- **Warm oil** may be placed in the ear to treat an earache or warm towels placed over the ear.
- **A hard knife (cold metal)** may be used to treat physical injuries such as bumps.
- **Clean** cuts and other wounds and cover with iodine. Kerosene is used to clean puncture wounds from nails.

Several over-the-counter remedies from Germany, such as *olbas* for colds and aches and pains, and *Magentropfen* for gastrointestinal ailments are available (Spector, 1983).

Current Health Problems

There do not appear to be any unusual health problems particular to German Americans.

■ Polish Americans

The first people immigrating to this country from Poland came with Germans in 1608 to Jamestown, Virginia, to help develop the timber industry. Since that time, Poland, too, has given America one of its largest ethnic groups, with over 9.5 million people claiming Polish ancestry. The peak year for Polish immigration was 1921, when well over 578,875 people immigrated here. Many of the people arriving before 1890 came for economic reasons. Those coming here since that time have come for both economic and political reasons and for religious freedom. Polish heroes include Casimir Pulaski and Thaddeus Kosciuszko, who were heroes in the American Revolution. The major influx of Poles to the United States began in 1870 and ended in 1913. The people who arrived were mainly peasants seeking food and release from the political oppression of three foreign governments in Poland. The immigrants who came both before and after this mass migration were better educated and not as poor. In the United States, Polish immigrants lived in poor conditions, either because they had no choice or because that was the way they were able to meet their own priorities. They were seen by other Americans to live as animals and were often mocked and called stupid. Quite often, the Polish people spoke and understood several European languages but had difficulty learning English and were therefore rejected by the outside society. Polish people shared the problem as a community and banded together in tight enclaves called "Polonia." They attempted to be as self-sufficient as possible. They worked at preserving their native culture, and voluntary Polish ghettos grew up in close proximity to the parish church (Green, 1980, pp. 787–803).

An example of the Polish experience in the United States is that of the Polish immigrants in Texas. The first Poles came to Texas in the second half of the 19th century, and most of them settled in Victoria, San Antonio, Houston, and Bandera. The first Polish colonies in America were located in Texas, the oldest being Panna Maria (Virgin Mary) in Karnes County, 50 miles southeast of San Antonio. Unlike other Polish people who wanted to return to Poland, the colonists who arrived in Texas after 1850 came to settle permanently and had no intention of returning to their homeland. Although these people came to Texas for economic, political, and religious reasons, severe poverty was their major reason for leaving Poland.

The first collective Polish immigration to America was in 1854, when 100 families came to Texas. They landed in Galveston, where a few in the party remained. The rest traveled in a procession northwestward, taking with them a few belongings such as featherbeds, crude farm implements, and a cross from their parish church. Their dream was to live on the fertile lands of Texas and raise crops, speak their own language, educate their children, and worship God as they pleased. This dream did not materialize, and members of the band grew discouraged. Some of the immigrants remained in Victoria and others went to San Antonio.

The people who went to San Antonio continued to travel; on Christmas Eve, 1854, they stopped at the junction of the San Antonio and Cibolo Rivers; there, under a live oak tree, they celebrated mass and founded Panna Maria. From 1855 to 1857, others followed this small group in moving to this part of Texas.

These settlers were exposed to many dangers from nature, such as heat, drought, snakes, and insects. The Polish settlers were not accepted by the other settlers in the area because their language, customs, and culture were different, but the immigrants survived and many moved to settle other areas near Panna Maria. Today, the people of Panna Maria continue to live simple lives close to nature and God and speak mainly Polish.

Much of the history of the Polish people in Texas is written around the founding and the location of the various church parishes. For example, in 1873, the Parish of the Nativity of the Blessed Virgin Mary was begun in Cestohowa. Above the main altar of this church is a large picture of the Virgin Mary of Czestochowa. This picture was taken to the church from Panna Maria. It is a copy of the famous Black Madonna of Czestochowa, Poland, a city 65 miles east of where the immigrants to Texas originated. The Black Madonna is a beloved, miraculous image and a source of faith to the Polish people. The Shrine of Our Lady in Czestochowa, Poland, is one of the largest shrines in the world. Since the 14th century, that picture has been the object of veneration and devotion of Polish Catholics. It is claimed to have been painted by Saint Luke the Evangelist. Its origin is traced to the 5th or 6th century and is the oldest picture of the Virgin in the world. The scars on the face date from 1430, when bandits struck it with a sword. The history, traditions, and miracles of Czestochowa are the heritage of the Polish people (Dworaczyk, 1979). One woman I interviewed said she had been ill with a fatal disease. The entire time that she lay close to death, she prayed to the Virgin. When she finally did recover, she made a pilgrimage back to her homeland in Poland and visited the shrine to give thanks to the Virgin. The woman was positive that this was the source of her recovery.

Health and Illness

The definitions of HEALTH among the Polish people I interviewed included "feeling okay—as a whole—body, spirit, everything a person cannot separate"; "happy, until war, do not need doctor, do not need medicine"; "active, able to work, feel good, do what I want to do"; and "good spirit, good to everybody, never cross." The definitions of ILLNESS may include "something wrong with body, mind, or spirit"; "one wrong affects them all"; "not capable of working, see the doctor often"; "not right, something ailing you"; "not active"; "feeling bad"; and "opposite of health, not doing what I want to do." The methods for maintaining HEALTH include maintaining a happy home, being kind and loving, eating healthy food, remaining pure, walking, exercising, wearing proper clothing, eating a well-balanced diet, trying not to worry, having faith in God, being active, dressing warmly, going to bed early, and working hard. The methods for preventing ILLNESS include cleanliness, the wearing of scapulars, avoiding drafts, following the proper diet, not gossiping, keeping away from people with colds, and wearing medals because "God is with you all the time to protect you and take care of you." Other ideas about ILLNESS include the beliefs that ILLNESSES are caused by poor diets and that the evil eye may well exist as a causative factor. This belief was attributed to the older generations and is not regarded as prevalent among younger Polish Americans.

The use of home remedies to treat illnesses and physical injuries continues to be practiced. The following are examples of commonly used home remedies:

- ■ **Teas** may be used, such as:
  - ■ **Peppermint, chamomile**, or **bess-plant**, to treat colic and cramps
  - ■ **Senna-leaf tea**, to treat constipation, and
  - ■ **Spearmint**, to treat indigestion.
- ■ **Poultices** made of **flaxseed, mustard**, or **oatmeal** may be used to treat a cold; or **goose fat** could be rubbed on the chest.
- ■ **"Gugel Mugel,"** a concoction made from warm milk with butter, whiskey, and honey, a mustard, or an onion poultice, or a few drops of turpentine and sugar, may be used to treat a cough.
- ■ **Urine** may be used to clean cuts and other injuries.
- ■ **Spider webs** may be used to clean scratches.
- ■ **Salt pork** is placed on puncture wounds; the wound is soaked in hot water.

One remedy is Swamp Root, a preparation that is used as a diuretic (Figure 13-4). Swamp Root is a liquid preparation used to flush the kidneys and bladder, thereby aiding in the elimination of waste matter. It contains 10.5% alcohol and various herbs such as peppermint, cape aloe, oil of juniper, and buchu leaves are incorporated into the syrup. The alcohol is said to be used for the purpose of preserving the ingredients (Spector, 1983).

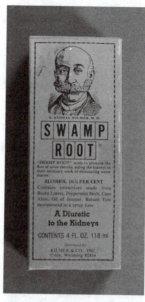

Figure 13-4   Swamp root.

Healthcare Problems

The Polish community has not tended to have any major problems with health-care providers. Language may be a barrier if members of the older generation do not speak English, and the taking of health histories is complicated when the providers cannot communicate directly with the informant. Again, problems may develop when there is difficulty finding someone who is conversant in Polish whom the informant can trust to reveal personal matters and who can translate medical terms accurately.

In Poland, there is a shortage of medical supplies, so the people tend to use faith healers and believe in miracle workers. On the main street of Warsaw, all sorts of folk medicine and miracle-worker paraphernalia are on sale: divining rods, cotton sacks filled with herbs to be worn over an ailing heart or liver, coils of copper wire to be placed under food to rid it of poisons, and pendulums (Letter from Poland, 1983).

■ Italian Americans

The Italian American community is made up of immigrants who came here from mainland Italy and from Sicily, Sardinia, and other Mediterranean islands that are part of Italy. Over 17.4% of the population claims Italian ancestry. Italian Americans have a proud heritage in the United States. America was "founded" by an Italian—Christopher Columbus; named for an Italian—Amerigo Vespucci; and explored by several Italian explorers, including Verrazano, Cabot, and Tonti (Bernardo, 1981, p. 26).

History of Migration

Between 1820 and 1990, over 5 million people from Italy immigrated to the United States (Lefcowitz, 1990, p. 6). The peak years were from 1901 to 1920, and only a small number of people continue to come today. Italians came to this country to escape poverty and to search for a better life in a country where they expected to reap rewards for their hard labor. The early years were not easy, but people chose to remain in this country and not return to Italy. Italians tended to live in neighborhood enclaves, and these neighborhoods, such as the North End in Boston and Little Italy in New York, still exist as Italian neighborhoods. Although the younger generation may have moved out, they still return home to maintain family, community, and ethnic ties (Nelli, 1980, pp. 545–560).

The family has served as the main tie keeping Italian Americans together because it provides its members with the strength to cope with the surrounding world and produces a sense of continuity in all situations. The family is the primary focus of the Italian's concern, and Italians take pride in the family and the home. Italians are resilient, yet fatalistic, and they take advantage of the present. Many upwardly mobile third- and fourth-generation Italian Americans often experience conflict between familial solidarity and society's emphasis on individualization and autonomy (Giordano & McGoldrick, 1996, p. 571). As mentioned, the home is a source of great pride, and it is a symbol of the family, not a status symbol per se. The church also is an important focus for the life of the Italian. Many of the festivals and observances continue to exist today, and in the summer, the North End of Boston is alive each weekend with the celebration of a different saint (Figure 13-5). *Madonna Della Cava* is another example of one of the saints for whom there is a summer festival. The prayers offered to her include prayers for health. Note the money that has been pinned on the statue's clothes and decorations.

The father traditionally has been the head of the Italian household, and the mother is said to be the heart of the household. The Italian population falls

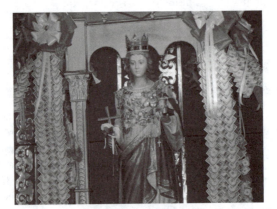

Figure 13-5   Madonna Della Cava.

into four generational groups: (1) the elderly, living in Italian enclaves; (2) a second generation, living both within the neighborhoods and in the suburbs; (3) a younger, well-educated group, living mainly in the suburbs; and (4) new immigrants (Ragucci, 1981, p. 216). More than 80% of Italian Americans have married people from a different ethnic group (Giordano & McGoldrick, 1996).

Health and Illness

Italians tend to present their symptoms to their fullest point and to expect immediate treatment for ailments. In terms of traditional beliefs, they may view the cause of illness to be one of the following: (1) winds and currents that bear diseases, (2) contagion or contamination, (3) heredity, (4) supernatural or human causes, and (5) psychosomatic interactions.

One such traditional Italian belief contends that moving air, in the form of drafts, causes irritation and then a cold that can lead to pneumonia. A belief an elderly person may express in terms of cancer surgery is that it is not a good idea to have surgery because surgery exposes the inner body to the air, and if the cancer is exposed to the air, the person is going to die more quickly. Just as drafts are considered to be a cause of illness, fresh air is considered to be vital for the maintenance of health. Homes and the workplace must be well ventilated to prevent illness from occurring.

The belief in contamination may manifest in the reluctance of people to share food and objects with people who are considered unclean, and often in not entering the homes of those who are ill. Traditional Italian women have a strong sense of modesty and shame, resulting in an avoidance of discussions relating to sex and menstruation.

Blood is regarded by some, especially the elderly, to be a "plastic entity" that responds to fluids and food and is responsible for many variable conditions. Various adjectives, such as *high* and *low* and *good* and *bad*, are used to describe blood. Some of the "old superstitions" include the following beliefs:

1. Congenital abnormalities can be attributed to the unsatisfied desire for food during pregnancy.
2. If a pregnant woman is not given food that she smells, the fetus will move inside and a miscarriage will result.
3. If a pregnant woman bends, turns, or moves in a certain way, the fetus may not develop normally.
4. A woman must not reach during pregnancy because reaching can harm the fetus.

Italians may also attribute the cause of illness to the evil eye (*malocchio*) or to curses (*castiga*). The difference between these two causes is that less serious illnesses, such as headaches, may be caused by *malocchio*, whereas more severe illnesses, which often can be fatal, may be attributed to more powerful *castiga*. Curses are sent either by God or by evil people. An example of a curse is the punishment from God for sins and bad behavior (Ragucci, 1981, p. 216).

Italians recognize that illness can be caused by the suppression of emotions, as well as stress from fear, grief, and anxiety. If one is unable to find an emotional outlet, one well may "burst." It is not considered healthy to bottle up emotions (Ragucci, 1981, p. 232).

Often, the care of the ill is managed in the home, with all members of the family sharing in the responsibilities. The use of home remedies ostensibly is decreasing, although several students have reported the continued use of rituals for the removal of the evil eye and the practice of leeching. One practice described for the removal of the evil eye was to take an egg and olive oil and to drip them into a pan of water, make the sign of the cross, and recite prayers. If the oil spreads over the water, the cause of the problem is the evil eye, and the illness should get better. Mineral waters are also used, and tonics are used to cleanse the blood. There is a strong religious influence among Italians, who believe that faith in God and the saints will see them through the illness. One woman whom I worked with had breast cancer. She had had surgery several years before and did not have a recurrence. She attributed her recovery to the fact that she attended mass every morning and that she had total faith in Saint Peregrine, whose medal she wore pinned to her bra by the site of the mastectomy. Italian people tend to take a fatalistic stance regarding terminal illness and death, believing that it is God's will. Death often is not discussed between the dying person and the family members. I recall when caring for an elderly Italian man at home that it was not possible to have the man and his wife discuss his impending death. Although both knew that he was dying and would talk with the nurse, to each other he "was going to recover," and everything possible was done to that end.

Italian families observe numerous religious traditions surrounding death, and funeral masses and anniversary masses are observed. It is the custom for the widow to wear black for some time after her husband's death (occasionally for the remainder of her life), although this is not as common with the younger generations.

Health-related Problems

Two genetic diseases commonly seen among Italians are: (1) favism, a severe hemolytic anemia caused by deficiency of the X-linked enzyme glucose-6-phosphate dehydrogenase and triggered by the eating of fava beans; and (2) the thalassemia syndromes, also hemolytic anemias that include Cooley's anemia (or beta-thalassemia) and alpha-thalassemia (Ragucci, 1981, p. 222).

Language problems frequently occur when elderly or new Italian immigrants are seeking care. Often, due to modesty, people are reluctant to answer the questions asked through interpreters, and gathering of pertinent data is very difficult.

Problems related to time also occur. Healthcare providers tend to diagnose emotional problems more often for Italian patients than for other ethnic groups because of the Italian pattern of reporting more symptoms and reporting them more dramatically (Giordano & McGoldrick, 1996, p. 576).

In general, Italian Americans are motivated to seek explanations with respect to their health status and the care they are to receive. If instructions and explanations are well given, Italians tend to cooperate with healthcare providers. It is often necessary to provide directions in the greatest detail and then to provide written instructions to ensure that necessary regimens are followed.

Health Status of the White (Non-Hispanic) Population

There are countless health status indicators wherein the White (non-Hispanic) cohort of the population differs from the total population, each of the racial groups, and Hispanics. Each of the preceding four chapters has included a table comparing the relevant group and all races. In this chapter, it is appropriate to compare the White non-Hispanic population to the total population (Tables 13-2, 13-3, and 13-4). In spite of the fact that only nine health indicators are listed as examples in the tables, the health differences and disparities in the overall populations are readily apparent.

Table 13-3 lists the 10 leading causes of death for Whites and compares them with the causes of death for the general population in 2013. There is no difference in the mortality rates between the White population and all persons for this year.

Table 13-2 Comparison of Selected Health Status Indicators: 2013 All Races and White

Health Indicator	All Races	White Only
Crude birth rate per 1,000 population by race of mother, 2013	12.4	12.0
Percentage of live births to teenage childbearing women—18–19 years, 2013	5.0	4.8
Percentage of low birth weight per live births >2,500 grams, 2013	8.02	7.0
Infant mortality per 1,000 live births, 2012	6.0	5.1
Respondent-reported prevalence percent of adults: Cancer—all sites, 2012–2013, 18 years and over	5.9	6.2
Respondent-reported prevalence percent of adults: Heart Disease—2012–2013, 18 years and over	10.6	10.8
Respondent-reported prevalence percent of adults: Stroke—2012–2013, 18 years and over	2.5	2.4
Male death rates from suicide, all ages, age adjusted per 100,000 resident population, 2013	20.3	**22.6**
Male death rates from homicide, all ages, age adjusted per 100,000 resident population.	8.2	4.4

Source: Health, United States, 2014: With Special Feature on Adults Aged 55–64, by National Center for Health Statistics, 2015, Hyattsville, MD: Author, pp. 58, 59, 62, 64, 76, 134, 135, 138, 139, 161.

Table 13-3 Comparison of Selected Health Status Indicators: All Races, American Indian and Alaska Native, Asian/Pacific Islander, Black or African American, Hispanic or Latino, and White Non-Hispanic: 2013

Health Indicator	All Races	American Indian and Alaska Native	Asian/Pacific Islander[1]	Black or African American	Hispanic or Latino	White Non-Hispanic
Crude birth rate per 1,000 population by race of mother, 2013	12.4	10.3	14.3	12.0	16.7	12.0
Percentage of live births to teenage childbearing women—18–19 years, 2013	5.0	8.7	0.5	4.8	7.1	4.8
Percentage of low birth weight per live births >2,500 grams, 2013	8.02	7.48	8.34	7.0	7.09	7.0
Infant mortality per 1,000 live births, 2012	6.0	8.4	4.1	5.1	5.1	5.1
Respondent-reported prevalence percent of adults Cancer—all sites, 2012–2013, 18 years and over	5.9	4.3	3.4	6.2	3.6	6.2
Respondent-reported prevalence percent of adults: Heart Disease—2012–2013, 18 years and over	10.6	10.1	6.4	10.8	8.0	10.8
Respondent-reported prevalence percent of adults: Stroke—2012–2013, 18 years and over	2.5	3.3	1.8	2.4	2.6	2.4
Male death rates from suicide, all ages, age adjusted per 100,000 resident population, 2013	20.3	18.1	9.2	22.6	9.3	22.6
Male death rates from homicide, all ages, age adjusted per 100,000 resident population, 2013						
Male death rates from homicide, all ages, age adjusted per 100,000 resident population, 2013	8.2	8.2	2.3	4.4	7.3	4.4

Source: Health, United States, 2014: With Special Feature on Adults Aged 55–64, by National Center for Health Statistics, 2015, Hyattsville, MD: Author, pp. 58, 59, 62, 64, 76, 134, 135, 138, 139, 161.

Table 13-4   Comparison of the 10 Leading Causes of Death for White and for All
Persons: 2013

White	All Persons
1. Diseases of heart	1. Diseases of heart
2. Malignant neoplasms	2. Malignant neoplasms
3. Chronic lower respiratory diseases	3. Chronic lower respiratory diseases
4. Unintentional injuries	4. Unintentional injuries
5. Cerebrovascular diseases	5. Cerebrovascular diseases
6. Alzheimer's disease	6. Alzheimer's disease
7. Diabetes mellitus	7. Diabetes mellitus
8. Influenza and pneumonia	8. Influenza and pneumonia
9. Nephritis, nephrotic syndrome, and nephrosis	9. Nephritis, nephrotic syndrome, and nephrosis
10. Suicide	10. Suicide

Source: Health, United States, 2014: With Special Feature on Adults Aged 55–64, by National Center for Health Statistics, 2015, Hyattsville, MD: Author, p. 97.

Both in this chapter, and in this entire book, I have attempted to open the door to the enormous diversity in HEALTH and ILLNESS beliefs that exists in White (European American) communities specifically and in the entire American population in general. I have only opened the door and invited you to peek inside. There is a richness of knowledge to be gained. It is for you to acquire it as you care for all patients. Ask them what they believe about health/HEALTH and illness/ILLNESS and what their traditional beliefs, practices, and remedies are. The students whom I am working with find this to be a very enlightening experience.

RESEARCH ON CULTURE

A great amount of research has been conducted among members of the White American populations. The following article describes one such study:

Hutson, S. P., Dorgan, K. A., Phillips, A. N., & Behringer, B. (2007, November). The mountains hold things in: The use of community research review work groups to address cancer disparities in Appalachia. *Oncology Nursing Forum*, 34(6), 1133–1139.

The purpose of this research study was to review regional findings about cancer disparities with grassroots community leaders in Appalachia and to discover what makes the experience of cancer unique in that part of the country. The study was community-based and information was gathered from focus groups. Four major themes emerged from the focus groups:

1. *Cancer storytelling.* One theme was the ubiquitous nature of cancer and that the members of the community expect to get cancer. Many participants believed that "cancer was more a hereditary thing" because of family histories.
2. *Cancer collectiveness.* Rural families tend to rely on themselves.

(continued)

RESEARCH ON CULTURE   *(continued)*

3. *Healthcare challenges.* Participants were doubtful about their ability to navigate and trust the healthcare system. They also told of the state's history of overlooking the people in this community.
4. *Cancer expectations.* Some rural people may not embrace what are seen as basic patients' rights.

The key discoveries were that the cancer experience in Appalachia appears to be affected uniquely by cultural, economic, and geographic influences; that healthcare professionals and researchers must respect and partner with existing social and familial community networks; and the use of community research review work is a viable method to examine cancer disparities in a marginalized population. Suggestions from this study supported the need for patient navigators and advocate services to reach communities and bridge the gaps between the healthcare system and laypeople. Cancer information should be tailored to individual patients' attributes, such as education and literacy levels and cultural and familial beliefs.

Explore ⬤ MediaLink

Go to the Student Resource Site at pearsonhighered.com/nursingresources for chapter-related review questions, case studies, and activities. Contents of the CulturalCare Guide and CulturalCare Museum can also be found on the Student Resource Site. Click on Chapter 13 to select the activities for this chapter.

■ References

Bernardo, S. (1981). *The ethnic almanac.* New York, NY: Doubleday.

Conzen, K. N. (1980). Germans. In S. Thernstrom (Ed.), *Harvard encyclopedia of American ethnic groups.* Cambridge, MA: Harvard University Press.

Dworaczyk, E. J. (1979). *The first Polish colonies of America in Texas.* San Antonio, TX: Naylor.

Giordano, J., & McGoldrick, M. (1996). Italian families. In M. McGoldrick, J. Giordano, & J. K. Pearce (Eds.), *Ethnicity and family therapy* (2nd ed.). New York, NY: Guilford.

Green, V. (1980). Poles. In S. Thernstrom (Ed.), *Harvard encyclopedia of American ethnic groups.* Cambridge, MA: Harvard University Press.

Hutson, S. P., Dorgan, K. A., Phillips, A. N., & Behringer, B. (2007, November). The mountains hold things in: The use of community research review work groups to address cancer disparities in Appalachia. *Oncology Nursing Forum, 34*(6), 1133–1139.

Lefcowitz, E. (1990). *The United States immigration history timeline.* New York, NY: Terra Firma Press.

Letter from Poland—of faith healers and miracle workers. (1983, August 21). *Boston Globe,* p. 15.

Lich, G. E. (1982). *The German Texan*. San Antonio: University of Texas Institute of Texan Cultures.

McDonnell-Smith, M. (2013). Asians are fastest-growing U.S. ethnic group, Blacks are slowest. *DiversityInc*. Retrieved from http://www.diversityinc .com/diversity-and-inclusion/asians-are-fastest-growing-u-s-ethnic-group-in -2012-blacks-are-slowest-reports-u-s-census-bureau/

National Center for Health Statistics. (2015). *Health, United States, 2014: With special feature on adults aged 55–64*. Hyattsville, MD: Author. Retrieved from http://www.cdc.gov/nchs/data/hus/hus14.pdf

Needleman, J. (2003). *The American soul*. New York, NY: Tarcher/Putman.

Nelli, H. S. (1980). Italians. In S. Thernstrom (Ed.), *Harvard encyclopedia of American ethnic groups*. Cambridge, MA: Harvard University Press.

Ragucci, A. T. (1981). Italian Americans. In A. Harwood (Ed.), *Ethnicity and medical care*. Cambridge, MA: Harvard University Press.

Spector, R. E. (1983). *A description of the impact of Medicare on health-illness beliefs and practices of White ethnic senior citizens in Central Texas* (Doctoral dissertation). University of Texas at Austin School of Nursing. Ann Arbor, MI: University Microfilms International.

U.S. Department of Commerce, U.S. Census Bureau. (2015a). *American Community Survey (ACS). 2014 ACS 1-year estimates*. Retrieved from https:// www.census.gov/programs-surveys/acs/technical-documentation/table-and -geography-changes/2014/1-year.html

U.S. Department of Commerce, U.S. Census Bureau. (2015b). *American Fact-Finder: Selected social characteristics in the United States*. Retrieved from http://factfinder.census.gov/faces/tableservices/jsf/pages/productview .xhtml?pid=ACS_13_5YR_DP02&src=pt

CHAPTER

14 CULTURALCOMPETENCY

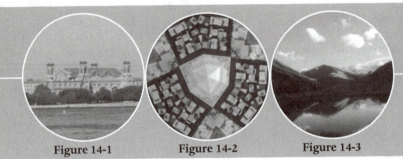

Figure 14-1　　　　　Figure 14-2　　　　　Figure 14-3

■ Objectives

1. Discuss the rationale for becoming CULTURALLYCOMPETENT.
2. Describe the components of the CULTURALCARE Circle.
3. Develop goals for integrating CULTURALCOMPETENCY into the scope of practice.

　　The closing link on the *HERITAGECHAIN* is that of CULTURALCOMPETENCY and it joins together all the links in the chain. The opening images for this chapter bring closure to the process of becoming CULTURALLYCOMPETENT. They both summarize and symbolize many of the concepts presented in the text. Each chapter opened with images representing the content of the chapter. Figure 14-1 is the main building in the Ellis Island museum in New York. We are a nation of immigrants, and this image of the location where so many people entered this country is a reminder. Figure 14-2 is a kaleidoscopic example of herbal remedies. The use of herbs—often those that can be grown in your own backyard—to treat many maladies is common. Countless people turn to herbs, usually as their first source of medication, and evidence indicates that the use of herbal remedies is prevalent among many people. Figure 14-3 represents the timelessness of the ongoing tensions between the allopathic and homeopathic philosophies and the conflict you may experience when you encounter people who prefer traditional HEALTH and ILLNESS beliefs and practices rather than modern healthcare therapies. Implicit in CULTURALCOMPETENCY is the understanding of a situation from a "person or patient's point of view."

The perplexing questions—

- *Why* must healthcare providers—nurses, physicians, public health and social workers, and other healthcare professionals—study culture, ethnicity, religion, and become culturally competent?
- *Why* must they know the difference between "hot" and "cold" and *yin* and *yang*?
- *Why* must they be concerned with the patient's failure to practice what professionals believe to be good preventive medicine, with the patient's failure to follow a given treatment regimen, or with the patient's failure to seek medical care during the initial phase of an illness?
- *Why* is there a difference between curing and HEALING?

—have now been explored and selected answers presented.

Figure 14-4, The CULTURALCARE Circle, serves as a summary of this book's theoretical content as it illustrates the following inherent factors:

- *Heritage*—culture, ethnicity, religion embraced in the processes of socialization
- *Demographics*—the changing picture of the United States and the challenges of the demographic factors
- *HEALTH*—physical, mental, and spiritual.

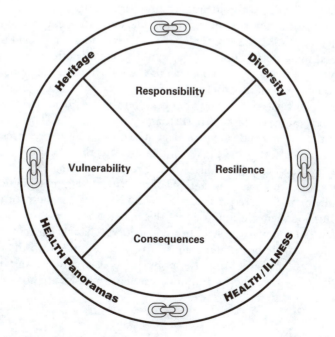

Figure 14-4 CULTURALCARE Circle.

The core focuses in the quadrants are:

1. *Vulnerability.* All humans are vulnerable, but their degrees of vulnerability and their responses to the challenges of vulnerability vary. One determining factor is the overall HEALTH of a given person, and that person's genetic makeup, socioeconomic status, the environmental challenges of where the person lives and works, and his or her resilience.

2. *Resilience.* This is the way by which a given person meets the challenges—physical, mental, and spiritual—that he or she confronts over a lifetime.

3. *Responsibility.* The responsibility of creating and maintaining a HEALTHY person and society are inherent factors in the scope of practice of all healthcare providers and of all people.

4. *Consequences.* The ongoing consequences for failing to meet the cultural needs of patients, families, and communities will be devastating—to both the providers of healthcare and those we serve.

The forthcoming text offers solutions to this vexing dilemma.

There is little disagreement that healthcare services in this country are unevenly distributed and that the poor and people of color—the "emerging majority[1]"—get the short end of the stick in terms of the care they receive (or do not receive). The apparent health disparities are a reality, as are the demographic and social disparities in areas of housing, employment, education, and opportunity. Just as there is the need to understand the people who comprise our multicultural society, there is also the need to understand new immigrants as more and more people flock to this country. Yet it is often maintained that when healthcare is provided, people fail to use it or use it inappropriately. Why does this seeming paradox exist?

The major focus of this book has been on the provider's and the patient's differing perceptions of health/HEALTH and illness/ILLNESS. These differences may account for the healthcare provider's misconception that services are used inappropriately and that people do not care about their health. What to the casual observer appears to be "misuse" may represent our failure to understand and to meet the needs and expectations of the patient. This possibility may well be difficult for healthcare providers to face, but careful analysis of the available information seems to indicate that this may—at least in part—be the case. How, then, can we, who are healthcare providers, change our method of operations and provide both safe and effective care for all—both the emerging majority and, at the same time, the population at large? The answer to this question is not an easy one, and some researchers think we are not succeeding.

---

[1]The United States is projected to become a majority–minority nation for the first time in 2042 or 2043 (Associated Press, 2015; National Urban Fellows, 2012).

A number of measures can and must be taken to ameliorate the current situation. CULTURALCARE and the educational preparation leading to this is a *process*, one that becomes a way of life and must be recognized as such. This is a philosophical issue. The changing of personal and professional philosophies, ideas, and stereotypes does *not* occur overnight, and the process, quite often, is neither direct nor easy. It is a multistep process, in which you, as a healthcare professional, must:

- ∞ Explore your own cultural identity and heritage and confront biases and stereotypes.
- ∞ Develop an awareness and understanding of the complexities of the modern healthcare delivery system—its philosophy and problems, biases, and stereotypes.
- ∞ Develop a keen awareness of the socialization process that brings the provider into this complex system.
- ∞ Develop the ability to "hear" things that transcend language, and to foster an understanding of the patient and his or her cultural heritage, and the resilience found within the culture that supports family and community structures.

Given the processes of acculturation, assimilation, and modernism, this is often difficult and painful. Yet, once the journey of exploring your own cultural heritage and prejudices is undertaken, the awareness of the cultural needs of others becomes more subtle and understandable. This is well accomplished by using the umbrella of HEALTH traditions as the point of entry.

A student I recently taught described the journey this way:

> I was born in 1994 to immigrant Korean parents. I understood a little bit of Korean culture and the way of thinking and did not question when my mother told me to drink a vile tasting brown liquid every morning to bring a healthy and long life. I went to a Caucasian school and was the only Korean student in my grade. I came to hate my heritage and wanted to scream that "I'm as White on the inside as you are." I was bitter and embarrassed by my heritage and blamed my family, who were proud of their ancestry. When my parents tried to teach me about Korean history, culture, and healthcare, I was not interested. I came to know, understand, and hate racism. On the inside I felt as "White American" as everyone else but I soon realized what I felt inside was not what other people saw. I now acknowledge who I am and I accept myself.

The voice of this young student speaks for many. In the course of having to explore the family's traditional HEALTH beliefs and practices, the student began to see, think through, understand, and accept herself.

Although curricula in professional education are quite full, CULTURALCARE studies must be taken by all people who wish to deliver healthcare. In the wake of September 11, 2001, and the recent acts of radical Islamic terrorism around the globe, it is obvious that it is no longer sufficient to teach a student in the health professions to "accept patients for who they are." The question arises: Who is the patient? Introductory sociology and psychology courses fail to provide this information unless tailored to include cultural aspects of HEALTH and ILLNESS. It is learned best by meeting with the people themselves and letting them describe who they are from their own perspective. I have suggested two approaches to the problem. One is to have people who work as patient advocates or as nurses and physicians come to the class setting and explain how people of their sociocultural or religious group view health/HEALTH and illness/ILLNESS and describe the given community's HEALTH traditions. Another approach is to accompany students out into the community and develop the opportunity to meet with people in their own settings. It is not necessary to memorize all the available lists of herbs, hot-cold imbalances, folk diseases, and so forth. The objective is to become more sensitive to the crucial fact that multiple factors underlie given patient and personal behaviors. One, of course, is that the patient may well perceive and understand HEALTH from quite a different perspective than that of the healthcare provider. *Each person comes from a unique culture and a unique socialization process.*

The healthcare provider must be sensitive to his or her own perceptions of health and illness and the professional health beliefs and practices he or she follows. Even though the perceptions of most health professionals are based on a middle-class and medical-model viewpoint, providers must realize that there are other ways to regard health and illness. Earlier chapters of this book are devoted to consciousness-raising about self-treatment and self-medication with the use of herbal and home remedies. It is always an eye-opening experience to publicly scrutinize ourselves in this respect. Quite often, we are amazed to see how far we stray from the system's prescribed methods of keeping healthy. The journals confirm that we, too, delay in seeking healthcare and fail to follow treatment regimens. Often, our ability to adhere to treatment recommendations rests on quite pragmatic issues, such as "What is it doing for me?" and "Can I afford to miss work and stay in bed for two days?" As we gain insight into our own health-illness attitudes and behaviors, we tend to be much more sympathetic to and empathetic with the person who fails to come to the clinic, who hates to wait for the physician, or who delays in seeking healthcare.

The healthcare provider should be aware of the complex issues that surround the delivery of healthcare from the patient's viewpoint. Calling the medical society for the name of a physician (because a "family member has a health problem") and visiting and comparing the services rendered in an urban and a suburban emergency department are exercises that can enable us to better appreciate some of the difficulties that the poor, the emerging majority, immigrants, and the population at large all too often experience when they attempt to obtain healthcare. Members of the healthcare team have a number of advantages in gaining access to the healthcare system. For example, they can choose a physician whom they know because they work with him or her or because someone they work with has recommended this physician. Healthcare providers must never forget, however, that most people do not have these advantages. It is indeed an unsettling, anxiety-provoking, and frustrating experience to be forced to select a physician from a list. It is an even more frustrating experience to be a patient in an unfamiliar location—for example, an urban emergency department, where, quite literally, anything can happen. The Michael Moore film *Sicko*, and the documentary series *Unnatural Causes* from California Newsreel, paint a most painful picture of the modern healthcare system and the unequal access and care many people receive. Books, such as J. P. Kassirer's *On the Take* (2005), which illustrates the complicity of the healthcare system and big business, and T. R. Reid's *The Healing of America: A Global Quest for Better and Cheaper, and Fairer Health Care* (2010), serve to illustrate other aspects of the complex healthcare system we live with today. Yet, people entering the system ought to be familiar with all aspects of it and many issues not mentioned, such as the costs of procedures and medications.

Another barrier to adequate healthcare is the financial burden imposed by treatments and tests. There are other issues as well. For example, a Chinese patient—who traditionally does not believe that the body replaces blood taken for testing purposes—should have as little blood work as necessary, and the reasons for the tests should be carefully explained. A Hispanic woman who believes that taking a Pap smear is an intrusive procedure that will bring shame to her should have the procedure performed by a female physician or nurse. When this is not possible, she should have a female chaperone and family member with her for the entire time that the male physician or nurse is in the room.

More members of the emerging majority must be represented in the health-care professions. Multiple issues are related to the problem of underrepresentation—the demographic disparity—that is ongoing because there are inadequate numbers of people from the emerging majority. Many of the programs designed to increase the number of emerging-majority students in the healthcare team have failed. Difficulties surrounding successful entrance into and completion of professional education programs are complex and numerous, having their roots in impoverished community structures, early educational deprivation, and family responsibilities. Although society is in some ways dealing with such issues—for example, initiating improvements in early education—we are faced with an *immediate* need to bring more emerging-majority people into healthcare services.

One method would be the more extensive use of patient advocates and outreach workers from the given racial or ethnic community who may be recognized by the community as HEALERS. The people can provide an overwhelmingly positive service to both the provider and the patient in that they can serve as the bridge in bringing healthcare services to the target community. The patient advocate can speak to the patient in the language that he or she understands and in a manner that is acceptable. Advocates are also able to coordinate medical, nursing, social, and even educational services to meet the patient's needs as the patient perceives them. In settings where advocates are employed, many problems are resolved to the convenience of both the healthcare member and, more importantly, the patient!

The persistent issue of language bursts forth with regularity. There are at least 350 languages spoken in American homes (U.S. Census Bureau, 2015), and there is frequently a problem when a non–English-speaking person tries to seek help from the English-speaking majority. The use of an interpreter or translator is always difficult because the translator generally "interprets" what he or she translates. To bring this thought home, the reader should recall the childhood game of "gossip": A message is passed around the room from person to person, and by the time it gets back to the sender, its content is usually substantially changed. This game is not unlike trying to communicate through an interpreter or translator, and the situation is even more frustrating when—as can frequently be the case—the translator is a young child. It is, obviously, far more satisfying and productive if the patient, nurse, and physician can all speak the same language. All institutions must follow the mandates of Title VI of the Civil Rights Law. In fact, in many institutions, there are professional interpreters available; however, they may not be present 24 hours a day, 7 days a week. Telephone devices and some computer-generated programs are available, but costly.

Health services must be made far more accessible and available to members of the emerging majority. I believe that one of the most important events in this modern era of healthcare delivery is the advent of neighborhood health centers. They are successful essentially because people who work in them know the people of the neighborhood. In addition, the people of the community can contribute to the decision making involved in governing and running the agency so that services are tailored to meet the needs of the patients. Concerned members of the healthcare team have a moral obligation to support the increased use of healthcare centers and not their decreased use, as currently tends to occur because of cutbacks in response to allegations (frequently politically motivated) of too-high costs or the misuse of funds. These neighborhood healthcare centers provide greatly needed personal services in addition to relief from the widespread depersonalization that occurs in larger institutions. When genuinely concerned healthcare providers face this reality, perhaps they will be more willing to fight for the survival of these centers and strongly urge their increased funding rather than acquiesce in their demise. In rural areas, the problem is even greater, and far more comprehensive health planning is needed to meet patient needs.

In the beginning of this text and throughout it, I used the metaphor of climbing stairs to reach CULTURALCOMPETENCY. However, this can be seen, too, as a journey. Thus, the *road*, or ascent, to CULTURALCOMPETENCY is similar to traveling on a road to anywhere, as depicted in Table 14-1, "The Journey to CULTURALCOMPETENCY." It takes time and thought and active participation. It is a learning experience wherein you discover countless facts (especially about yourself), a dynamic *process* in which you face a number of obstacles on the road:

CULTURALCARE is the term I have coined to express all that is inherent in this text. Countless conflicts in the healthcare delivery arenas are predicated on cultural misunderstandings. Although many of these misunderstandings are related to universal situations, such as verbal and nonverbal language misunderstandings, the conventions of courtesy, sequencing of interactions,

Table 14-1   The Journey to CULTURAL COMPETENCY

Collisions	Head-ons—meeting dense cultural conflicts and barriers—can be fatal
	Rear-enders—come at you from behind to sabotage efforts
	Fender benders—slips and blunders
	Side swipes—minor, but hurtful frustrations
Conditions	Culture + Climate—Social/Institutional attitudes
	Weather (rain, snow, fog, sun)—Heritage—Race/Ethnicity/Religion/ Socialization
Curves	The unknown—inability to anticipate the real responses, verbal vs. nonverbal
Destination	Physical, Mental, Spiritual—a realization of and respect for holistic HEALTH
Hills	The process of gaining CULTURAL COMPETENCY—content and experience— an up and down experience
Lights	Slow, and controls the progress
No Signs	Road twists and turns and no identifying markings
Open Highway	Cruise along—but not too fast
Other Drivers	Slow you down or speed you up on the road to CULTURAL CARE
Pot Holes	Frequent blocks to smooth movement, often unseen, filled with water or covered with ice
Rush Hour	Institutional and provider clogs
Ruts	When cruising along, the unexpected hits and it is often difficult to break free
Speed Limits	Analogous to Institutional and Professional restraints—do not go too fast or too slow or you are in trouble and everyone is behind you
Tolls	Expensive—pay for books, travel, objects, admissions, tools
Unexpected Events	Negative—radar, accidents, ice—anger, "isms"
	Positive—enduring friendships with people you may have never met
	Knowledge far deeper than ever anticipated
	Wisdom
	Deep love of life and people

phasing of interactions, objectivity, and so forth, many cultural misunderstandings are unique to the delivery of healthcare. The necessity to provide CULTURAL CARE—professional healthcare that is culturally sensitive, culturally appropriate, and culturally competent—is essential as we live in this millennium, and it demands that providers be able to assess and interpret a given patient's health/HEALTH beliefs and practices. CULTURAL CARE alters the perspective of healthcare delivery as it enables the provider to understand, from a cultural perspective, the manifestations of the patient's HEALTHCARE beliefs and practices. Note that the terms CULTURAL COMPETENCY and CULTURAL CARE are written in small capitals to indicate that the view is holistic—three-dimensional rather than two.

■ CULTURALCOMPETENCY

You will know you are on the road to CULTURALCOMPETENCY when you understand that:

- Even when you are a part of a group, social or professional, you are a person who has your own HERITAGE—your own culture, ethnicity, and religion.
- You have been socialized—first by your parents, then by schools/ teachers, and later by society at large—to be who you are.
- You have your own HEALTH and ILLNESS beliefs and practices.
- There are countless ways to protect and maintain your HEALTH other than those prescribed by the dominant culture.
- Amulets may be commonly used by people from many heritages to protect or restore their HEALTH.
- There are countless ways to restore your HEALTH other than those prescribed by the dominant culture's allopathic healthcare system.
- Herbal remedies, teas, aromatherapy, and so on are used by people from countless traditional heritages.
- Religion plays a profound role in the HEALTH and HEALING beliefs and practices of traditional people from all walks of life.
- Shrines, either secular or religious, are inherent in the HEALING process of countless people.

I should like to reiterate that this book was written with the hope that by sharing the material I have learned and taught for over 45 years, some small changes will be made in the thinking of all healthcare providers who read it. There is nothing new in these pages. Perhaps it is simply a recombination of material with which the reader is familiar, but I hope it serves its purpose: the sharing of beliefs and attitudes, and the stimulation of purposeful consciousness raising concerning issues of vital concern to healthcare providers who must confront the needs of patients with diverse cultural backgrounds.

Explore ◉ MediaLink

Go to the Student Resource Site at pearsonhighered.com/nursingresources for chapter-related review questions, case studies, and activities. Contents of the CULTURALCARE Guide and CULTURALCARE Museum can also be found on the Student Resource Site. Click on Chapter 14 to select the activities for this chapter.

■ References

Associated Press. (2015, November 19). Census considers more race choices. *The Boston Globe*, 2015, p. A-2.

Kassirer, J. P. (2005). *On the take*. Oxford, England: Oxford University Press.

National Urban Fellows. (2012). *Diversity counts: Racial and ethnic diversity among public service leadership* (p. 2). Retrieved from http://www.nuf.org/sites/default/files/Documents/NUF_diversitycounts_V2FINAL.pdf

Reid, T. R. (2010). *The healing of America: A global quest for better and cheaper, and fairer health care*. New York, NY: Penguin.

U.S. Census Bureau. (2015). *Census Bureau reports at least 350 languages spoken in U.S. homes*. Retrieved from http://www.census.gov/newsroom/press-releases/2015/cb15-185.html

Appendix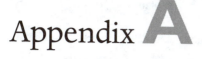

Selected Key Terms Related to Cultural Diversity in Health and Illness

The following terms have been defined to help you in the development of CULTURALCOMPETENCY. They are the "bricks" that comprise the "steps" to climb; or the linked terms necessary in the process of developing CULTURALCOMPETENCY. They are the language of CULTURALCARE.

Aberglaubish or *aberglobin*—The traditional German term for the "evil eye."

Access—Gaining entry into a system; the term used in this text refers to access into the modern healthcare system. *Access* also means entry into a profession, education, employment, housing, and so forth.

Acculturation—The process of adapting to another culture; to acquire the majority group's culture.

Acupuncture—The traditional Chinese medical way of restoring the balance of *yin* and *yang* that is based on the therapeutic value of cold. Cold is used in a disease where there is an excess of *yang*.

Ageism—Being against people of a certain age.

Alcoholismo—Traditional Hispanic word for alcoholism.

Alien—Every person applying for entry to the United States; anyone who is not a U.S. citizen.

Allopathic philosophy—Health beliefs and practices that are derived from current scientific models and involve the use of technology and other modalities of present-day healthcare, such as immunization, proper nutrition, and resuscitation.

Allopathy—The treatment of a disease by using remedies that cause the opposite effects of the disease.

Alternative health system—A system of healthcare a person may use that is not predicated within his or her traditional culture but is not allopathic.

Amulet—An object with magical powers, such as a charm, worn on a string or chain around the neck, wrist, or waist to protect the wearer from both physical and psychic illness, harm, and misfortune.

Anamnesis—The traditional Chinese medical way of diagnosing a health problem by asking questions.

Apparel—Traditional clothing worn by people for cultural or religious beliefs on a daily basis, such as head coverings.

Aromatherapy—Ancient science that uses essential plant oils to produce strong physical and emotional effects in the body.

Assimilation—To become absorbed into another culture and to adopt its characteristics; to develop a new cultural identity.

Ataque de nervios—Traditional Hispanic term for an attack of nerves, or a nervous breakdown.

Average charge—Average amount of monetary charge in hospital bills for discharged patients.

Average length of stay—The typical number of days a patient stays in the hospital for a particular condition.

Ayurvedic—A 4,000-year-old method of healing that originated in India, the chief aim of which is longevity and quality of life. It is the most ancient existing medical system that uses diet, natural therapies, and herbs.

Balance (or equilibrium)—Each aspect of the person—physical, mental, and spiritual—carries equal magnitude.

Bankes—Small, bell-shaped glass that is used to create a vacuum, placed on a person's chest, to loosen chest secretions.

Biofeedback—The use of an electronic machine to measure skin temperatures. The patient controls responses that are usually involuntary.

Biological variations—Biological differences that exist among races and ethnic groups in body structure, skin color, biochemical differences, susceptibility to disease, and nutritional differences.

Borders—Legal, geographic separations between nations.

Botanica—Traditional Hispanic pharmacy where amulets, herbal remedies, books, candles, and statues of saints may be purchased.

Bruja—Traditional Hispanic word for a witch.

Caida de la mollera (fallen fontanelle)—Traditional Hispanic belief that the fontanelle falls if the baby's head is touched.

Calendar—Dates of religious holidays. Many of these dates of observance can change from year to year on the Julian calendar.

Care—Factors that assist, enable, support, or facilitate a person's needs to maintain, improve, or ease a health problem.

Celos—Traditional Hispanic word for jealousy.

Census—The U.S. Census Bureau counts every resident in the United States. The data collected by the decennial census determine the number of seats each state has in the U.S. House of Representatives and is also used to distribute billions in federal funds to local communities.

Charm—Objects that combine the functions of both amulets and talismans but consist only of written words or symbols.

Chinese doctor—Physician educated in China who uses traditional herbs and other therapeutic modalities in the delivery of healthcare.

Chiropractic—A form of healthcare that believes in the use of "energy" to treat diseases.

Complementary medicine—Treatment modalities used to complement allopathic regimens.

Citizen—A citizen of the United States is a native-born, foreign-born child of citizens, or a naturalized person who owes allegiance to the United States and who is entitled to its protection.

Conjure—To effect magic.

Coraje—Traditional Hispanic word for rage.

Costs—The monetary price of an item, or the consequences of ignoring social factors.

CULTURALCARE—A concept that describes holistic HEALTHCARE that is culturally sensitive, culturally appropriate, and culturally competent. CULTURALCARE is critical to meeting the complex nursing care needs of a person, family, and community. It is the provision of healthcare across cultural boundaries, and it takes into account the context in which the patient lives as well as the situations in which the patient's health problems arise.

Culturally appropriate—Implies that the healthcare provider applies the underlying background knowledge that must be possessed to provide a given patient with the best possible healthcare.

CULTURALLYCOMPETENT—Implies that within the delivered care, the healthcare provider understands and attends to the total context of the patient's situation. CULTURALCOMPETENCE is a complex combination of knowledge, attitudes, and skills.

Culturally sensitive—Implies that the healthcare providers possess some basic knowledge of and constructive attitudes toward the HEALTH traditions observed among the diverse cultural groups found in the setting in which they are practicing.

Culture—Nonphysical traits, such as values, beliefs, attitudes, and customs, that are shared by a group of people and passed from one generation to the next; a meta-communication system.

Culture shock—A disorder that occurs in response to transition from one cultural setting to another. Former behavior patterns are ineffective in such a setting, and basic cues for social behavior are absent.

Curandera(o)—Traditional Hispanic holistic healer.

Curing*—A two-dimensional phenomenon that results in ridding the body or mind (or both) of a given disease.

Decoction—A simmered tea made from the bark, root, seed, or berry of a plant.

Demographic disparity—A variation below the percentages of the profile of the total population with a specific entity, such as poverty, or professional, such as nursing. Comparison with the demographic profile of the total population.

Demographic parity—An equal distribution of a given entity, such as registered nurses, and the demographic profile of the total population.

Demographics—The population profile of the nation, state, county, or local city or town.

Demography—The statistical study of populations, including statistical counts of people of various ages, sexes, and population densities for specific locations.

*Terms with an asterisk (*), such as this one, are defined with their traditional connotations, rather than with modern denotations (compiled over time by R. Spector).

Determinism—Believing that life is under a person's control.

Diagnosis—The identifying of the nature or cause of something, especially a problem.

Disadvantaged background—Both educational and economic factors that act as barriers to an individual's participation in a health professions program.

Discrimination—Denying people equal opportunity by acting on a prejudice.

Divination—Traditional American Indian practice of calling on spirits or other forces to determine a diagnosis of a health problem.

Documentation—The papers necessary to prove one's citizenship or immigration status.

Duklij—A turquoise or green malachite amulet that may be used among American Indians to ward off evil spirits.

Dybbuk—Wandering, disembodied soul that enters another person's body and holds fast.

Emerging majority—People of color—Blacks; Asians/Pacific Islanders; American Indians, Eskimos, or Aleuts; and Hispanics—who are expected to constitute a majority of the American population by the year 2020.

Emic—Person's way of describing an action or event; an inside view.

Empacho—Traditional Hispanic belief that a ball of food is stuck in the stomach.

Envidia—Traditional Hispanic belief that the envy of others can be the cause of illness and bad luck.

Environmental control—Ability of a person from a given cultural group to actively control nature and to direct factors in the environment.

Epidemiology—The study of the distribution of disease.

Epilepsia—Traditional Hispanic word for epilepsy.

Ethnicity—Cultural group's sense of identification associated with the group's common social and cultural heritage.

Ethnocentrism—Tendency of members of one cultural group to view the members of other cultural groups in terms of the standards of behavior, attitudes, and values of their own group. The belief that one's own cultural, ethnic, professional, or social group is superior to that of others.

Ethnomedicine—Health beliefs and practices of indigenous cultural development, not practiced in many of the tenets of modern medicine.

Etic—The interpretation of an event by someone who is not experiencing that event, an outside view.

Evil eye—Belief that someone can project harm by gazing or staring at another's property or person.

Excessism—Desiring to live with numerous possessions and material goods.

Exorcism—Ceremonious expulsion of an evil spirit from a person.

Faith—Strong beliefs in a religious or other spiritual philosophy.

Fatalism—Believing that life is not under a person's control.

Fatigue—Traditional Hispanic word for asthma-like symptoms.

Folklore—Body of preserved traditions, usually oral, consisting of beliefs, stories, and associated information of people.

Fundamentalism—Strict belief in the traditions of a heritage.

Garments—Sacred clothing that a person may wear.

Gender-specific care—Care provided to another person by a person of the same gender—may be a religious mandate or personal preference.

Geophagy—Eating of nonfood substances, such as starch.

Glossoscopy—Traditional Chinese medical way of diagnosing a health problem by examining the tongue.

Green card—Documentation that a person is a legally admitted immigrant and has permanent resident status in the United States.

Gris-gris—Symbols of voodoo. They may take numerous forms and be used either to protect a person or to harm that person.

Halal—A designation for meat from animals that has been slaughtered in the ritual way by Islamic law so that it is suitable to be eaten by traditional Islamic people and follows Islamic dietary laws.

Haragei—Japanese art of using nonverbal communication.

HEALING*—Holistic, or three-dimensional, phenomenon that results in the restoration of balance, or harmony, to the body, mind, and spirit, or between the person and the environment.

HEALTH*—The balance of the person, both within one's being—physical, mental, and spiritual—and in the outside world—natural, communal, and metaphysical.

Herbrias—Traditional Hispanic word for a person who sells herbs.

Heritage—The family culture, ethnicity, and/or religion into which one is born.

Heritage consistency—Observance of the beliefs and practices of one's traditional cultural belief system.

Heritage inconsistency—Observance of the beliefs and practices of one's acculturated belief system.

Hex—Evil spell, misfortune, or bad luck that one person can impose on another.

Histeria—Traditional Hispanic word for hysteria.

Homeopathic philosophy—Health beliefs and practices derived from traditional cultural knowledge to maintain health, prevent changes in health status, and restore health.

Homeopathic medicine—In the practice of homeopathic medicine, the person, not the disease, is treated.

Homeopathy—System of medicine based on the belief that a disease can be cured by minute doses of a substance, which, if given to a healthy person in large doses, would produce the same symptoms that the person being treated is experiencing.

Hoodoo—A form of conjuring and a term that refers to the magical practices of voodoo outside New Orleans.

Hydrotherapy—The use of water in the maintenance of health and treatment of disease.

Hypnotherapy—The use of hypnosis to stimulate emotions and control involuntary responses, such as blood pressure.

Iatrogenic—The unexpected symptom or illness that can result from the treatment of another illness.

ILLNESS*—State of imbalance among the body, mind, and spirit; a sense of disharmony both within the person and with the environment.

Immigrant—Alien entering the United States for permanent (or temporary) residence.

Indigenous—People native to an area.

Intangible cultural heritage—The traditions or living expressions inherited from ancestors such as oral traditions and *traditional* HEALTH/ILLNESS/HEALING beliefs and practices.

Kineahora—Word spoken by traditional Jewish people to prevent the "evil eye."

Kosher—A designation for food that has been prepared so that it is suitable to be eaten by traditional Jewish people and follows Jewish dietary laws.

Kusiut—A reference term for an American Indian medicine man; a "learned one."

Lay midwife—A person who practices lay midwifery.

Lay midwifery—Assisting childbirth for compensation.

Legal Permanent Resident (LPR)—A green card recipient; a person who has been granted lawful permanent residence in the United States.

Limpia—Traditional Hispanic practice of cleansing a person.

Locura—Traditional Hispanic word for craziness.

Macrobiotics—Diet and lifestyle from the Far East adapted for the United States by Michio Kushif. The principles of this vegetarian diet consist of balancing *yin* and *yang* energies of food.

Magico-religious folk medicine—Use of charms, holy words, and holy actions to prevent and cure illness.

Mal ojo (bad eye)—Traditional Hispanic belief that excessive admiration by one person can bring harm to another person.

Massage therapy—Use of manipulative techniques to relieve pain and return energy to the body.

Materialism—Taking great pleasure from having more than is necessary.

Medically underserved community—Urban or rural population group that lacks adequate healthcare services.

Melting pot—The social blending of cultures.

Mental—The aspect of the person that is related to thinking and cognition.

Meridians—Specific points of the body into which needles are inserted in the traditional Chinese medical practice of acupuncture.

Mesmerism—Healing by touch.

Metacommunication system—Large system of communication that includes both verbal language and nonverbal signs and symbols.

Milagros—Traditional Hispanic word for small figures of body parts or other objects that are offered to saints for thanksgiving.

Minimalism—Knowing how to live with few possessions and material goods.

Miracle—Supernatural, unexplained event.

Modern—Present-day health and illness beliefs and practices of the providers within the American, or Western, healthcare delivery system.

Modernism—Adherence to modern ways and a belief that other values no longer exist.

Motion in the hand—An example of a traditional American Indian practice of moving the diagnostician's hands in a ritual of divination.

Moxibustion—Traditional Chinese medical way of restoring the balance of *yin* and *yang* that is based on the therapeutic value of heat. Heat is used in a disease where there is an excess of *yin*.

Multicultural nursing—Pluralistic approach to understanding relationships between two or more cultures to create a nursing practice framework for broadening nurses' understanding of health-related beliefs, practices, and issues that are part of the experiences of people from diverse cultural backgrounds.

Mysticism—Aspect of spiritual healing and beliefs.

Natural folk medicine—Use of the natural environment and use of herbs, plants, minerals, and animal substances to prevent and treat illness.

Naturalization—The process by which U.S. citizenship is conferred upon foreign citizens or nationals after fulfilling the requirements established by Congress.

Nonimmigrant—People who are allowed to enter the country temporarily under certain conditions, such as crewmen, students, and temporary workers.

Occult folk medicine—The use of charms, holy words, and holy actions to prevent and cure illness.

Orisha—Yoruba, African, god or goddess.

Osphretics—Traditional Chinese medical way of diagnosing a health problem by listening and smelling.

Osteopathic medicine—School of medical practice that directs recuperative power of nature that is within the body to cure a disease.

Overheating therapy (hyperthermia)—Used since the time of the ancient Greeks, this treatment involves stimulating the natural immune system with heat to kill pathogens.

Partera—A Mexican American or Mexican lay midwife.

Pasmo—Traditional Hispanic disease of paralysis of the face or limbs.

Physical—The aspect of a person one can see, such as the face, eyes, ears, and so forth; and internal organs such as the heart, liver, spleen, and so forth.

Pluralistic society—A society comprising people of numerous ethnocultural backgrounds.

Poultice—A hot, soft, moist mass of herbs, flour, mustard, and other substances spread on muslin and placed on a sore body part.

Powwow—A form of traditional HEALING practiced by German Americans.

Prejudice—Negative beliefs or preferences that are generalized about a group and that leads to "prejudgment."

Promesa—Traditional Hispanic word for a deep and serious promise.

Racism—The belief that members of one race are superior to those of other races.

Rational folk medicine—Use of the natural environment and use of herbs, plants, minerals, and animal substances to prevent and treat illness.

Raza-Latina—A popular term used as a reference group name for people of Latin American descent.

Reflexology—Natural science that manipulates the reflex points in the hands and feet that correspond to every organ in the body in order to clear the energy pathways and the flow of energy through the body.

Refugee—Any person who is outside his or her country of nationality, who is unable or unwilling to return to that country because of persecution or a well-founded fear of persecution.

Religion—Belief in a divine or superhuman power or powers to be obeyed and worshipped as the creator(s) and ruler(s) of the universe.

Remedies—Natural folk medicines that use the natural environment—herbs, plants, minerals, and animal substances—to treat illnesses. Natural remedies have come to the United States from every corner of the world—the East and the West. They may be purchased in pharmacies, markets, and natural food stores.

Resident alien—A lawfully admitted alien.

Resiliency—The state of being strong and able to resist the consequences of an adverse event or emotional or physical danger.

Restoration—Process used by a person to return to health.

Risk adjustment—Complex sets of data are put into terms whereby they are comparing apples to apples.

Sacred objects—Objects, such as amulets and *milagros*, that have a spiritual purpose.

Sacred places—Places where people take petitions for favors or offer prayers of thanksgiving for the granting of a request.

Sacred practices—Religious practices, such as dietary taboos or lighting of candles, that a person is commanded to follow.

Santeria—Traditional Hispanic word for a syncretic religion comprising both African and Catholic beliefs.

Santero(a)—Traditional Hispanic word for the traditional priest and healer in the religion of *Santeria*.

Secular—Beliefs and practices that are not under the auspices of a religious body.

Self-denialism—Taking great pleasure from having less than is necessary.

Senoria—Traditional Hispanic word for a woman who is knowledgeable about the causes and treatment of illness.

Sexism—Belief that members of one sex are superior to those of the other sex.

Shrine—A place—natural, secular, and/or affiliated with a religious tradition—where people make spiritual journeys or pilgrimages for the purposes of giving thanks or petitioning for favors. They are related to magico-religious folk medicine, and the use of charms, holy words, and holy actions, such as prayer, may be observed.

Singer—A type of traditional American Indian healer who is able to practice singing as a form of treating a health problem.

Skilly—An agent that is believed to cause disease by traditional Cherokee people.

Social organization—Patterns of cultural behavior related to life events, such as birth, death, childrearing, and health and illness, that are followed within a given social group.

Socialization—Process of being raised within a culture and acquiring the characteristics of the group.

Soul loss—Belief that a person's soul can leave the body, wander around, and then return.

Space—Area surrounding a person's body and the objects within that area.

Spell—A magical word or formula or a condition of evil or bad luck.

Sphygmopalpation—Traditional Chinese medical way of diagnosing a health problem by feeling pulses.

Spirit—The noncorporeal and nonmental dimension of a person that is the source of meaning and unity. It is the source of the experience of spirituality and every religion.

Spirit possession—Belief that a spirit can enter people, possess them, and control what they say and do.

Spiritual—Ideas, attitudes, concepts, beliefs, and behaviors that are the result of a person's experience of the spirit.

Spirituality—The experience of meaning and unity.

Stargazing—Example of a traditional American Indian practice of praying the star prayer to the star spirit as a method of divination.

Stereotype—Notion that all people from a given group are the same.

Superstition—Belief that performing an action, wearing a charm or an amulet, or eating something will have an influence on life events. These beliefs are upheld by magic and faith.

Susto (soul loss)—Traditional Hispanic belief that the soul is able to leave a person's body.

Szatan—The traditional Polish term for the "evil eye."

Taboo—A culture-bound ban that excludes certain behaviors from common use.

Talisman—Consecrated religious object that confers power of various kinds and protects people who wear, carry, or own them from harm and evil.

Tao—Way, path, or discourse; on the spiritual level, the way to ultimate reality.

Time—Duration, interval of time; instances, or points in time.

Tirisia—Traditional Hispanic word for anxiety.

Title VI—Under the provisions of Title VI of the Civil Rights Act of 1964, people with Limited English Proficiency (LEP) who are cared for in such healthcare settings as extended care facilities, public assistance programs, nursing homes, and hospitals and are eligible for Medicaid, other healthcare, or human services cannot be denied assistance because of their race, color, or national origin.

Tradition—The handing down of statements, beliefs, legends, customs, and information from generation to generation, especially by word of mouth or by practice.

Traditional—Ancient, ethnocultural-religious beliefs and practices that have been handed down through the generations.

Traditional epidemiology—Belief in agents other than those of a scientific nature, causing disease. These could be such agents as "envy," "jealousy," and "hate."

Traditionalism—Belief in the traditional HEALTH, ILLNESS, and HEALING methods of a given cultural cohort.

Tui Na—A complex Chinese system of massage, "pushing and pulling," using meridian stimulation used to treat orthopedic and neurological problems.

Undocumented alien—Person of foreign origin who has entered the country unlawfully by bypassing inspection or who has overstayed the original terms of admission.

Universalism—Open beliefs in many domains that may not be part of a given personal heritage.

Unlocking—Steps taken to help break down and understand the definitions of the terms *health*/HEALTH and *illness*/ILLNESS in a living context. It consists of persistent questioning: What is health? No matter what the response, the question "What does that mean?" is asked. Initially, this causes much confusion, but as each term is analyzed, the process makes sense.

Voodoo—A religion that is a combination of Christianity and African Yoruba religious beliefs.

Vulnerability—The state of being weak or prone to an adverse event or emotional or physical danger.

Witched—Example of a traditional American Indian belief that a person is harmed by witches.

Xenophobia—Morbid fear of strangers.

Yang—Male, positive energy that produces light, warmth, and fullness.

Yin—Female, negative energy that produces darkness, cold, and emptiness.

Yoruba—The African tribe whose myths and rites are the basis of *Santeria*.

Appendix **B**

CULTURALCARE Assessments

The *HERITAGECHAIN* links in this appendix provide guidelines for working with and caring for people from diverse heritages, and assessment tools for gathering information about their personal heritage, family's heritage, and ethnocultural community.

Preparing

Before you begin:

- Be aware of your own cultural values, biases, and traditional health/HEALTH beliefs and practices.
- Develop basic knowledge about the cultural values and health/HEALTH beliefs and practices for the people and populations you work with and care for.

Communication

- Be respectful of, interested in, and understanding of other peoples' health/HEALTH beliefs and practices without being judgmental. Be aware that health/HEALTH beliefs and practices vary both within and between ethnic, cultural, and religious communities.
- Assess the person's ability to speak, comprehend, and read English; arrange for an interpreter if necessary.
- Ask the person how they prefer to be called—"Mr.," "Mrs.," and so forth. Do not call the person by their first name or by diminutive or generic terms such as "honey" or "guy."
- Make the person comfortable and ensure personal space and eye contact. If the person prefers not to establish eye contact, do not become upset. In many cultures, it is considered polite to avoid eye contact.
- Avoid body language and gestures that may be offensive or misunderstood.
- Speak directly, respectfully, distinctly, and quietly to the person, whether an interpreter is present or not, and do not use jargon, slang, or colloquialisms.
- Provide reading material that is easily read in the person's native language. Do not use cartoons and cartoon characters for illustrations.

Heritage Assessment

This set of questions is used to determine a person's (or your own) ethnic, cultural, and religious background. The *heritage assessment* is helpful to determine how deeply a person identifies with his or her *traditional* heritage. This assessment is very useful in setting the stage for understanding a person's traditional HEALTH and ILLNESS beliefs and practices and in helping determine the family and community resources that will be appropriate for support when necessary. The greater the number of positive responses, the greater the degree to which the person may identify with his or her traditional heritage. The one exception to positive answers is the question about whether a person's name was changed. The respondent is credited one point for answering "no." The background rationale for the development of this tool is found in Chapter 2.

1. Where was your mother born? _____

2. Where was your father born? _____

3. Where were your grandparents born? _____

    A. Your mother's mother? _____

    B. Your mother's father? _____

    C. Your father's mother? _____

    D. Your father's father? _____

4. How many brothers _____ and sisters _____ do you have?

5. What setting did you grow up in? Urban _____ Suburban _____ Rural _____

6. What country did your parents grow up in?

    Father _____

    Mother _____

7. How old were you when you came to the United States?

8. How old were your parents when they came to the United States?

    Mother _____

    Father _____

9. When you were growing up, who lived with you? _____

    _____

10. Have you maintained contact with:

A. Aunts, uncles, cousins?	(1) Yes ____	(2) No ____
B. Brothers and sisters?	(1) Yes ____	(2) No ____
C. Parents?	(1) Yes ____	(2) No ____
D. Your own children?	(1) Yes ____	(2) No ____

11. Did most of your aunts, uncles, and cousins live near your home?
    (1) Yes ____
    (2) No ____

12. Approximately how often did you visit family members who lived outside of your home?
    (1) Daily ____
    (2) Weekly ____
    (3) Monthly ____
    (4) Once a year or less ____
    (5) Never ____

13. Was your original family name changed?
    (1) Yes ____
    (2) No ____

14. What is your religious preference?
    (1) Catholic ____
    (2) Jewish ____
    (3) Protestant ____ Denomination ____
    (4) Islam ____
    (5) Buddhist ____
    (6) Hindu ____
    (7) Other ____
    (8) None ____

15. Is your spouse/partner the same religion as you?
    (1) Yes ____
    (2) No ____

16. Is your spouse/partner the same ethnic background as you?
    (1) Yes ____
    (2) No ____

17. What kind of school did you go to?
    (1) Public ____
    (2) Private ____
    (3) Parochial ____

18. As an adult, do you live in a neighborhood where the neighbors are the same religion and ethnic background as you?
    (1) Yes ____
    (2) No ____

19. Do you belong to a religious institution?
    (1) Yes ____
    (2) No ____

20. Would you describe yourself as an active member?
    (1) Yes ____
    (2) No ____

21. How often do you attend your religious institution?
    (1) More than once a week ____
    (2) Weekly ____
    (3) Monthly ____
    (4) Special holidays only ____
    (5) Never ____

22. Do you practice your religion in your home?
    (1) Yes ____ (if yes, please specify by checking activities below)
       Praying ____
       Bible reading ____
       Diet ____ Celebrating religious
       holidays ____
    (2) No ____

23. Do you prepare foods special to your ethnic or religious background?
    (1) Yes ____
    (2) No ____

24. Do you participate in ethnic activities?
    (1) Yes ____ (if yes, please specify by checking activities below)
       Singing ____
       Holiday celebrations ____
       Dancing ____
       Festivals ____
       Costumes ____
    (2) No ____

25. Are your friends from the same religious background as you?
    (1) Yes ____
    (2) No ____

26. Are your friends from the same ethnic background as you?
    (1) Yes ____
    (2) No ____

27. What is your native language other than English? ____

28. Do you speak this language?
    (1) Yes ____
    (2) Occasionally ____
    (3) No ____

29. Do you read your native (other than English) language?
    (1) Yes ____
    (2) No ____

EthnoHEALTH Family Interview

Interview your *maternal* grandmother, your mother, or a *maternal* aunt to learn your traditions; in clinical practice, interview the patient or an older family member to learn about the HEALTH traditions in their family of origin. The mother is suggested because she is usually the person who is the gatekeeper and person who passes the health/HEALTH beliefs and practices to the next generation.

1. Ethnic background ____

   Country of origin ____

   Religion ____

   Number of generations in U.S. ____

2. What does she do to *maintain* HEALTH? Also, if she can remember, what did her mother do?

3. What does she do to *protect* HEALTH? Also, if she can remember, what did her mother do?

4. What "home remedies" does she use to *restore* HEALTH? Also, if she can remember, what did her mother do?

5. How do her religious/spiritual beliefs define *birth*? What rituals accompany this event?

6. How do her religious/spiritual beliefs define *illness*? What rituals accompany this event?

7. How do her religious/spiritual beliefs define *healing*? What rituals accompany this event?

8. How do her religious/spiritual beliefs define *death*? What rituals accompany this event?

Ethnocultural Community Assessment

One way to learn about the community you, your colleague, or your patient comes from is to participate in an "urban hike"—taking skills, knowledge, and curiosity applied to the great outdoors and applying it to peopled areas. It is an extraordinary way to tantalize your senses as you:

1. See—the infrastructure of a new or familiar place, the housing stock, the stores and small businesses, the markets, the transportation system, the pharmacies, houses of worship, and so forth.

2. Hear—listen to the symphony of voices, traffic, and music.

3. Taste—new foods by eating in neighborhood restaurants.

4. Smell—food as it is prepared on the streets, in homes, or in restaurants.

5. Feel—the textures of different fabrics and objects.

It is a way to witness and learn about cultural diversity and the New America and to erase fears of the unknown social and cultural phenomena that may hinder your ability to embrace the demographic changes occurring in the United States.

The following is an assessment guide to adapt for the community you wish to explore. Using it will facilitate your understanding and delivery of CULTURALCARE. Gather the following demographic data:

- Total population size of entire city or town
- Focus on demographics of the target community
- Population breakdown by race, ages, education, occupations, income, nations of origin, ancestry, and so forth.

(This information is readily available from the U.S. Census Website).

Question community people to discover traditional health/HEALTH and illness/ILLNESS beliefs and practices such as:

- Traditional causes of illness/ILLNESS, such as poor eating habits, wrong food combinations, punishment from God, the evil eye, hexes, spells, or envy and so forth as discussed in Chapter 5.
- Traditional methods of maintaining health/HEALTH, protecting health/ HEALTH, and restoring health/HEALTH
- Resources for allopathic and homeopathic home remedies, such as:
  - Neighborhood health centers and hospitals
  - Sources of traditional medicines such as grocery stores, *botanicas*, Asian pharmacies, and so forth
- Childbearing beliefs and practices
- Childrearing beliefs and practices
- Rituals and beliefs surrounding death and dying.

These assessment tools will serve to enhance your level of CULTURALCOMPETENCY and help you have an ever-growing understanding for the diversity that is an indelible part of the American whole.

Appendix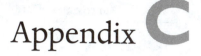

Calendar: Cultural and Religious Holidays That Change Dates

There are many Holy Days observed by people from many different cultural and religious heritages that do not fall on the same dates of the Julian calendar on an annual basis. This is because some religions, such as Judaism, follow the lunar calendar; and others, such as Islam, follow both the lunar and solar calendars. Given the increasing amount of cultural and religious diversity in this country, it is imperative that this fact be considered. Religious leaders of a given faith community must be contacted regarding the Julian dates of a given holiday. Cultural and religious holidays have a significant impact on the lives of both patients and workers. Surgical procedures and extensive tests ought to be avoided on holidays, and large professional meetings and other activities must not be scheduled at that time to cause conflict.

Heritage	Holiday	Approximate Date
Islam	Eid al-Fitr and Al Hisrah (New Year)	Varies
Chinese	Sending Off the Kitchen God Day	January
Islam	Laylat al-Qadr	January
Sikh	Guru Gobind Singh Ji's Birthday	January
Hindu	Makara Sakranti/Pongal	January
Chinese	New Year: Chinese, Korean, Tibetan, Vietnamese	February
Chinese	Lantern Festival	February
Baha'i	Intercalary Days	February or March
Christian	Shrove Monday	February or March
Christian	Shrove Tuesday	February or March
Christian	Ash Wednesday	February or March
Eastern Orthodox	Beginning of Lent, Eastern Orthodox Christian	March
Hindu	Maha Shivaratri (Shiva's Night)	March
Hindu	Holi	March
Iranian	Now Rouz	March
Christian	Palm Sunday	March or April
Jewish	Passover begins at sundown	March or April
Jewish	Passover	March or April

Heritage	Holiday	Approximate Date
Christian	Good Friday	March or April
Christian	Easter	March or April
Eastern Orthodox	Palm Sunday	March or April (a week after Christian Palm Sunday)
Christian	Easter Monday	March or April
Eastern Orthodox Christian	Good Friday	March or April (a week after Christian Good Friday)
Eastern Orthodox	Easter: Eastern Orthodox, also known as Pascha	March or April
Chinese	Respect for Ancestors (Ch'ing-ming)	April
Islam	Muharram	April
Vietnamese	Thanh Minh (Respect for Ancestors Day)	April
Hindu	Ramanavami	April
Cambodian	New Year	April
Hindu	Vaisakhi (Solar New Year)	April
Sikh	Baisakhi (New Year)	April
Jain	Mahavir Jayanti	April
Baha'i	Festival of Ridvan	April
Buddhist	Visakaha Day	May
Jewish	Shavuoth begins at sundown	May or June
Chinese	Dragon Boat Festival	June
Eastern Orthodox	Ascension Day	June
Christian	Pentecost	June
Islam	Maulid an-Nabi	June
Eastern Orthodox	Pentacost	June
Jewish	Tisha B' Av Fast Day	July or August
Chinese	Seventh Night	August
Hindu	Janmashtami	August
Korean	Chusok	September
Coptic Christian	Coptic New Year	September
Chinese	Midautumn Moon Festival—Chung-ch'iu	September
Jewish	Rosh Hashanah begins at sundown	September or October
Jewish	Yom Kippur begins at sundown	September or October
Jewish	Yom Kippur	September or October
Jewish	Sukkoth begins at sundown	September or October
Jewish	Shmini Atzeret begins at sundown	September or October

Heritage	Holiday	Approximate Date
Jewish	Simchat Torah begins at sundown	September or October
Hindu	Durga Puja	October
Baha'i	Birthday of the Bab	October
Hindu	Diwali	October
Sikh	Nanak's Birthday	November
Baha'i	Birthday of Baha'u'llah	November
Jewish	Chanukah	December
Islam	Ramadan	Varies

Source: Adapted from *Multicultural resource calendar.* (2011). Amherst, MA: Amherst Educational Publishing, 800-865-5549 or visit http://www.diversityresources.com/index.php. An annual calendar is available with the exact dates and explanations for the given holidays. There is an electronic version of this calendar that has numerous features including global religious, cultural, commemorative, and public holidays, pronunciations, food information, and resource information.

There are numerous observances that must also be considered. The following is a list of these observances:

■ African American History Month (February)
■ Women's History Month (March)
■ Irish American Heritage Month (March)
■ Asian/Pacific American Heritage Month (May)
■ Older Americans Month (May)
■ Anniversary of Americans with Disabilities Act (July 26)
■ Hispanic Heritage Month (September 15–October 15)
■ American Indian/Alaska Native Heritage Month (November)

These are available from the U.S. Census Bureau's Facts for Features series and can be accessed from http://www.census.gov/newsroom/releases/archives/facts_for_features_special_editions/cb11-ff13.html

Appendix D

Selected Data Resources

Countless invaluable resources are available on the internet. It is important to note that the URLs change; however, the new addresses are usually linked to the old site. The focus here is on the agencies within the federal government that are useful for information regarding health and diversity.

1. *The U.S. Census Bureau* provides information related to the decennial Census, Statistical Abstract, Census Maps, and so forth. American Community Survey and American FactFinder are sources for population, housing, economic, and geographic data with annual estimates to update the information.

2. *The U.S. Citizenship and Immigration Services (USCIS)* provides immigration information, grants benefits, promotes awareness and understanding of *citizenship*, and ensures the integrity of the immigration process.

3. *The U.S. Department of Homeland Security* has responsibility for information regarding immigration, commerce and trade, and emergency preparedness.

4. *The Office for Civil Rights*, located within the U.S. Department of Health and Human Services, is responsible for enforcing the nondiscrimination requirements of **Title VI of the Civil Rights Act of 1964.**

5. *The National Center for Health Statistics—Healthy People 2020*—describes the ways in which it plans to improve the health of all Americans in the years between 2010 and 2020.

6. *The National Center for Health Statistics* provides U.S. public health statistics including diseases, pregnancies, births, aging, and mortality.

7. *The Health Resources and Services Administration (HRSA)* is the primary federal agency for improving access to healthcare services for people who are uninsured, isolated, or medically vulnerable.

8. *The Office of Minority Health (OMH)* advises the Secretary and the Office of Public Health Science on public health issues affecting American Indians and Alaska Natives, Black and African Americans, Asian Americans, and Hispanic Americans, as well as the elimination of racial and ethnic health disparities.

9. *The National Center for Complementary and Integrative Health (NCCIH)*, part of the U.S. National Institutes of Health, undertakes research, training, and dissemination of data relevant to the public and professionals on the use and efficacy of complimentary and alternative medicine.

10. *HealthFinder* is the U.S. government directory of online publications, clear-inghouses, databases, Websites, and support and self-help groups.

11. *The Center for Medicare & Medicaid Services* has as its mission to ensure effective, up-to-date healthcare coverage and to promote quality care for beneficiaries.

12. *The Centers for Disease Control (CDC)* has as its mission to save lives, protect people, and save money through prevention. The CDC seeks to accomplish its mission by working with partners throughout the nation and the world to monitor health, detect and investigate health problems, conduct research to enhance prevention, and so forth.

Credits

FRONT MATTER

p. 9: From The Shadow of the Wind by Carlos Ruiz Zafon. Published by Penguin Books, © 2005; **p. 16:** Pablo Picasso.

CHAPTER 1

p. 1: Pearson Education, Inc.; **p. 3:** From A Life in Medicine: A Literary Anthology by Robert Coles and Randy-Michael Testa. Published by The New Press, © 2002; **p. 7:** Rachel E. Spector, Cultural Diversity in Health and Illness, 9th Ed., © 2017, Pearson Education, Inc., New York, NY; **pp. 9–10:** National Standards for Culturally and Linguistically Appropriate Services in Health Care, Think Health, U.S Department of Health and Human Services; **p. 10:** Title VI of the 1964 Civil Rights Act, U.S Department of Justice; **p. 11:** From "Language Barriers to Health Care in the United States" by Glenn Flores in The New England Journal of Medicine, Volume: 355, Issue: 03, pp: 229–231. Published by The New England Journal of Medicine, © 2006; **p. 12:** From Advancing Effective Communication, Cultural Competence, and Patient- and Family-Centered Care: A Roadmap for Hospitals. Published by The Joint Commission, © 2010; **pp. 13–15:** Rachel E. Spector, Cultural Diversity in Health and Illness, 9th Ed., © 2017, Pearson Education, Inc., New York, NY.

CHAPTER 2

p. 18: From Heritage Consistency as a Consideration in Counseling Native Americans. Paper read at the National Indian Education Association Convention by Darryl Zitzow and George Estes. Published by ERIC, © 1980; **p. 19:** Rachel E. Spector, Cultural Diversity in Health and Illness, 9th Ed., © 2017, Pearson Education, Inc., New York, NY; **p. 20:** From Medicine and Anthropology by Iago Galdston. Published by International Universities Press, © 1959; **pp. 20–21:** By permission. From Merriam-Webster's Collegiate® Dictionary,

11th Edition © 2016 by Merriam-Webster, Inc. (www.Merriam-Webster.com); **p. 22:** From Harvard Encyclopedia of American Ethnic Groups by Stephan Thernstrom. Published by Harvard University Press, © 1980; **p. 22:** By permission. From Merriam-Webster's Collegiate® Dictionary, 11th Edition © 2016 by Merriam-Webster, Inc. (www.Merriam-Webster.com); **p. 29:** A Blueprint for Reform: The Reauthorization of the Elementary and Secondary Education Act, US Department of Education, 2010; **p. 29:** Rachel E. Spector, Cultural Diversity in Health and Illness, 9th Ed., © 2017, Pearson Education, Inc., New York, NY; **p. 31:** Rachel E. Spector, Cultural Diversity in Health and Illness, 9th Ed., © 2017, Pearson Education, Inc., New York, NY.

CHAPTER 3

p. 34: From The New Colossus by Emma Lazarus, 1886; **p. 35:** Population by Hispanic or Latino Origin and by Race for the United States: 2000 and 2010; Selected Characteristics of the Native ad Foreign-Born Populations 2014 American Community Survey 1-year Estimates, U.S. Census Bureau; **p. 38:** Population Estimates; American Community Survey; Selected Population Profile in the United States 2014 American Community Survey 1-year Estimates, U.S. Census Bureau; **p. 40:** Learn About the United States Quick Civics Lessons for the Naturalization Test, U.S Citizenship and Immigration Services, 2011; **p. 41:** U.S. Lawful Permanent Residents, 2013; Department of Homeland Security, 2014; **p. 42:** Rachel E. Spector, Cultural Diversity in Health and Illness, 9th Ed., © 2017, Pearson Education, Inc., New York, NY; **p. 45:** Rachel E. Spector, Cultural Diversity in Health and Illness, 9th Ed., © 2017, Pearson Education, Inc., New York, NY; **p. 46:** Rachel E. Spector, Cultural Diversity in Health and Illness, 9th Ed., © 2017, Pearson Education, Inc., New York, NY.

CHAPTER 4

p. 48: Chief Seattle Suqwamish; **p. 49:** Florence Nightingale; **p. 49:** Rachel E. Spector, Cultural Diversity in Health and Illness, 9th Ed., © 2017, Pearson Education, Inc., New York, NY; **p. 49:** By permission. From Merriam-Webster's Collegiate® Dictionary, 11th Edition © 2016 by Merriam-Webster, Inc. (www.Merriam-Webster.com); **p. 54:** Vision Statement of Healthy People 2020, Office of Disease Prevention and Health promotion, 2015; **p. 57:** By permission. From Merriam-Webster's Collegiate® Dictionary, 11th Edition © 2016 by Merriam-Webster, Inc. (www.Merriam-Webster.com); **p. 62:** Rachel E. Spector, Cultural Diversity in Health and Illness, 9th Ed., © 2017, Pearson Education, Inc., New York, NY; **p. 63:** Rachel E. Spector, Cultural Diversity in Health and Illness, 9th Ed., © 2017, Pearson Education, Inc., New York, NY.

CHAPTER 5

p. 64: Rachel E. Spector, Cultural Diversity in Health and Illness, 9th Ed., © 2017, Pearson Education, Inc., New York, NY; **p. 72:** From Library of Health: Complete Guide to Prevention and Cure of Disease, Containing Practical Information on Anatomy by Benjamin Franklin Scholl. Published by History Publishing Company, © 1924; **p. 76:** Rachel E. Spector, Cultural Diversity in Health and Illness, 9th Ed., © 2017, Pearson Education, Inc., New York, NY; **p. 77:** Rachel E. Spector, Cultural Diversity in Health and Illness, 9th Ed., © 2017, Pearson Education, Inc., New York, NY; **p. 79:** From Dybbuk by Gershon Winkler. Published by Judaica Press, © 1981; **pp. 81–82:** Rachel E. Spector, Cultural Diversity in Health and Illness, 9th Ed., © 2017, Pearson Education, Inc., New York, NY; **pp. 85–86:** Rachel E. Spector, Cultural Diversity in Health and Illness, 9th Ed., © 2017, Pearson Education, Inc., New York, NY; **p. 86:** Copyright © 2011 by Houghton Mifflin Harcourt Publishing Company. Adapted and reproduced by permission from The American Heritage Dictionary of the English Language, Fifth Edition; **p. 88:** From Health and Healing: Understanding Conventional and Alternative Medicine by Andrew Weil. Published by Houghton Mifflin, © 1983; **p. 90:** Rachel E. Spector, Cultural Diversity in Health and Illness, 9th Ed., © 2017, Pearson Education, Inc., New York, NY; **p. 93:** From Science and Health with Key to the Scriptures by Mary Baker Eddy. Published by Christian Scientist Publishing Company, 1875; **p. 93:** NCCIH Facts-at-a-Glance and Mission, National Center for Complementary and Integrative Health; **p. 95:** Rachel E. Spector, Cultural Diversity in Health and Illness, 9th Ed., © 2017, Pearson Education, Inc., New York, NY.

CHAPTER 6

pp. 98–99: From Aspects of Malaysian Magic by William Shaw. Published by Muzium Negara, © 1975; **p. 99:** From Depth Psychology and Modern Man: A New View of the Magnitude of Human Personality, Its Dimensions & Resources by Ira Progoff. Published by McGraw-Hill, © 1959; **p. 99:** From The Realms of Healing by Stanley Krippner and Alberto Villoldo. Published by Celestial Arts, © 1976; **p. 99:** From Faith Healing - God or Fraud by George Victor Bishop. Published by Sherbourne Pr, © 1967; **p. 99:** From Healing In His Wings by A J Russell. Published by Methuen, © 1937; **p. 99:** From Shaman's Path: Healing, Personal Growth & Empowerment by Gary Doore. Published by Shambhala, © 1988; **p. 99:** From Health and Healing by Naegele Kaspar. Published by Jossey-Bass, © 1970; **p. 101:** Exodus 15:26, The Holy Bible; **p. 101:** Deuteronomy 32:39, The Holy Bible; **p. 107:** Rachel E. Spector, Cultural Diversity in Health and Illness, 9th Ed., © 2017, Pearson Education, Inc., New York, NY; **p. 108:** From The Rites of Birth, Marriage, Death, and Kindred Occasions Among the Semites by Julian Morgenstern. Published by Hebrew Union College Press, © 1966; **p. 111:** From Muslim Customs and Traditions Relating to Childbirth by Michelle Lee. Published by Demand Media, © 2015; **p. 114:** Rachel E. Spector, Cultural Diversity in Health and Illness, 9th Ed., © 2017, Pearson Education, Inc., New York, NY; **p. 115:** Rachel E. Spector, Cultural Diversity in Health and Illness, 9th Ed., © 2017, Pearson Education, Inc., New York, NY.

CHAPTER 7

p. 117: From Folk Medicine-Fact and Fiction: Age-old cures, Alternative Medicine, Natural Remedies by Frances Kennett. Published by Crescent Books, ©1976; **pp. 122–123:** Rachel E. Spector, Cultural Diversity in Health and Illness, 9th Ed., © 2017, Pearson Education, Inc., New York, NY; **pp. 124–125:** Rachel E. Spector, Cultural Diversity in Health and Illness, 9th Ed., © 2017, Pearson Education, Inc., New York, NY; **p. 128:** Rachel E. Spector, Cultural Diversity in Health and Illness, 9th Ed., © 2017, Pearson Education, Inc., New York, NY.

CHAPTER 8

p. 130: From Fortune Magazine, Issue 79, Published by Fortune Magazine. © January 1970; **p. 133:** From For Profit Enterprise in Health Care: Can it Contribute to Health Reform by Eleanor D. Kinney. Published American Journal of Law and Medicine, © 2010; **p. 134:** Health, United States, 2014: With Special Feature on Adults Aged 55-64, U.S. Department of Health and Human Services; **pp. 137–138:** Rachel E. Spector, Cultural Diversity in Health and Illness, 9th Ed., © 2017, Pearson Education, Inc., New York, NY; **p. 140:** Rachel E. Spector, Cultural Diversity in Health and Illness, 9th Ed., © 2017, Pearson Education, Inc., New York, NY; **p. 145:** Rachel E. Spector, Cultural Diversity in Health and Illness, 9th Ed., © 2017, Pearson Education, Inc., New York, NY.

CHAPTER 9

p. 147: Rachel E. Spector, Cultural Diversity in Health and Illness, 9th Ed., © 2017, Pearson Education, Inc., New York, NY; **p. 150:** Wooden Leg; **p. 153:** From More and More Claiming American Indian Heritage by Zuckoff, Mitchell. Published by Boston Globe © 1995; **p. 154:** From An American Indian looks at health care by H. Bilagody in The ninth annual training institute for psychiatrist-teachers of practicing physicians by R. Feldman and D. Buch. Published by Western Interstate Commission for Higher Education, © 1969; **pp. 158–159:** Littlejohn, Hawk. (1979). Personal interview. Boston, MA; **p. 160:**

From Encyclopedia of Native American Healing, 2e by William S. Lyon. Published by W.W. Norton Company, © 1996; **pp. 162, 185:** Rachel E. Spector, Cultural Diversity in Health and Illness, 9th Ed., © 2017, Pearson Education, Inc., New York, NY; **pp. 163, 185:** Rachel E. Spector, Cultural Diversity in Health and Illness, 9th Ed., © 2017, Pearson Education, Inc., New York, NY; **p. 164:** From The Broken Cord, 1e by Michael Dorris and Louise Erdrich. Published by Harper & Row, © 1989; **pp. 167–168:** Rachel E. Spector, Cultural Diversity in Health and Illness, 9th Ed., © 2017, Pearson Education, Inc., New York, NY; **p. 168:** Rachel E. Spector, Cultural Diversity in Health and Illness, 9th Ed., © 2017, Pearson Education, Inc., New York, NY.

CHAPTER 10

p. 171: From The English Studies Book: An Introduction to Language, Literature and Culture by Rob Pope. Published by Routledge Publishers, © 2015; **p. 173:** From The Religions of Man, 1e by Huston Smith. Published by Harper & Row, © 1958; **p. 177:** From Chinese folk medicine by Heinrich Wallnofer and Anna von Rottauscher. Published by New American Library, © 1972; **pp. 187–188:** Rachel E. Spector, Cultural Diversity in Health and Illness, 9th Ed., © 2017, Pearson Education, Inc., New York, NY; **p. 188:** Rachel E. Spector, Cultural Diversity in Health and Illness, 9th Ed., © 2017, Pearson Education, Inc., New York, NY.

CHAPTER 11

p. 190: Frederick Douglass; **p. 191:** From There Are No Children Here: The Story of Two Boys Growing Up in the Other America by Alex Kotlowitz. Published by Anchor Books, © 1991; **p. 192:** From Resiliency in Ethnic Minority Families: African-American families by Hamilton I McCubbin. Published by The University of Wisconsin System, © 1995; **p. 194:** Brunner, B. and Haney, E., Civil Rights Timeline: Milestones in the modern civil rights movement. © 2000-2012. Reprinted by permission of Pearson Education, Inc.; **pp. 201–202:** Rachel E. Spector, Cultural Diversity in Health and

Illness, 9th Ed., © 2017, Pearson Education, Inc., New York, NY; **p. 203:** Rachel E. Spector, Cultural Diversity in Health and Illness, 9th Ed., © 2017, Pearson Education, Inc., New York, NY; **p. 205:** Rachel E. Spector, Cultural Diversity in Health and Illness, 9th Ed., © 2017, Pearson Education, Inc., New York, NY; **p. 209:** Rachel E. Spector, Cultural Diversity in Health and Illness, 9th Ed., © 2017, Pearson Education, Inc., New York, NY; **p. 210:** Rachel E. Spector, Cultural Diversity in Health and Illness, 9th Ed., © 2017, Pearson Education, Inc., New York, NY.

CHAPTER 12

pp. 224–226: Based on information from Texas Department of State Health Services, 2012; **p. 226:** From Division of Health Related Professions by J. Castillo, © 1982; **p. 227:** Rachel E. Spector, Cultural Diversity in Health and Illness, 9th Ed., © 2017, Pearson Education, Inc., New York, NY; **pp. 229–230:** Rachel E. Spector, Cultural Diversity in Health and Illness, 9th Ed., © 2017, Pearson Education, Inc., New York, NY; **p. 233:** Rachel E. Spector, Cultural Diversity in Health and Illness, 9th Ed., © 2017, Pearson Education, Inc., New York, NY; **p. 234:** Rachel E. Spector, Cultural Diversity in Health and Illness, 9th Ed., © 2017, Pearson Education, Inc., New York, NY; **p. 235:** Rachel E. Spector, Cultural Diversity in Health and Illness, 9th Ed., © 2017, Pearson Education, Inc., New York, NY.

CHAPTER 13

p. 237: From The American Soul: Rediscovering the Wisdom of the Founders by Jacob Needleman. Published by TarcherPerigee, © 2003; **p. 239:** Selected Social Characteristics In the United States 2009-2013 American Community Survey 5-Year Estimates, U.S. Census Bureau; **p. 241:** From The German Texans by Glen E. Lich. Published by University of Texas, © 1982; **p. 249:** Rachel E. Spector, Cultural Diversity in Health and Illness, 9th Ed., © 2017, Pearson Education, Inc., New York, NY; **p. 250:** Rachel E. Spector, Cultural Diversity in Health and Illness, 9th Ed., © 2017, Pearson Education, Inc., New York, NY; **p. 251:** Rachel E. Spector, Cultural Diversity in Health and Illness, 9th Ed., © 2017, Pearson Education, Inc., New York, NY; **pp. 251–252:** Rachel E. Spector, Cultural Diversity in Health and Illness, 9th Ed., © 2017, Pearson Education, Inc., New York, NY.

CHAPTER 14

p. 255: Pearson Education, Inc.; **p. 261:** Rachel E. Spector, Cultural Diversity in Health and Illness, 9th Ed., © 2017, Pearson Education, Inc., New York, NY.

APPENDIX

pp. 281–283: Based on data from the Multicultural resource calendar. (2011). Amherst, MA: Amherst Educational Publishing; **p. 283:** Profile America Facts for Features, U S Census Bureau.

Index